Veterinary Neuropathology

Companion website

This book is accompanied by a companion website which is maintained by the Division of Diagnostic Imaging, Dept. clinical veterinary medicine, Vetsuisse Faculty, University of Bern, Switzerland.

www.wiley.com/go/vandevelde/veterinaryneuropathology

The website includes

- Interactive MRI – Neuropathology Atlas
- A range of different pathologies
- Complete sequences to scroll through
- Matching gross images
- Microscopic images of selected lesion sites

Website editors:

Johann Lang, Dr.med.vet, DECVDI Division of Diagnostic Imaging, Department of Clinical Veterinary Medicine, Vetsuisse Faculty, University of Bern, Switzerland

Eric R. Wiesner, DVM DACVR Department of Surgical & Radiological Sciences, School of Veterinary Medicine University of California, Davis, USA

Veterinary Neuropathology
Essentials of Theory and Practice

Marc Vandevelde
Neurocenter, Vetsuisse Faculty, University of Bern, Switzerland.

Robert J. Higgins
Department of Pathology, Microbiology & Immunology, School of Veterinary Medicine, University of California, Davis, USA.

Anna Oevermann
Neurocenter, Vetsuisse Faculty, University of Bern, Switzerland.

WILEY-BLACKWELL
A John Wiley & Sons, Ltd., Publication

This edition first published 2012 © 2012 by John Wiley & Sons, Ltd

Wiley-Blackwell is an imprint of John Wiley & Sons, Ltd formed by the merger of Wiley's global Scientific, Technical and Medical business with Blackwell Publishing.

Registered office: John Wiley & Sons, Ltd, The Atrium, Southern Gate, Chichester, West Sussex, PO19 8SQ, UK

Editorial offices: 9600 Garsington Road, Oxford, OX4 2DQ, UK
    The Atrium, Southern Gate, Chichester, West Sussex, PO19 8SQ, UK
    2121 State Avenue, Ames, Iowa 50014-8300, USA

For details of our global editorial offices, for customer services and for information about how to apply for permission to reuse the copyright material in this book please see our website at www.wiley.com/wiley-blackwell.

The right of the author to be identified as the author of this work has been asserted in accordance with the UK Copyright, Designs and Patents Act 1988.

Library of Congress Cataloging-in-Publication Data

Vandevelde, Marc, 1947–
  Veterinary neuropathology : essentials of theory and practice / Marc Vandevelde, Robert J. Higgins, Anna Oevermann.
    p. cm.
  Includes bibliographical references and index.
  ISBN 978-0-470-67056-9 (hardback : alk. paper) 1. Veterinary neurology. 2. Veterinary pathology. 3. Nervous system–Diseases. I. Higgins, Robert J., 1941– II. Oevermann, Anna, 1974–
III. Title.
  SF895.V36 2012
  636.089'607–dc23

               2012005850

A catalogue record for this book is available from the British Library.

Wiley also publishes its books in a variety of electronic formats. Some content that appears in print may not be available in electronic books.

Cover design by Meaden Creative

Set in 10.5/12.5 pt Minion by Toppan Best-set Premedia Limited

1 2012

Contents

This book is accompanied by a companion website: which is maintained by
the Division of Diagnostic Imaging, Dept of Clinical Veterinary Medicine,
Vetsuisse Faculty, University of Bern, Switzerland.

www.wiley.com/go/vandevelde/veterinaryneuropathology

Preface

This book has evolved in the frame of a veterinary neuropathology course of the European School of Advanced Veterinary Studies (ESAVS), which has been taught regularly at the University of Bern in Switzerland since the early 1990s. The original participants were veterinary pathologists seeking practical training in diagnostic neuropathology. Over the years, along with the introduction of MRI in veterinary neurology, more and more neurologists and even diagnostic imaging specialists visited the course. Based on our experience to teach neuropathology to such a mixed audience, we decided to expand and edit our course notes into a compact book. This is a didactic book teaching a practical approach to diagnostic neuropathology starting from the very basics for pathologists and clinicians with a special interest in neuropathology. It is also intended to support neurologists, radiologists, other MRI users, and residents in these disciplines who wish to deepen their knowledge of the pathology and pathogenesis of neurological diseases.

While the factual information in this book is up to date, we did not intend to present a detailed account of the accumulated veterinary neuropathological knowledge. Complete and detailed coverage of the veterinary neuropathological literature up to the mid 1990s is provided in the excellent book of Brian Summers, John Cummings and Alexander de Lahunta: *Veterinary Neuropathology*, Mosby St. Louis, 1995. This book, unfortunately out of print, is the last of its kind and has been complemented with a good image database on the Cornell university website. Since 1995, the veterinary neurological knowledge has continued to expand and the internet now allows easy and often free access to original publications. Those who study this book should be able to target additional information very quickly with a few mouse clicks. Still, at the end of each chapter of our book a few selected references are listed, mostly reviews, recent case reports listing the literature on a particular subject and examples of good neuropathological practice. These are not meant to be a comprehensive reference base but intended as "further reading" and to make the users of this book familiar with the current literature on the subject.

The coverage of the pathology of the peripheral nervous system and muscles is limited to the most common lesions as encountered in a routine neuropathological examination. As neuromuscular pathology has become a highly specialized field beyond the scope of this book we listed some key literature references on this subject where appropriate. We thank all collegues who contributed MRI and other images shown in this book in particular Rosemarie Fatzer (Bern, Switzerland) and Rick Hayes (UC Davis) for preparing the line drawings.

How to use this book

The first chapter of this book covers the nuts and bolts of neuropathology including basic neuroanatomy, necropsy and sampling techniques as well as general reaction patterns in the nervous system. At the end of this chapter is a very important section on classification of neurological diseases and recognition of major lesion patterns, the stepping stone for the subsequent chapters which each address a certain disease category, for example " inflammation" or "neoplasia".

In each of these following chapters we first present general common features and disease mechanisms, different lesion patterns encountered within the major category and strategies to solve diagnostic problems. Subsequently we discuss the specific disease entities.

Since advanced diagnostic imaging techniques and neuropathology increasingly overlap the reader will also find MRI images in this book. However to do this field justice, far more information is needed. Therefore this book is linked to a companion website on interpretation of MRI images from a representative series of neurological cases which also went to necropsy (www.wiley.com/go/vandevelde/veterinaryneuropathology). The MRI images are compared to the gross and microscopic findings of the very same cases with cross-referencing to the corresponding sections in the book. This MRI–pathology atlas has been prepared by our colleagues of the diagnostic imaging departments in Bern and Davis, with whom we have enjoyed an excellent collaboration for many years.

Marc Vandevelde
Robert J. Higgins
Anna Oevermann

Foreword

Marc Vandevelde, Robert J. Higgins and Anna Oevermann have collaborated to write a very thorough treatise on veterinary neuropathology. "Essentials of theory and practice" in the title does not provide the credit this book deserves. This is a textbook by all definitions.

It seems most appropriate that the authors based the origin of this text on the course material presented each year at the European School of Advanced Veterinary Studies at the University of Bern, Switzerland. This annual event was originally designed for the purpose of training veterinary pathologists in diagnostic neuropathology. In 1930, the University of Bern established the Institute of Comparative Neurology which was led by Prof. Walden Hoffman, a veterinarian, and Prof Ernst Frauchiger, a physician. This work was later continued by Prof. Rudolph Fankhauser and then Prof. Marc Vandevelde in the Institute of Animal Neurology at the Veterinary Faculty, University of Bern. Historically, the first major textbook of neuropathology of use to veterinarians was written by Ernst Frauchiger and Rudolph Fankhauser in 1957. This was: "Vergleichende Neuropathologie des Menschen and der Tiere". This textbook served well the German speaking scholars and forced those of us dependent on English to revive our German language training. I recall many occasions of discovering what I thought was a unique malformation in the necropsy room only to find a beautiful photograph of that same lesion in this textbook by Frauchiger and Fankhauser. In 1962, Comparative Neuropathology was published by JRM Innes and LZ Saunders. No further textbook publications occurred that covered this subject until 1995 when Summers, Cummings and de Lahunta published "Veterinary Neuropathology".

The three authors of this new textbook have carried on this tradition of excellence in neuropathology. They have many years of hands on experience in neuropathology and are well-recognized as experts in this specialty. With the Summer's textbook out of print, this is the only current textbook of neuropathology in English available to the veterinary profession today.

This text is well organized with many excellent illustrations and is easy to read and understand. It will be useful to all veterinary practitioners, neurologists and pathologists and will be especially welcomed by the residents in specialty training in neurology and pathology.

I congratulate Marc Vandevelde, Robert J. Higgins and Anna Oevermann for their fine contribution to the veterinary literature.

Alexander de Lahunta

1

General neuropathology

In this chapter, we will introduce the basic tools for diagnostic neuropathology starting with practical neuroanatomy and neurohistology. In the following, we will describe the process of collecting and sampling tissues and subsequently the basic histological reaction patterns to injury of the different cell types of the nervous system. Based on this information, we then describe a number of basic lesion types or patterns of disease. We also show how neurological diseases are classified into different disease categories (e.g. inflammation, tumors, etc.) and which of the basic patterns can be expected to occur in each of these categories. Recognizing these patterns and histological responses, together with a basic understanding of the classification system, provides a critical diagnostic guide for classification of specific disease categories, each of which is covered in one of the subsequent chapters.

1.1 Principles of neuroanatomy for diagnostic neuropathologists

The nervous system is anatomically immensely complex with important structural and biochemical differences between its various regions. As a result these different regions have, to a certain extent, their own diseases. Therefore, some basic understanding of neuroanatomy is essential for diagnostic neuropathologists. This includes the recognition of the major anatomic regions of the central nervous system (CNS) and how they interact both topographically and functionally. Such information will help to interpret the clinical information, to examine the brain in a standardized way and serve as a basis for using a brain atlas. Excellent concise and schematic information in these topics can be found in current text books of veterinary neurology.

1.1.1 Anatomical orientation by using the ventricular system

An effective approach to learning neuroanatomy is to identify and correlate all of the CNS regions by their relationship to the ventricular system of the brain (Fig. 1.1). The CNS in the adult animal develops after closure of the neural tube. This tubular structure is still preserved in both the central canal of the spinal cord and the aqueduct in the midbrain. During further development of the brain the neural tube forms specific evaginations caudally to rostrally: the fourth ventricle, the third ventricle and, in the forebrain, bilateral ventricles originating from two vesicles bulging at the rostral end of the neural tube (Fig. 1.1A). This basic structure undergoes further bending and distortion during subsequent development but remains recognizable in the postnatal animal. All anatomical structures originate from the subependymal zone of the ventricular system. This development is depicted in Fig. 1.1A. The lateral wall of the lateral ventricle develops into the cortex and the basal nuclei. As a result of unequal growth the lateral ventricles assume a half-moon shape (Fig. 1.1B) and the forebrain expands to cover the thalamus and midbrain. The thalamus–hypothalamus develops around the third ventricle; the third ventricle becomes ring shaped because the two halves of the thalamus connect in the midline (*interthalamic adhesion*) forming the dorsal and ventral lumens of the third ventricle. The midbrain develops around the aqueduct, the medulla oblongata from the ventral part of the fourth ventricle. Dorsally it gives rise to both a thin layer of tissue (the *medullary velum*) and to the cerebellum, which forms above the fourth ventricle (Fig. 1.1C). The spinal cord develops from the central canal after closure of the caudal part

Veterinary Neuropathology: Essentials of Theory and Practice, First Edition. Marc Vandevelde, Robert J. Higgins, and Anna Oevermann.
© 2012 John Wiley & Sons, Ltd. Published 2012 by John Wiley & Sons, Ltd.

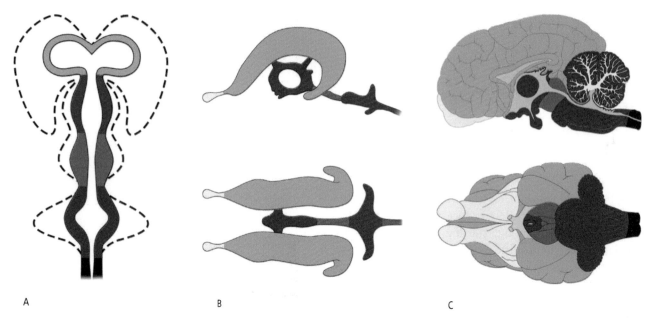

A   B   C

Fig. 1.1 Major divisions of the brain in relation to the ventricular system. A: Schematic drawing of the neural tube and its extensions (dorsal view). The dotted line indicates developmental growth of the periventricular tissues with the cerebral hemispheres overlapping the thalamus and midbrain. B: Schematic drawing of ventricular system dorsal and lateral view; different divisions of the ventricles are color coded. C: Medial and ventral view of an adult brain. The different colored areas arose from their respective color-coded sections of the ventricular wall. Yellow: olfactory bulb, tract and cortex; green: cerebral cortex; red: thalamus; dark blue: midbrain; brown: pons, medulla and cerebellum; black: spinal cord; light blue: cerebrospinal fluid. (Adapted from M. Stoffel: Funktionelle Neuroanatomie für die Tiermedizin, Enke, Stuttgart, 2011.)

of the neural tube. Additionally, there are several other extensions from within the ventricular system such as the olfactory canal extending from the lateral ventricles into the olfactory bulb, the *infundibular recess* extending ventrally from the third ventricle into the infundibulum, the lateral recesses of the fourth ventricle and the *suprapineal recess* dorsally from the third ventricle, which is best detected in sagittal magnetic resonance imaging (MRI) images. The choroid plexi in the walls of the lateral, III and IV ventricles develop from evaginations containing vessels and modified ependyma (*telea choroidea*) into the wall of the appropriate neural tube vesicles.

Thus when we transversely section the brain we can always identify some part of the ventricular system. Keeping in mind a three-dimensional concept of the ventricular system, as illustrated in Fig. 1.1, in each section we can thus correlate the shape of the ventricular system with the corresponding level of the CNS and also identify the relevant anatomical landmarks.

1.1.2 Major anatomical regions of interest

In this section we introduce the most diagnostically useful neuroanatomical sites of the CNS. The major regions of the CNS are the cerebral cortex and associated white matter, basal nuclei, thalamus/hypothalamus,

midbrain, cerebellum, medulla oblongata and spinal cord. To perform a competent neuropathological evaluation, one should have at least a concept of how these major regions relate to each other topographically, preferably in all three dimensions, and be able to recognize the major landmarks.

This level of neuroanatomy is sufficient to start. Further information can be found in neuroanatomy textbooks and atlases, which should be consulted during the neuropathological examination to acquire a more detailed anatomical knowledge. This knowledge also needs to include the functional connections between certain structures, which are essential for the interpretation of secondary changes.

The CNS on external gross examination

External views of the brain are illustrated in Fig. 1.2.

Dorsally the cerebral cortex of the cerebral hemispheres is separated along the midline by the longitudinal cerebral fissure and divided into frontal, occipital, parietal and temporal lobes, the vermis of the cerebellum and the brainstem. Ventral and lateral views illustrate the olfactory bulb and tract extending into a bulbous structure, the piriform lobe representing the

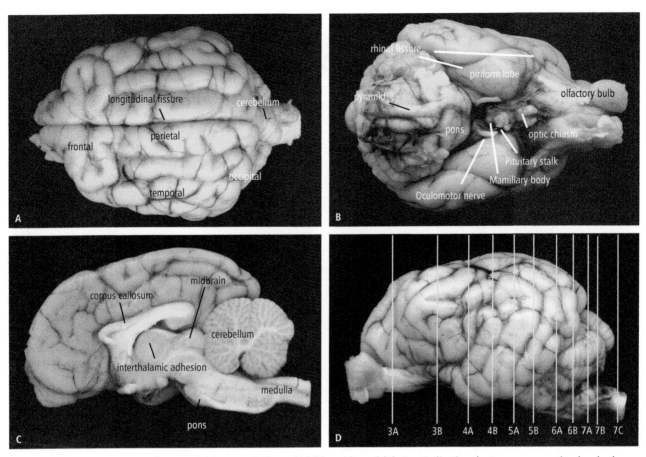

Fig. 1.2 Brain as seen externally. Dorsal (A), ventral (B), medial (C) and lateral (D) view indicating the transverse section levels shown in the subsequent figures (Figs.1.3–1.7).

most ancient part of the cortex (paleocortex) which is demarcated from the neocortex by the rhinal fissure. We need to recognize the optic chiasm, the pituitary stalk and the oculomotor nerves arising from the midbrain. The pons is the ventral bulge of white matter connecting the two cerebellar hemispheres, and also on the ventral aspect of the brainstem are the prominent pyramids, which are white matter tracts connecting the forebrain with the spinal cord. A medial view (Fig. 1.2C) following sagittal sectioning reveals the details of the ventricular system (as explained above), the corpus callosum, the interthalamic adhesion, the midbrain, brainstem and cerebellum. Fig. 1.2 D illustrates the levels at which the brain has been transversely sectioned to produce Fig. 1.3, Fig. 1.4, Fig. 1.5, Fig. 1.6 and Fig. 1.7.

The CNS in transverse sections

Serial transverse sections are illustrated in Fig. 1.3, Fig. 1.4, Fig. 1.5, Fig. 1.6 and Fig. 1.7. These brain slices have been stained to enhance the contrast between white and gray matter: the myelin content of the white matter is stained black. This is usually how brain sections are presented in a brain atlas and is somewhat reminiscent of T2W MRI images (see explanation below).

On transverse sections of the forebrain we can roughly discern three divisions according to the subcortical structures we can see: the frontal one-third containing the largest extent of the basal nuclei (Fig. 1.3), the middle one-third containing the thalamus/hypothalamus (Fig. 1.4) and the caudal one-third containing the midbrain (Fig. 1.5). Note that the caudal parts of the basal nuclei overlap with the thalamus and the caudal parts of the thalamus with the midbrain. Caudally to the forebrain we identify the brainstem, covered on its dorsal aspect by the cerebellum (Fig. 1.6 and Fig. 1.7). While studying the following transverse sections, keep the three-dimensional structure of the ventricular system in mind as the major feature for orientation to the major anatomical landmarks. In Fig. 1.3, Fig. 1.4, Fig. 1.5, Fig. 1.6 and Fig. 1.7 the colored drawing of the lateral view of the ventricular system (Fig. 1.1B) is shown indicating the level of sectioning.

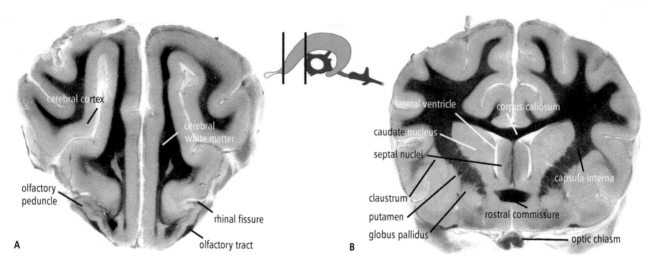

Fig. 1.3 A and B: Transverse sections frontal lobe and basal nuclei. Levels of sectioning shown in schematic drawing of the ventricles from Fig. 1.1.

Area of the basal nuclei (Fig. 1.3)

- Section A transversely slices the prefrontal area; the ventricles at this level consist of very narrow canals in the olfactory bulb (not visible). Section B transversely slices the rostral part of the lateral ventricles.
- Section A, ventral aspect, illustrates the olfactory bulb and associated tract (thin layer of white matter on the outside) extending caudally into the piriform lobe, a prominent bulbous structure best seen on ventral views (Fig 1.2B).
- The cerebral cortex is the gray matter on the surface of the hemispheres folded into gyri separated by sulci above the subcortical white matter. It has many functions associated with conscious perception of sensory input, voluntary control of movement and behavior.
- The basal nuclei consist of the caudate nucleus as a large convex structure protruding in the lateral ventricle and the putamen/pallidum/claustrum, distinct gray matter areas on the lateral side of the capsula interna. They all play a role in the control of motor function as part of the extrapyramidal system.
- Along the midline ventrally and bulging into the lateral ventricles are the septal nuclei, which belong to the limbic system and are involved in emotion.
- The corpus callosum is a large white matter tract connecting both hemispheres.
- The capsula interna, a wide white matter tract, bisects the deep gray matter nuclei of the hemispheres. It contains most connections from and to the cerebrum.
- The rostral commissure is a horseshoe-shaped band of white matter connecting both hemispheres ventrally.

Area of the thalamus (Fig. 1.4)

- Both sections show the lateral ventricles and the third ventricle. Section B slices through the lateral ventricles at the level where they curve back ventrally and rostrally; thus we see a dorsal and a ventral part. In addition to the lateral ventricles we see the third ventricle in the midline with – in section A slicing through the ring-shaped ventricle – a dorsal and a ventral portion.
- We can still see cortex, capsula interna and corpus callosum. In the wall of the lateral ventricle we see the caudal extension (the "tail") of the caudate nucleus; lateral to the capsula interna the caudal portions of the other basal nuclei. Section A shows the full extent of the piriform lobes which contain the amygdala, nuclear areas belonging to the limbic system.
- In section B the hippocampus appears, the particular shape of which results from inward folding of the cerebral cortex in the medial wall of the lateral ventricle. Envisage it as a sausage-shaped structure following the half moon of the lateral ventricle. At this level the hippocampus is exposed in its dorsal and ventral aspect. The hippocampus is part of the limbicsystem and plays an important role in memory.
- The fornix forms flattened bands of white matter attached to and containing the major connections of the hippocampus. They appear to be floating in the lateral ventricles.
- The gray matter in the centre is the thalamus, the major relay station for all sensory input, before it is projected in the cortex. The thalamus consists of many nuclear areas, some of which are anatomically quite distinct, notably the geniculate bodies (see below). Other prominent structures are the habenula

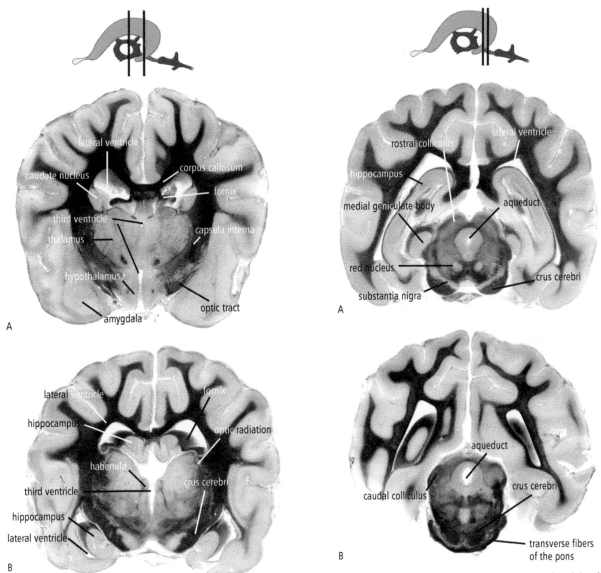

Fig. 1.4 A and B: Transverse sections at the level of the thalamus.

Fig. 1.5 A and B: Transverse sections at the lel of the midbrain.

protruding medially into the third ventricle; they play a role in control of circadian rhythms, emotional and social behavior and movement.

- The ventral extension of the gray matter on either side of the ventral portion of the third ventricle is the hypothalamus which regulates endocrine and vegetative functions. Ventrally is the pituitary gland (not present), attached to the hypothalamus via the infundibulum. When the latter is removed we can look directly into the third ventricle from the ventral surface.

- The optic tracts are the caudal and flattened extensions of the optic nerves and optic chiasm (easily seen on the ventral view), which can be recognized as distinct white matter structures; the optic tract eventu-

ally terminates at the lateral geniculate body, the primary visual centre in the thalamus.

- In section B of the thalamus we can see how the crura cerebri are starting to form from the internal capsule. The crura cerebri contain motor fibers, which continue into the spinal cord.

Area of the midbrain (Fig. 1.5)

- The ventricular system is limited here to the mesencephalic aqueduct, around which the midbrain developed. The lateral ventricles in the surrounding occipital lobes reach their maximal size at this level.

- This area contains the midbrain with, in its rostral part, the attached caudal extensions of the thalamus, the lateral and medial geniculate bodies, which are involved in visual and acoustic function respectively. Section A shows the medial geniculate bodies. Note that the forebrain is no longer merged together with the subcortical structures: the midbrain is separated from the hemispheres by a meningeal space.

- In the lateral ventricle we can see the major extent of the hippocampus, which now appears as a continuous oval structure because it is sliced in its caudal part.
- The colliculi are four rounded protrusions on the roof of the midbrain and are associated with visual and acoustic orientation.
- The crura cerebri (corticospinal tract) at the base of the midbrain in the first section are the continuation of the internal capsule containing connections between forebrain and brainstem. In section B, these tracts traverse the pons.
- The red nucleus and the substantia nigra are prominent well demarcated nuclei in the ventral part of the midbrain, which play an important role in control of motor function (extrapyramidal system).
- In the caudal portion of the midbrain we discern the transverse fibers of the pons, a transverse protrusion at the base of the brainstem, and white matter connection between both cerebellar hemispheres. It also contains the large pontine nuclei, the relay station between forebrain and cerebellum.

Area of the pons, medulla and cerebellum (Fig. 1.6)

- The ventricular system expands into the fourth ventricle seen in sections A and B. In section B it has a lateral extension on either side (the lateral recesses).
- The cerebellar cortex is a strongly convoluted structure. It plays an important role in coordination of movement. The center of the cerebellum consists of white matter, and the embedded cerebellar nuclei.
- In the brainstem, white and gray matter are intimately mixed. The brainstem contains cranial nerve nuclei, which are responsible for motor and sensory function of the head, e.g. chewing, swallowing, movement of the lips. On either side of the midline is the reticular formation, which plays an important role in controlling the level of consciousness.
- Further useful white matter landmarks are the caudal cerebellar peduncle, the pyramids and the spinal tract of the trigeminal nerve. The pyramids are prominent triangular white matter tracts at the base on either side of the midline. They are the continuation of the crura cerebri containing motor connections between brain and spinal cord.

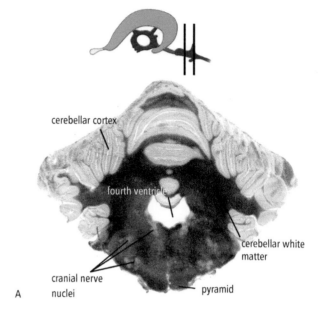

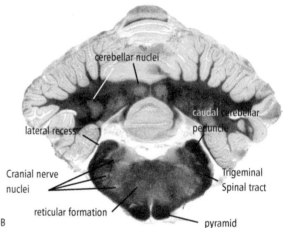

Fig. 1.6 A and B: Transverse sections through brainstem and cerebellum.

Area of medulla and spinal cord (Fig. 1.7)

- In section A we can see the thin roof of the fourth ventricle: the medullary velum. The ventricle becomes again surrounded by parenchyma in section B. At the level of the cord the ventricular system assumes a tubular configuration: the central canal.
- Further prominent gray matter structures in the medulla are the nuclei of the dorsal columns, the relay station for conscious proprioceptive impulses from the spinal cord, and the olivary nuclei, connecting the cerebellum with the extrapyramidal system, on either side of the midline just above the pyramids. The latter are quite large, triangular and can be easily recognized.

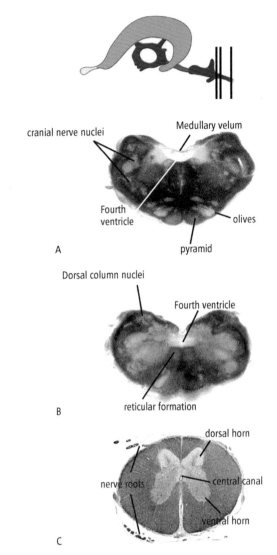

cranial nerve nuclei

Medullary velum

Fourth ventricle

olives

pyramid

A

Dorsal column nuclei

Fourth ventricle

reticular formation

B

dorsal horn

nerve roots

central canal

ventral horn

C

Fig. 1.7 A, B and C: Transverse sections through brainstem and spinal cord.

- In the cord, the gray matter is in the center with dorsal and ventral horns containing neurons responsible for movement of the limbs; especially important are the cervical and lumbar swellings associated with the fore and hind limbs.
- The white matter on the outside of the gray matter contains all connections between brain and spinal cord neurons.
- Note also the spinal nerve roots as the origin of the peripheral nerves; the dorsal nerve roots also contain dorsal root ganglia.

1.1.3 Histological neuroanatomy

Basic histological structure of the gray matter

There is a huge diversity in the histological appearance of the various anatomical areas of gray matter

exemplified by the different sizes and shapes of neurons and their arrangement in layers and nuclei. The basic histological features of neurons as well as glial cells are, however, very similar throughout the CNS.

Neurons are generally the largest cells and are distinguished by their cytoplasmic content of clumps of chromatin, called *Nissl substance*, formed by aggregations of rough endoplasmic reticulum with ribosomes. In some neuron subtypes (e.g., pontine nuclei, inferior olivary nuclei), the Nissl substance is normally marginated (not to be confused with *chromatolyis*, discussed in Section 1.3). The *neuropil* is the tissue between neurons formed of countless neuronal cell processes (dendrites and axons) and synapses, which cannot be visualized on hematoxylin and eosin (HE)-stained formalin-fixed, paraffin-embedded (FF-PE) sections. In the neuropil are glial cells (oligodendrocytes, astrocytes and microglia), of which there are almost ten times the number of neurons. On routine HE stain, we usually only see their nuclei. Oligodendroglia have small, strictly round and hyperchromatic nuclei resembling nuclei of lymphocytes (Fig. 1.8A, small arrows), and their processes form myelinated internodal segments around axons (Fig. 1.9E,G). They are much more numerous in white matter. Astrocytes have round to oval nuclei that are larger, more irregular and paler than those of oligodendrocytes with less dense chromatin (Fig. 1.8A, thick arrows). The *astrocytes* and their processes basically occupy any remaining space in the neuropil, cover the surface of neurons and synapses, and form a continuous superficial layer (*glial limiting membrane*) of endfeet processes under the pia mater of the CNS. Either oligodendroglia and/or astrocytes can normally be located peripherally around neuronal cell bodies in the process of *neuronal satellitosis*. Microglia are small, thin, elongated cells without apparent cytoplasm in both white and gray matter and comprise up to 15% of all glial cells.

The gray matter is densely vascularized. The blood vessels in both the gray and white matter consist of an inner layer of endothelial cells connected by tight impermeable junctions, covered by a basement membrane and surrounded by pericytes and the *endfeet* of astrocytic processes. Together these structures form the *blood–brain barrier* (BBB). Large arteries penetrating the cortex have a perivascular space, called the *Virchow-Robin (VR) space*, formed by an extension of the arachnoid membrane, and which is continuous with the subarachnoid space. The VR space is no longer present at the level of capillaries and its function is unknown.

In the peripheral nervous system (PNS), the gray matter consists of ganglia (sensory and autonomic) and

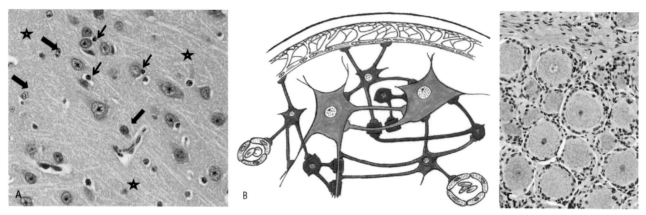

Fig. 1.8 Microanatomy of gray matter. A: Dog. Cerebral cortex with several neurons and glial cells, of which only the nuclei are visible. Small dark nuclei: oligodendrocytes (small arrows); the larger clear ones: astrocytes (large arrows). Most of the space between the neurons consists of neuropil (stars) and blood vessels. HE. B: Schematic drawing of gray matter structure with neurons (green), astrocytes (blue) making contact with neurons, blood vessels, oligodendrocytes and meninges. Oligodendrocytes (red) make contact with neuronal perikarya and particularly with the axons, where their processes form myelin sheaths. The surface is covered by meninges. C: Dog. Spinal ganglion. Neurons are surrounded by satellite cells. HE.

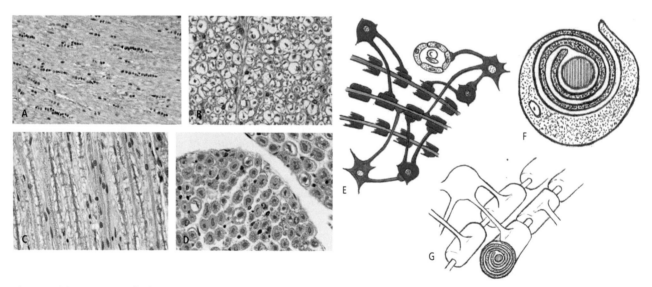

Fig. 1.9 Microanatomy of white matter. A: Dog. Longitudinal section of corpus callosum. HE. B: Dog. Transverse spinal cord section. The structure of the fibers of central white matter is discernible. Oligodendroglial nuclei in corpus callosum aligned in rows. HE. C: Dog. Longitudinal section of peripheral nerve. Note fishbone structure of myelin sheaths due to the Schmidt-Lantermann clefts. HE. D: Dog. Peripheral nerve cross-section showing individual axons surrounded by myelin sheath. HE. E: Schematic drawing of white matter structure with oligodendrocytes (red) covering axons (green) with myelin sheath segments separated by nodes of Ranvier, astrocytes (blue) and blood vessels. F: Schematic drawing of Schwann cell wrapping around an axon. G: More detailed drawing of CNS white matter showing oligodendroglial processes wrapping around axons to form myelin sheaths.

other less well demarcated accumulations of neurons (e.g. *Auerbach's and Meissner's myenteric plexus* in the gut). These ganglionic neurons are each surrounded by a layer of specialized Schwann cells called *satellite cells*.

Basic histological structure of the white matter

The white matter consists largely of tightly packed axons surrounded by myelin sheaths. On HE sections the myelin stains dark pink, although it is normally difficult to identify individual axons and their myelin sheaths. The sheaths are produced by oligodendrocytes, which wrap their processes around the axons in a spiral fashion creating segments of myelin called *internodes*, which are interrupted by the *nodes of Ranvier*. One oligodendrocyte can produce up to 60 internodes on regional axons. In the white matter, most oligodendrocytes are arranged in longitudinal rows along axonal tracts (Fig. 1.9). The white matter also contains many astrocytes, whose processes cover the axons at the nodes of Ranvier.

In the peripheral nerves, the myelin sheaths are produced by *Schwann cells*, with each cell contributing only one internode. Thinner non-myelinated axons are also wrapped by Schwann cell processes. The peripheral nerves also contain connective tissue with the *endoneurial fibroblasts* with their collagenous processes separating individual axons, the perineurium formed by modified Schwann cells isolating groups of axons as *fascicles* and fibroblast-derived *epineurium* wrapped around all the fascicles forming the peripheral nerve. In histological sections, the individual nerve fibers can be more easily identified than in the CNS. In longitudinal FF-PE sections the normal myelin sheaths often exhibit a "fishbone" structure due to *Schmidt-Lanterman's clefts* within the myelin internodes (Fig. 1.9C).

Intra- and extraventricular space and cerebrospinal fluid

The leptomeninges form the outer (*arachnoid membrane*) and inner (*pia mater*) border of the cerebrospinal fluid (CSF)-filled *subarachnoid space* around the brain and spinal cord (Fig. 1.10). Surrounding the leptomeninges is the pachymeninges or *dura mater* separated from the arachnoid membrane by the sudural space. In the calvarium the inner periosteum is formed by the dura mater but in the spinal cord the dura mater is separated from the vertebral bodies.

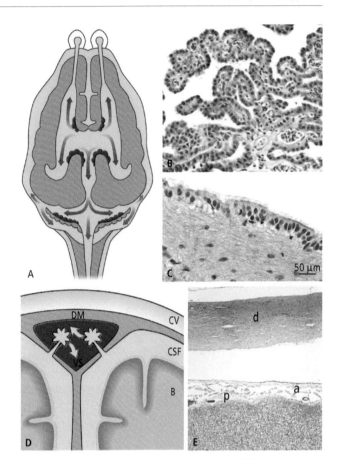

Fig. 1.10 CSF spaces. A: Schematic drawing of CSF flow (arrows). CSF produced by choroid plexus (red) flows caudally through the ventricles, and leaves the fourth ventricle into the arachnoidal space. B: Dog. Choroid plexus with vascular stroma covered by epithelial cells. HE. C: Dog. Fourth ventricle. Ciliated ependymal cells lining the ventricle. HE. D: Schematic drawing of CSF resorption via the arachnoidal granulations protruding into the venous sinuses (DM, dura mater; CV, bony cranial vault; CSF, cerebrospinal fluid in the subarachnoid space; B, brain lined by pia mater [yellow]). E: Dog. Meninges over the spinal cord d, dura mater or pachymeninges; a, arachnoid membrane with multiple trabecula; p, pia mater immediately overlying the neuropil. HE. The space between dura and arachnoidea is arteficial.

The ventricular walls are generally lined by a single layer of ciliated *ependymal cells*. The *choroid plexus* consists of a vascular stroma covered by epithelial cells of ependymal origin evaginated into specific sites within the ventricular system. CSF produced by the choroid plexus through filtration from the blood flows caudally within the ventricular system and gains access to the extraventricular subarachnoid space through the lateral foramina within the fourth ventricle. CSF is reabsorbed into the blood through the arachnoidal villi protruding in the extracerebral veins and sinuses.

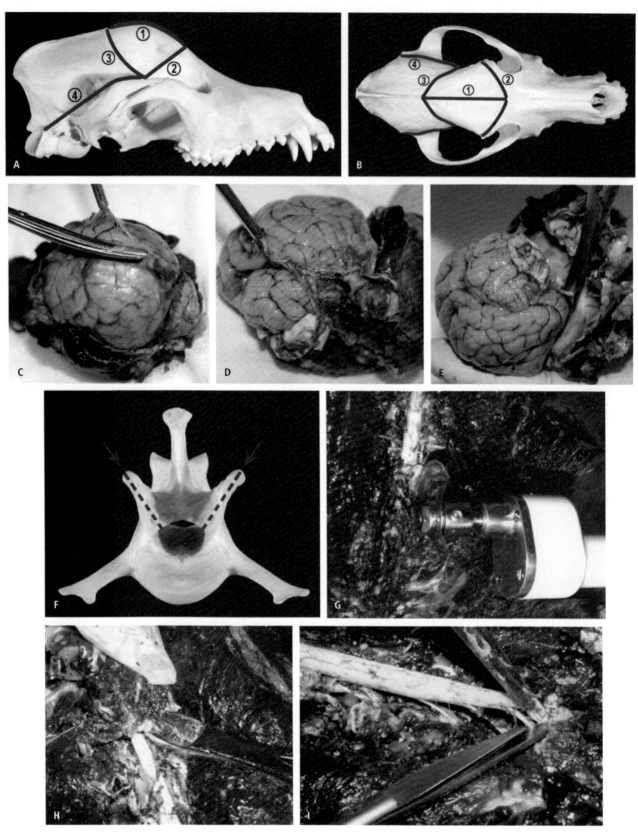

Fig. 1.11 Necropsy technique. Lateral (A) and dorsal (B) view of canine skull with lines marked in order (1, 2, 3 and then 4) for cuts using an autopsy saw, for partly removing the skull to easily access the brain : #1, 2 and 3 are to remove the frontal sinuses when present and #4 to remove the dorsal surface of the cranial vault. C: Removing the dura. D: Cutting the tentorium. E: Cutting cranial nerves with head upsidedown. F: Lumbar vertebral body indicating the site of the cut (using a Stryker saw) starting at the articular process (arrows) and extending down at an angle of about 30 degrees bilaterally resulting in a dorsal laminectomy and exposure of the spinal cord. G: Using the Stryker saw. H: Removing the roof of the vertebral column with rongeurs. I: Removing spinal cord by cutting spinal nerves.

1.2 Neuropathological techniques

1.2.1 Necropsy techniques

The CNS is protected by a solid bony calvarium and by the vertebral bodies. Thus, the skull and vertebral column have to be opened by considerable mechanical force to access the delicate CNS tissue. The latter is very soft and friable and should always be handled with care to avoid the many possible resultant artifactual changes. The brain therefore needs to be minimally touched, pressed or stretched during removal. Additionally, the spinal cord should not be folded or bent, nor should excessive pressure be placed on nerve roots during excision from the spinal canal. Post-mortem degeneration progresses rapidly within a few hours in nervous tissue. Thus, longer postmortem intervals considerably add to a range of artifactual changes.

Removal of the brain

Decapitate the animal by cutting ventrodorsally through the exposed soft tissues after extending the neck, opening the atlanto-occipital joint, separating the brain from the spinal cord before removing the head completely. Remove all skin and muscle from the head to expose the calvarium. Remove the dorsal cranial vault by using a saw (e.g. electric Stryker saw or Dremmel high-speed drill) cutting along the lines, as indicated in Fig. 1.11A and B, while avoiding contact with the underlying brain tissue. In very small animals, one can use a pair of rongeurs, starting at the medial side of one orbit until the dura mater is exposed; than remove the bone towards the foramen magnum. Always try to minimize touching the surface of the brain by cutting outwards from the brain. Then incise and remove the dura mater, falx and tentorium by using forceps and scissors or a scalpel (Figs 1.11C,D).

Then turn the head upsidedown, tilt to one side and shake gently to detach the brain from the skull and expose the cranial nerves; cut these cranial nerves transversely on the exposed side as close as possible to their exit foramina (Fig. 1.11E). Repeat for the other side.

Keeping the head upsidedown, hold the nose and shake gently; cut the remaining cranial nerves including the optic nerve and infundibulum and any other meningeal adhesions; detach the olfactory bulbs by arching the scissors or a wooden tongue depressor gently between bone and brain tissue; then shake gently to extract the brain completely.

Immediately after removal of the brain always examine the cranial vault, meninges, pituitary gland and fossa, the cranial nerves and their foramina to detect any relevant abnormalities. Sample the trigeminal (Gasserian) ganglia, and in ruminants the *rete mirabile caroticum*, which are both easily accessible at the base of the skull lateral to the pituitary fossa. Examine the whole brain for external gross lesions after removal and before fixation. Further detailed examination follows transverse sectioning of the brain.

Removal of the spinal cord

Expose the dorsal aspect of the spinal vertebrae by removing the paraspinal muscles. In small dogs and cats use rongeurs to remove the bone of the dorsal arch at the lumbosacral junction until you can see the cauda equina. Then, proceed cranially and remove the roof of each consecutive vertebra by cutting the lamina laterally on both sides without touching the cord (Fig. 1.11F–I). In large dogs, use an electric Stryker saw and perform a dorsal laminectomy by cutting through the lateral articular facets as an external guide, at approximately 30 degrees, to remove the dorsal arch and upper part of the vertebral arch. Once the cord is exposed, clamp the meninges over the cauda equina with a forceps and pull it gently horizontally, then, segment by segment in a cranial direction, cut the spinal nerve roots on each side with a scalpel blade or scissors, progressively lifting the cord (which remains confined within the dura mater) out of the spinal canal. When required for subsequent histological examination remove the dorsal root ganglia, which occur as tan, nodular thickenings of the nerve roots.

In large animals, suspend the eviscerated animal head down with the hind limbs maximally spread. Cut the vertebral column parasagittally with an electric saw to leave the cord intact and avoid damaging the nerve roots (at least on one side). Alternatively use a band saw after removal of the vertebrae from the carcass and again cut the vertebral bodies parasagittally. Remove the cord by cutting the spinal nerve roots on the remaining intact side of the canal. Avoid excessive bending of the labeled spinal cord segments for immersion fixation by placing labeled sections in a large rectangular flat container.

Depending on the neurological diagnosis, evaluate the vertebral canal and intervertebral foramina for any lesions that might cause stenosis; examine each intervertebral disc sagittally and the associated ligaments within the floor of the vertebral canal.

Evaluation of the neuromuscular system

In neurologically well documented cases in which neuromuscular disease is suspected, clinical biopsies of muscle and nerve, or at postmortem, selected tissues are sampled and processed for appropriate evaluation (e.g. frozen sections for histochemistry, resin-embedding for semi-thin and subsequent thin transmission electron microscope (TEM) sections, teased fiber preparations for examining individual nerve fibers) in specialized neuromuscular laboratories.

For initial histological examination, small pieces of muscle and nerve can be immersion-fixed in formalin and embedded in paraffin. The orientation and quality of such nerve and muscle samples can be optimized by attaching them (e.g. suturing) outstretched on a solid (e.g. cardboard or a nerve biopsy apparatus) support while fixing. For most effective evaluation by any technique, it is most important to include longitudinal as well as transversely oriented sections from muscle and nerve samples.

Fixation procedures

For routine diagnostic neuropathological evaluation, immersion fixation of brain or spinal cord in 10:1 v/v of 10% buffered formalin solution to tissue is optimal. A single sheet of absorbent paper between the brain and the bottom of the container will prevent adherence of the brain and severe artifactual changes. Adequate immersion fixation of brains in 10% formalin takes between 5 and 10 days for small and large animal brains respectively. For specialized laboratory techniques other fixatives or procedures (e.g. freeze drying) may be used. Certain histological techniques require unfixed tissue, snap frozen and sectioned in a cryostat. Such frozen sections have an inferior morphological resolution as compared with FF-PE sections.

For TEM or scanning electron microscope (SEM) small pieces of fresh tissue can be immersion-fixed in buffered 3% glutaraldehyde, although more specialized ultrastructural studies require perfusion fixation for optimal preservation of detail.

1.2.2 Brain sectioning, macroscopic inspection and sampling for histology

Macroscopic inspection

Section the brain and cord only after an appropriate fixation time. Use a very sharp knife to avoid compression during sectioning. Specialized wide-blade brain knives are not necessary but do ensure a smoother cut surface which can be important for optimal photography. Always use the same standardized procedure: with the exception of very specific indications, make only transverse 3–4 mm thick slices starting at the frontal lobe and ending at the medulla so that one can always identify anatomical landmarks and reconstruct the brain for

reexamination if necessary. Never make random cuts. Lay out the brain slices in their consecutive anatomical order for macroscopic inspection and for selection of areas for histological examination. Following autopsy and brain cutting after fixation, all regions must be examined (cerebral cortex, corpus striatum, thalamus, hippocampus, midbrain, cerebellum, brainstem and spinal cord). Pay attention to the following points, particularly when MRI is available:

- Check the ventricular system for stenosis, dilatation, compression and exudate. Examine the choroid plexi for swelling and congestion.
- During the entire examination look for alterations of all structures in size (e.g. aplasia, hypoplasia, atrophy, swelling), shape (e.g. cerebellar coning) and symmetry of both sides of the brain.
- Look for space-occupying changes (e.g. a tumor, abscess).

Other questions to consider are:

- Is there loss of substance (e.g. a cavity)?
- Is there a change of color (e.g. red indicates hemorrhage, white or yellow necrosis)?
- Is there a change of consistency (hardening or softening)?
- Are changes well demarcated from surrounding normal tissue?
- What is the pattern of distribution of the changes (single, multiple, bilateral or unilateral, anatomical localization)?

Often one may find very little change on macroscopic examination of the brain even when severe histological lesions are present.

Sampling for histological examination

When a definitive localization is suggested by neurological examination and confirmed by MRI, the examination can be concentrated on that specific anatomical area. However, representative sampling is the standard approach if no macroscopic lesions are present. Neurological disease is almost never the result of a small isolated single lesion except in the spinal cord. Small lesions are clinically often silent and even large lesions can remain unnoticed. When lesions of the CNS are the cause of neurological signs they are usually large or widespread. Still, often only specific regions are affected and in order to detect them a systematic approach with appropriate sampling is needed. Thus, where there are no grossly detectable lesions identified we aim to examine all the major divisions of the CNS histologically. These (depicted in Fig. 1.12) include: the area of the basal nuclei (roughly rostral one third of the fore-brain), the thalamus (roughly in the middle of the fore-brain), the midbrain (roughly the caudal third), the cerebellum–pontine area and the medulla oblongata. The first two areas include cerebral cortex. Make sure to include some hippocampus in the section of thalamus. A somewhat more extensive survey additionally includes occipital and frontal cortex which would be included, e.g. with either blindness or behavioral or/and cognitive deficits respectively detected clinically.

The spinal cord should be always examined when there are relevant clinical deficits. A representative survey of the cord in the dog and cat includes at least one transverse and longitudinal section from each of the following segments: upper cervical segments C1 and C4, cervical intumescence (C7), upper thoracic (T4), lower thoracic (T12), lumbar intumescence (L5) and sacral segments (S1).

Depending on the size of the brain and the capabilities of the histology laboratory, several alternative approaches are possible. Nowadays few laboratories can process full transverse sections. Therefore, from the large brain slices, take alternating halves; e.g. basal nuclei left, thalamus right. Always routinely mark one side of the brain sections, either the left or right side, with an incision. These halves can be further divided in order to fit the size of the tissue cassettes; however, always standardize the system you use to cut the smaller sec-tions so that you consistently recognize where you are anatomically. For documented cases of primary cerebellar disease we recommend sagittally sectioning the vermis prior to transverse sectioning of the cerebellar hemispheres.

Histological technique

The routine technique consists of paraffin embedding of the formalin-fixed tissues. Briefly, fixed tissue samples are dehydrated in graded ethanols, cleared in xylene and infiltrated with paraffin. Sections are cut 3–5 μm thick from the paraffin blocks and stained. The standard routine stain is HE, which allows the detection of lesions in nearly all cases. Special histochemical and immunocytochemical stains are used to define and characterize the detected lesions more precisely. Reliable methods are: Nissl stain (cresyl Echt violet) for neurons, luxol fast blue for myelin (best combined with HE), Bielschowsky silver-based stain for axons, trichrome (Gomorri) stain for connective tissue. However, special silver impregnations for neurons and glial cells are often difficult to reproduce and extremely cumbersome. Much more specific and reliable is the demonstration of cell-specific antigens with immunohistochemical labeling by relevant antibodies. The latter are referred to in the section on basic tissue reaction patterns. For special purposes, fresh unfixed tissues are snap-frozen but the

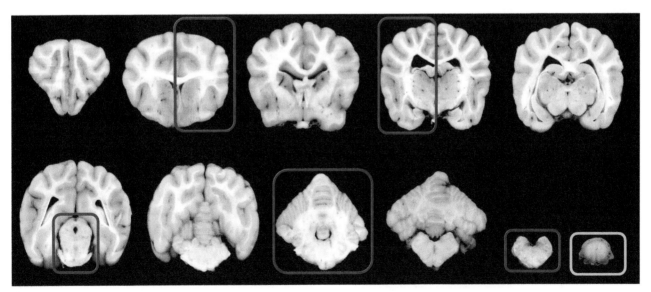

Fig. 1.12 Representative sampling. Serial sections of a fixed canine brain. The red boxes include the minimal areas of the brain which must be trimmed in for histological processing. Appropriate levels of the spinal cord (green box) should be included whenever possible.

morphological resolution of such frozen sections is of much lower quality than paraffin sections.

More precise structural resolution can be obtained by resin embedding (in which there is no fat extraction) for transmission electron microscopy. From such material so-called semi-thin sections can be cut and stained with toluidine blue for microscope study.

Examining microsopic slides histologically

At the microscopic level, scan all sections systematically, most effectively initially with low- and then medium-power magnification. In view of the great anatomical variations between the different regions, familiarity with the normal histological structure of all these regions helps to detect lesions. This familiarity comes only with experience, best started in a mentored one-on-one setting. When scanning slides it helps to consciously and constantly register microanatomical details. The morphology of reactions of the different cell types to injury is described in Section 1.3.

1.3 Basic tissue reaction patterns

The wide range of neuropathological entities in animals and man is due mainly to both the anatomical complexity and to inherent differences in vulnerability to injury in different areas of the nervous system. Cells in the CNS can mount a relatively limited number of reactions in response to injury: the same basic reactions can occur in different anatomical locations and combinations, thus giving the impression of a large variety of reaction patterns. As with any other organ system in the body, the CNS is subject to pathologic changes depending on genetic background (endogeneous causes: disease susceptibility, inborn degenerative diseases) of an individual, and external causes (exogeneous: e.g. trauma, viral, bacterial or protozoal infections, and metabolic–toxic agents). We will briefly discuss the reactive changes in the major CNS cell populations of neurons, oligodendrocytes, astrocytes, ependymal/choroid plexus cells, microglial cells and blood vessels to injury.

1.3.1 Reactions of neurons to injury

Microscopically the nervous system consists in part of neurons whose axons can extend over enormous distances. This creates the problem of neurons having to provide metabolic support in dendritic and axonal processes of the cell that are far removed from the perikaryon. Neurons are also highly differentiated and functionally specialized cells, which are not capable of regeneration to any significant extent. Another special feature of the CNS is the generation of action potentials and conduction of such signals along the axons. The

efficiency of this process is greatly enhanced by the presence of segmented myelin sheath internodes allowing saltatory conduction across these segments.

A variety of molecular mechanisms have been unraveled, which can impair structural and functional integrity of neurons. Two important ones are *excitotoxicity* and *oxidative change*. Neuronal excitotoxicity depends on the excessive sustained release from neurons of certain excitatory neurotransmitters (e.g. glutamate, aspartate) and their decreased removal by astrocytes in the CNS in response to such factors as ischemia, anoxia or hypoglycemia. Subsequent binding of excessive glutamate to various types of ionotropic receptors (e.g. for N-methyl-d-aspartate, NMDA) on neurons results in transmembrane ionic fluxes with rising intracellular levels of calcium leading to activation of proteolytic enzymes, which then damage cell organelles. *Acidophilic neuronal necrosis* is considered to be the final common pathway resulting from neurotransmitter-induced neuronal excitotoxicity. Neurons are also particularly prone to oxidative damage, a final common pathway of cell pathology in many different diseases. During respiration mitochondria produce superoxide anions which, under normal circumstances, are reduced by *superoxide dismutases* (SOD) to H_2O_2. Under pathological circumstances H_2O_2 can be converted to hydroxyl (OH) radicals, which are highly reactive, particularly with lipids (in which the nervous system is very rich) inducing membrane damage and ultimately tissue destruction. Another class of reactive oxygen species includes the *nitric oxides* (NO) generated by *nitric oxide synthetases*. Reaction of NO with H_2O_2 can lead to the formation of the highly toxic peroxynitrite. Cells have developed defense systems such as SOD against such toxic events. Breakdown of the equilibrium between oxygen radicals and such defense mechanisms leads to cell pathology.

A wide spectrum of neuronal changes to injury has been described but here we will describe only a few common patterns.

Intraneuronal inclusions

Intracytoplasmic and intranuclear inclusion bodies, often with distinctive characteristic morphological, biochemical and ultrastructural features, can accumulate in neurons/glial cells as a result of certain degenerative, metabolic and viral diseases, and have often received the names of their discoverers (e.g. Negri and Lafora bodies).

Their usually distinctive morphology, intracellular localization (intranuclear versus intracytoplasmic or both) and biochemical and ultrastructural composition can be diagnostically important for specific diseases (Fig. 1.13A). Since most neurons are postmitotic, are

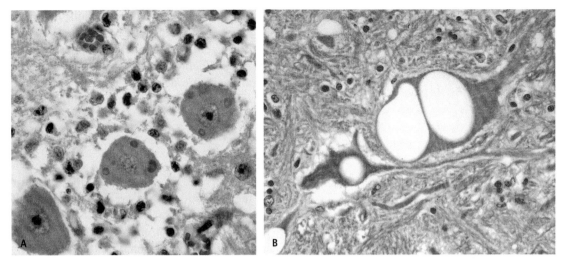

Fig. 1.13 A: Dog with rabies virus infection. Cerebellum. Multiple intraneuronal intracytoplasmic inclusion bodies (Negri bodies) in Purkinje cells. HE. B: Sheep with scrapie. Brainstem. Multiple intracytoplasmic intraneuronal vacuoles. HE.

usually not replaced and have no exocytic capability, neuronal or glial cytoplasmic storage of metabolites within hyperplastic lysosomes as a result of genetic or acquired lysosomal enzyme defects can be quite spectacular in the CNS (see Chapter 8). Empty cytoplasmic vacuoles in the neuronal cell body (Fig. 1.13B) and its processes are characteristic of prion-induced transmissible spongiform encephalopathies in animals, e.g. scrapie, bovine spongiform encephalopathy. However, they may occur in limited numbers also as incidental finding in normal cattle (e.g. in the red nucleus).

Eosinophilic inclusion bodies (pseudo-Negri bodies) of unknown significance are often found in neurons of the lateral geniculate body and hippocampus in cats and occasionally in other species. Similar small inclusions can occur in thalamic and cerebellar Purkinje cells in dogs. Widespread neuronal intranuclear inclusions were reported in a horse, resembling intranuclear neuronal inclusion body disease in humans.

Dark brown neuromelanin granules are normally found in the hypothalamus and sometimes in other neurons but rarely to the extent that it becomes grossly visible as in certain human neuroanatomical regions.

Chromatolysis

Central chromatolysis is a frequent reactive response in neurons. Histologically, there is an initial swelling of the cell body and processes, perinuclear dispersion of Nissl substance with loss of ribosomes from the rough endoplasmic reticulum (RER), a thin intact cytoplasmic border of Nissl substance and peripheral margination and flattening of the nucleus (Fig. 1.14). It can be commonly seen in lower motor neurons of the spinal cord in ruminants with postnatally acquired copper defi-

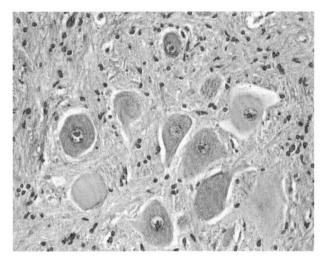

Fig. 1.14 Sheep with copper deficiency. Spinal cord. Various stages of chromatolysis in ventral horn motor neurons. HE.

ciency. It is also the result of a retrograde axonal reaction to nerve root injury, e.g. after brachial plexus avulsion. The histochemical stain, cresyl Echt violet, is very useful for visualization of the Nissl substance dispersion. This process can be either functionally and morphologically reversible with treatment or eventually lead to neuronal necrosis depending on the cause and severity of injury. The process of chromatolysis should not be confused with the normal morphology of cranial nerve nuclei (e.g. V, VII) which normally have only a peripheral rim of Nissl substance but a centrally placed nucleus.

Acidophilic neuronal necrosis

Cell death of neurons can be either necrotic or non-necrotic. *Necrosis* is solely due to external factors

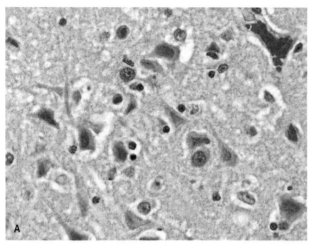

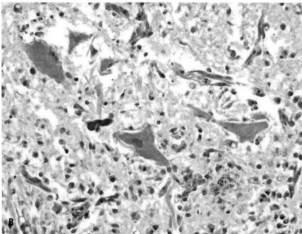

Fig. 1.15 A: Sheep with polioencephalomalacia. Cerebral cortex. Acidophilic (ischemic) neuronal necrosis with shrunken eosinophilic neurons. HE. B: Dog with spinal cord infarct. Myelomalacia with acidophilic neuronal necrosis. HE.

leading to membrane damage and cell swelling. Neurons, being primarily dependent on glycolysis for energy, are extremely sensitive to conditions interfering with glucose metabolism including ischemia, hypoglycemia or thiamin deficiency. Their morphologic reaction to anoxia/ischemia is acidophilic (ischemic) neuronal necrosis with marked granular change and eosinophilia of the cytoplasm in HE sections, acute swelling and later shrinkage of the cell body, as well as nuclear pyknosis of the centrally placed nucleus (Fig. 1.15). This is an irreversible lesion. Importantly from a diagnostic view, this change can only be detected after 6–8 hours following the triggering injury. The underlying mechanism (e.g. ischemia, hypoglycemia, anoxia, trauma, virus infection etc.) is thought to be mediated by excessive sustained release of various excitotoxic neurotransmitters (e.g. glutamate, aspartate), irrespective of the inciting event.

Global ischemia results in acidophilic neuronal necrosis in specific neuroanatomical sites: cerebral cortex, hippocampus and Purkinje cells. Anatomically defined sites of selective neuronal susceptibility to ischemia as in the pyramidal neurons of the CA1 and CA2 sectors may be explained by their high concentration of dendritic glutamate receptors.

Apoptosis

In non-necrotic cell death such as *apoptosis*, components of the regulation of the cell cycle control the events leading to programmed cell death. Neuronal apoptosis is particularly common during fetal CNS development, in degenerative and some viral diseases. The two most important categories of molecules regulating apoptosis are the *Bcl2 family* and the *caspases*. Morphologically it is characterized by chromatin condensation, cytoplasmic blebbing, nuclear fragmentation and presence of so-called "apoptotic bodies". However, in HE-stained sections it might be difficult to definitely distinguish between necrosis and apoptosis and hence apoptosis is best confirmed with positive immunoreactivity to, for example, activated caspase 3.

Neuronal loss

Irrespective of etiology, individual necrotic neurons in the neuropil are removed by the process of *neuronophagia* mediated by activated phagocytic microglia, which accumulate around the neuron as microglial nodules (Fig. 1.16). Such focal microgliosis is also one characteristic histological feature of the triad of meningoencephalitis (perivascular cuffing, neuronal degeneration/necrosis, microglial nodules) that are hallmarks of neurotropic viral infections.

Neurons do not regenerate as a general rule. Thus typically in the CNS, neuronal damage frequently results in permanent loss of cells termed neuronal loss. There is a characteristic regional selective susceptibility of neurons or nuclei to different etiologic agents. A combination of irreplaceable loss of certain nerve cell populations and Wallerian degeneration of their axons results in neuropathological patterns which are highly typical of certain acquired or inherited degenerative diseases. Atrophy mainly occurs as a result of loss of trans-synaptic afferent input in anterograde and retrograde degeneration (see below) or geriatric change.

Trans-synaptic degeneration

Neurons form interconnected networks, whereby axon terminals of one neuron make synapses with other

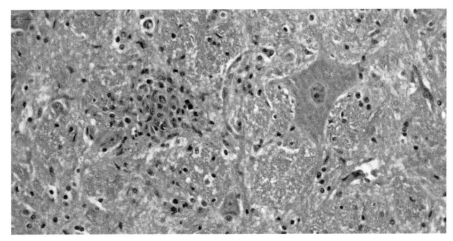

Fig. 1.16 Dog with neurotropic canine distemper virus encephalitis. Brainstem. Neuronophagia. Microglial nodule removing degenerated neuron. HE.

neurons. When a neuron and its processes degenerate, afferent and efferent synaptic contacts from neurons in both anterograde and retrograde locations are also lost (Fig. 1.17). This bidirectional process results in trans-synaptic neuronal degeneration, which maybe reversible depending on the primary injury. With a basic knowledge of neuroanatomical pathways between

nuclear groups the concept of trans-synaptic degeneration can help to interpret certain lesion distribution patterns, e.g. Purkinje cell loss leads to anterograde trans-synaptic atrophy and eventually degeneration of the cerebellar nuclei and retrograde trans-synaptic atrophy of the cerebellar granule cells (see Chapter 8).

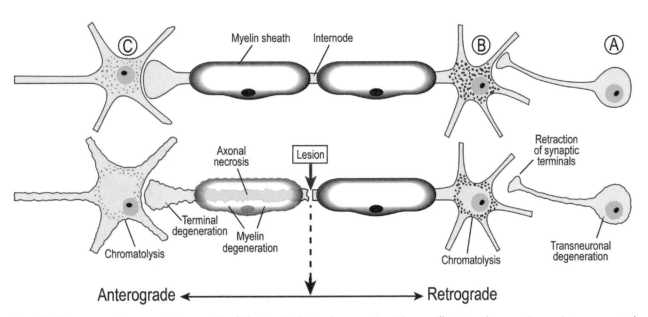

Fig. 1.17 Trans-synaptic neuronal degeneration following Wallerian degeneration. Diagram illustrates three contiguous interconnnected neurons A, B and C. Distal to the site of the transecting lesion is axonal necrosis and myelin degeneration with retraction of the synaptic junction and chromatolysis of the downstream neuron (C) in an *anterograde* direction. Upstream there is neuronal chromatolysis (B) and retraction of synaptic contacts from A in a *retrograde* direction.

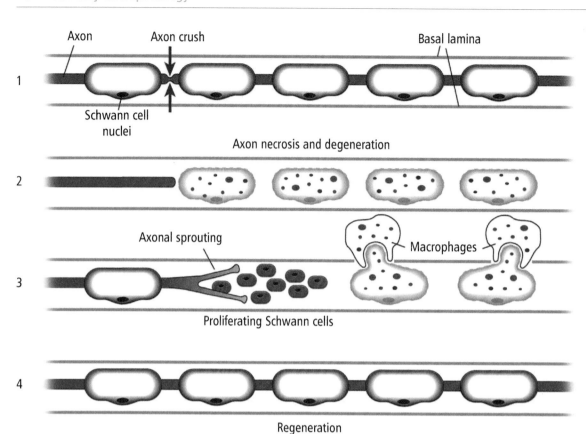

Fig. 1.18 A: Schematic drawing of Wallerian degeneration. 1. Peripheral axon covered by myelin sheath formed by Schwann cells. 2. Axon and myelin sheath distal to injury undergo degeneration. 3. Macrophages of blood monocyte origin ingest the axonal and myelin debris. Schwann cells proliferate within the persisting endoneurial tube forming densely packed cell chains, so-called Büngner's bands, providing support for axon sprouts arising from the damaged axon. 4. New myelin segments are formed around regenerating axon.

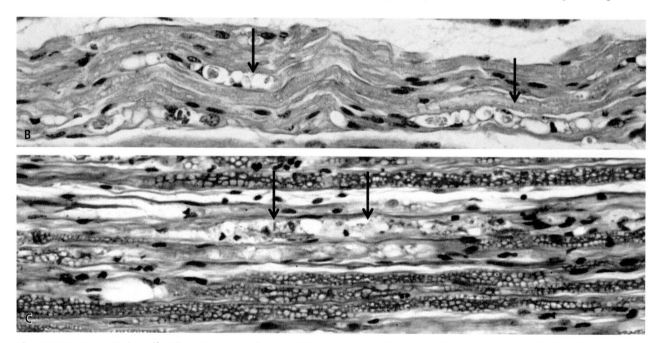

Fig. 1.18 B: Brown Swiss calf with motor neuron disease. Wallerian degeneration in peripheral nerve, longitudinal section: segments of fragmented axons in several fibers (arrows). HE. C: Dog with peripheral nerve injury. Longitudinal section. Wallerian degeneration, intact myelin sheaths are stained red. Degenerated fibers are replaced by macrophages containing myelin debris (arrows). Masson's trichrome stain.

Axonal and dendritic changes

The axonal and dendritic processes of neurons can undergo degeneration independent of the neuronal cell body. A typical reaction of the axon to a variety of insults is *Wallerian* (or *Wallerian-like*) *degeneration*. This process consists of a series of degenerative and reparative histological events which occur to the axon and myelin sheath classically following primary traumatic injury to the axon or dendrite (Wallerian degeneration) but may also occur following any other type of axonal damage, e.g. ischemia, degenerative axonal disorders (so called Wallerian-like degeneration). Though these changes occur also in the CNS, they are best studied in peripheral nerve injury. When a nerve fiber is focally damaged, the nerve process distal to the lesion undergoes anterograde degeneration due to interference with the vital mechanism of bidirectional axonal transport systems. In Wallerian degeneration, the axons undergo focal segmental swelling forming axonal spheroids due to interference with axonal transport and subsequent proximate metabolite accumulation, followed by distension of the myelin sheath, necrosis of both structures and their ingestion by macrophages of blood monocyte origin or of microglial cells in the CNS (Fig. 1.18). In peripheral nerves, Schwann cells proliferate within the persisting endoneurial tube and form densely packed cell chains, so-called *Büngner's bands* (Fig. 1.18). Complete functional regeneration following axonal sprouting and segmental remyelination is possible in the peripheral nervous system but rarely happens in the CNS. The most conspicuous feature in the neuron whose nerve fiber has been injured close to the cell body can be retrograde chromatolysis (see above).

The axon can swell segmentally many times its normal size and these axonal spheroids can be easily detected in a histological preparation (Fig. 1.19). Such swellings can also result from intrinsic metabolic hereditary disorders known as axonal dystrophies. Since there is little regeneration in the CNS, axonal damage usually ends as axonal loss, generally with a reactive astrogliosis, and can be best detected by using a combination of axonal and myelin stains.

Immunohistochemical identification of neurons and their processes

For routine diagnostic purposes, currently the most widely used antibodies for the immunocytochemical identification of neurons and their processes are those to synaptophysin; triple neurofilaments (NF-L, NF-M, NF-H molecular weights) either individually or in various cocktails, and also as phosphorylated or non-phosphorylated neurofilaments; and to Neu-N. There are, however, many more neuronal specific antigens, e.g. neural cell adhesion molecules (NCAM) and microtubule associated proteins (MAPs), often requiring strict fixation techniques; these are mainly for experimental use. Cells of the neuroendocrine system express synaptophysin, chromogranin A and neuron-specific enolase, which can all be visualized immunocytochemically.

Axons (both normal and undergoing pathological changes) in the CNS/PNS are best visualized immunocytochemically by antibodies to NF-200, and triple neurofilaments either in a phosphorylated or non-phosphorylated state. Amyloid precursor protein (APP) is a robust marker of early axonal injury.

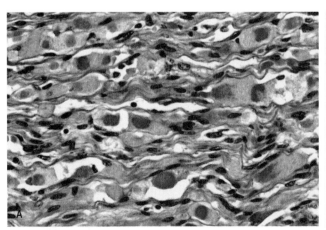
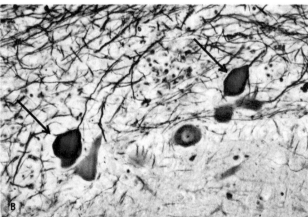

Fig. 1.19 A: Horse. Trigeminal nerve compressed by an abscess. Many swollen eosinophilic and fragmented axons. HE. B: Bovine with axonal dystrophy. Cerebellar cortex, axon swellings depicted by arrows. Holmes' silver stain.

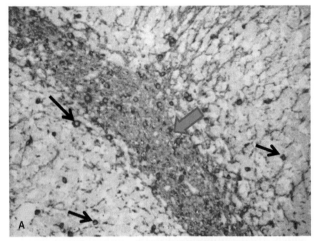

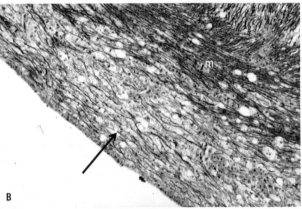

Fig. 1.20 A: Dog. Normal cerebellar white matter and adjacent granular layer. Oligodendrocytes (arrow) and myelin sheaths (big arrow) are labeled with an anti-CNP antibody. B: Dog. Brainstem. Demyelinating lesion in canine distemper infection (m, unaffected white matter with dark-staining axons covered by green/blue-stained intact myelin). In the demyelinating lesion there is focal loss of myelin staining but preservation of axons (arrow). Luxol fast blue–Holmes' silver stain.

1.3.2 Oligodendrocytes

These are highly specialized glial cells with small round dark basophilic nuclei and short processes, the distal ends of which flatten into wide membranous sheets that form myelin sheaths as explained above or clusters around neurons in the gray matter as normal satellitosis.

Demyelination – primary or secondary

When oligodendrocytes are damaged (e.g. by virus infection or ischemia), their complex membranous structures forming myelin internodes undergo degeneration and phagocytosis in the process of primary demyelination (Fig. 1.20B). In contrast to Wallerian degeneration, there is selective degeneration of the myelin sheath or oligodendrocyte in this primary demyelinating process with axons remaining intact for a long time. Secondary demyelination occurs after primary axonal necrosis with an obligatory loss of the myelin sheath. Functional remyelination by oligodendrocytes can occur in the CNS but not to the same degree as from their myelinating counterparts of Schwann cells in the PNS. To demonstrate demyelination histochemically the luxol fast blue/Holmes silver stain can distinguish between primary and secondary demyelination. In primary demyelination there is an absence of blue-staining myelin sheaths but the black silver-impregnated axons remain intact (Fig. 1.20B). In secondary demyelination there is a concommitant loss both of axons and then of their myelin sheaths. In the luxol fast blue/cresyl Echt violet/PAS stain (Klüver-Barrera) macrophages in the demyelinated area are demonstrated to contain myelin debris. Alternatively immunocytochemical procedures can be used to demonstrate specific antigenic markers for either axons (see above) or myelin.

Leukodystrophy is the term applied to an intrinsic dysfunction in oligodendrocytes with formation of unstable myelin in contrast to demyelination where there is an acquired lesion affecting myelin from normal oligodendrocytes.

Immunohistochemical staining

For routine diagnostic purposes (FF-PE tissue) there are many antigenic markers for oligodendrocytes/myelin sheath although no single specific unequivocal marker for oligodendrocytes. Some antigens expressed by oligodendrocytes include myelin basic protein (MBP), myelin associated glycoprotein (MAG), and proteolipid protein (PLP), galactocerebroside (GC), 2'-3'-cyclic nucleotide-3'-phosphatase (CNP) (Fig. 1.20A), transferrin and the transcription factor Olig2, as well as many antibodies that are useful for more specialized experimental purposes. Normal oligodendrocytes can be definitively labeled using *in situ hybridisation* for PLP mRNA.

1.3.3 Astrocytes

Astrocytes play a critical role in many normal functions including intercellular homeostasis of ions, glutamine and neurotransmitters and the detoxification of, for example, oxidants and ammonia. They insulate and isolate white matter tracts and are involved in inflammatory and immune responses, expressing cytokines, growth factors and adhesion molecules. Astrocytes provide intrinsic structural support and guidance for fetal brain development. They form the glia limitans and perivascular foot processes, an integral component of the blood–brain barrier. They are morphologically described as protoplasmic or fibrillary in normal gray or white matter respectively. The distinction between the two forms requires special stains.

Gliosis

Both protoplasmic and fibrillary astrocytes react similarly and non-specifically to almost any kind of damage (e.g. edema, viral infections, malacia, degeneration) to the CNS by either hypertrophy (astrocytosis) or proliferation (astrogliosis). There are basically two reactive forms: in acute injury the *gemistocytic astrocyte*, in which there is substantial homogeneous eosinophilic enlarge-ment of the perikaryon with multiple thick short processes on HE sections (Fig. 1.21D) and chronically a morphological transformation to the *fibrillary astrocyte* with large numbers of glial fibrillary acidic protein (GFAP)-containing thin elongate cell processes (Fig. 1.21C). Chronic fibrillary astrogliosis is also called *sclerosis*. On routine HE stains, astrocytosis is apparent as an increased number of cell nuclei in the affected area (Fig. 1.21B).

Fluid accumulation in the CNS, edema, is associated with a spongy vacuolated appearance of the tissue (see Section 1.3.7). In cytotoxic edema there is an accumulation of fluid within and marked swelling of astrocytic cell bodies and processes. A special kind of reactive astrocyte is the so-called Alzheimer type II cell found in clusters in gray matter in metabolic encephalopathy

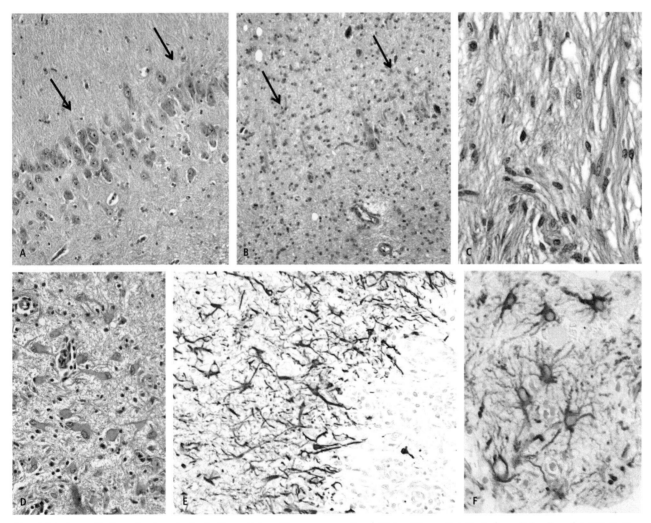

Fig. 1.21 Astrogliosis and astrocytosis. A: Normal dog. Hippocampus. Pyramidal cell layer. Relatively few glial cell nuclei. HE. B: Dog with hippocampal sclerosis. Same area as in A with nearly complete loss of neurons and massive increase in number of astrocytic nuclei. HE. C: Dog. Edge of old infarct. Fibrillary astrogliosis. HE. D: Dog with necrotizing encephalitis. Brainstem. Reactive gemistocytic astrocytes. HE. E: Dog. GFAP immunostaining of reactive fibrillary astrocytes around an oligodendroglioma. IHC. F: Dog. GFAP immunoreactive gemistocytic astrocytes with thickened processes. IHC.

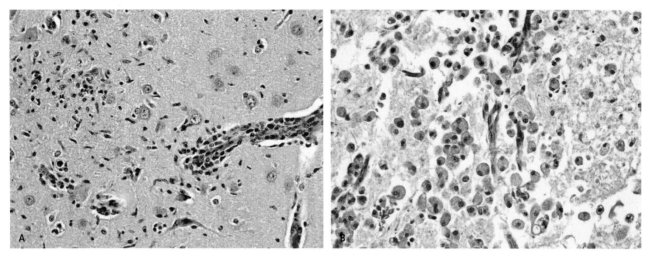

Fig. 1.22 A: Dog with viral encephalitis. Brainstem. Rod-shaped activated microglial cells. HE. B: Dog with cerebral infarct. Phagocytic gitter cells. HE.

associated with hepatic and less often renal disease (see Chapter 6). These cells have large pale nuclei with minimal cytoplasm. *Rosenthal fibers* are eosinophilic bodies found within processes of fibrillary astrocytes in tumors, sites of chronic injury and in **Alexander's disease** in the dog and sheep (see Chapter 8).

Immunohistochemical stains

The most widely used antigen detected immunocytochemically for normal, reactive and neoplastic astrocytes is glial fibrillary acidic protein (GFAP) (Fig. 1.21E,F). *Vimentin* and *nestin* can also be co-expressed with GFAP in reactive and neoplastic astrocytes. There is some cross-reactivity of GFAP with normal and neoplastic Schwann cells in the PNS.

1.3.4 Microglia/macrophages
Microglia and neuronophagia

The CNS contains a population of resident phagocytes, the so-called *resting microglia*, derived from monocytes of bone marrow origin entering the CNS during fetal development. These cells are capable of reactive proliferation in a variety of conditions. Activated reactive microglia, also called *rod cells*, appear as elongated, often twisted nuclei with very scant cytoplasm (Fig. 1.22A). This type of reaction occurs in more subtle lesions such as in retrograde neuronal degeneration and often in some protozoal and viral infections. These reactive microglia are mainly involved in removal of individual neurons in the process of neuronophagia mediated by chemokine-induced clusters of microglial cells forming microglial nodules.

Gitter cells and malacia

Acute necrosis of large areas of neuropil leads to almost complete loss of the original architecture of the affected area. This necrotic tissue is called *malacia*, which can be macroscopically visible when the lesion is large enough. The necrotic (malacic) tissue is initially infiltrated by densely packed actively phagocytic macrophages, also called gitter cells, which remove cell debris, axons and myelin (Fig. 1.22B). These cells are largely derived from blood-borne monocytes and to a much lesser extent from residential microglial cells.

Within weeks to months, a malacic area is completely cleared of all necrotic tissue and is replaced by a fluid-filled cystic cavity. Chronically reparative attempts with neovascularization and astrogliosis result in a fibrillary astroglial scar in and around the lesion and sometimes additional fibrous connective tissue formed by perivascular mesenchymal cells.

Identification by immunohistochemically detected markers

Both resting and activated microglia and macrophages derived from blood monocytes in the canine CNS can be broadly identified immunocytochemically by antibodies to both CD18 and CD11d in conventional FF-PE tissue. A fraction of microglia and macrophages may stain with antibodies to CD68, lysozyme and MAC (*myeloid/histiocyte antigen*). However antibodies capable of discriminating between these functional cell types in the CNS (resting or activated microglia, macrophages) are not yet available in the dog. Both activated microglia

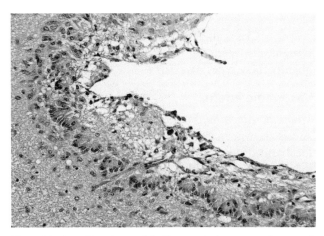

Fig. 1.23 Dog. Fourth ventricle. Traumatic damage to the ependyma leads to rosette formation, supra-ependymal astrocytosis and partial occlusion of mesencephalic aqueduct. HE.

and blood-borne macrophages express MHC class I and II antigens, various adhesion molecules, chemokines and cytokines and can act as antigen-presenting cells in modulating both inflammatory and immune responses.

1.3.5 CSF spaces

Ependymal cells

A single layer of usually ciliated ependymal cells lines the ventricles, mesencephalic aqueduct and central canal of the spinal cord, and allows for the regulated bidirectional flow of proteins and fluid between the ventricles and the interstitial space of the brain. Viral cytolysis, inflammation (*ependymitis*) or traumatic loss of these cells can lead to attempts at repair with rosette formation, sub- and supra-ependymal astrogliosis (Fig. 1.23) and occlusion with partial or complete obstruction of CSF flow at critical stricture points and subsequent non-communicating hydrocephalus. Atrophy with loss of cilia can occur with increased and sustained hydrostatic pressure of hydrocephalus. Normal and neoplastic ependymal cells are variably immunoreactive for GFAP and more consistently positive for vimentin. The subependymal zone around the lateral ventricles is a niche environment for neural stem cell populations.

Choroid plexus

The choroid plexus develops from evaginations of blood vessels covered by modified ependymal cells into specific sites within the lateral, third and fourth ventricles. The modified ependymal epithelial cells secrete CSF that fills both the ventricular system and subarachnoid space. The CSF delivers nutrients to and removes waste metabolites from the CNS. There is a tight-junction-mediated barrier between epithelial cells of the choroid plexus and

the CSF (blood-cerebrospinal fluid-barrier). Bacteria, protozoa and viruses commonly invade the CNS by infecting the choroid plexus and disseminating within the ventricular system once the integrity of tight junctions between the epithelial cells is compromised. Canine distemper virus gains access to the CSF after productive viral infection of the plexus epithelium and subsequent dispersion of high titers of infectious viral particles into the CSF. Normal and neoplastic choroid plexus epithelium is usually immunohistochemically reactive for both low and high molecular weight *cytokeratins* while the lamina is immunoreactive for collagen IV. Neoplastic choroid plexus epithelium variably expresses GFAP.

Meninges

Leptomeninges (pia mater and arachnoid membrane) and the pachymeninges (dura mater) can be involved mainly as meningitis in bacterial or viral infections of the CNS associated with infection of the subarachnoid space. The major reactive change of the leptomeninges consists of fibroblastic proliferation and fibrous collagenous thickening. In chronic inflammatory disease, the latter may become very extensive and potentially occlusive.

Osteomyelitis, trauma and skull fractures may impinge on the contiguous dura mater and focal fibroblastic proliferation of the inner surface of the dura can occur in response to chronic dural irritation (tumors, vertebral subluxation, meningitis etc.). *Dural metaplastic ossification* can occur incidentally and mainly in large-breed dogs particularly in cervical and lumbar segments with formation of elongated bony plaques, often containing hematopoietic bone marrow.

Meningothelial cells express vimentin and variably cytokeratin.

1.3.6 Blood vessels

Blood–brain barrier

The CNS is extremely well vascularized with a very dense capillary network.

In contrast to other organs, the endothelial cells of the blood vessels in the nervous system are connected by *tight junctions* creating an effective protective mechanical and biochemical barrier between the blood and the nervous tissue. Lipid-mediated passive diffusion of small molecules is possible but most traffic across the BBB is by rate-limited, receptor- and carrier-mediated transport of nutrients, proteins and electrolytes. Also involved in the BBB as a functional system are the pericytes, which – together with the endothelial cells – form a *basement membrane*, and the astrocytic foot processes, which cover most of the external surface of the vessels.

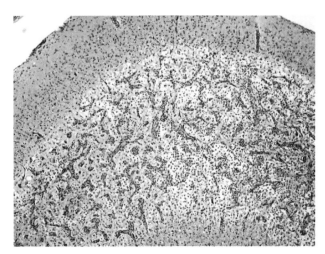

Fig. 1.24 Dog with chronic band-like (pseudolaminar) polioencephalomalacia. Cerebral cortex. Marked neovascular proliferation. HE.

In the normal state, little protein and a few inflammatory cells cross the BBB. Because of this blood–brain barrier the nervous system has been considered to be an *immunologically privileged site*. However, as we will see, this barrier can be breached rendering the CNS vulnerable to many immunopathologically mediated events. In infectious/inflammatory diseases, the BBB plays a very important role, regulating access of immune cells to the CNS. Endothelial cells are very active when homeostasis is lost: they react by upregulating MHC antigens and adhesion molecules, and can express various cytokines such as IL-1, IL-6 and IL-8, hence mediating inflammation in the CNS as explained in depth in Chapter 3.

Reactive blood vessels

The endothelial cells of the blood vessels of the CNS react in a variety of conditions by hypertrophy and proliferation (Fig. 1.24) initiated by hypoxia and resulting in upregulation of expression of vascular growth factors such as *vascular endothelial growth factor* (VEGF). Such growth factors are important in development and homeostasis and they can be affected by or participate in tissue damage and repair. Proliferation of endothelial cells results in neovascularization, which is easily recognized in routinely stained HE sections and immunohistochemically by antibodies to either CD31 or von Willebrand factor VIII related antigen.

1.3.7 Disturbance of water balance: edema

Homeostasis of exchange of water and electrolytes between the blood and the CNS depends on complex mechanisms in which the BBB plays an important regulatory role. Edema is the result of excess fluid accumulation in the CNS parenchyma and is frequently associated with most disease categories described in subsequent chapters. Classically, three different types of edema are recognized depending on their pathogenesis, but frequently these types co-exist.

Vasogenic edema

Vasogenic edema is the most common form of edema and is seen in many types of injuries such as trauma, focal and diffuse inflammatory processes, tumors and infarcts. The physical breakdown of the tight junctions between endothelial cells of the BBB causes increased vascular permeability with leakage of serum proteins into the intercellular space of the neuropil (Fig. 1.25A). The resulting increased osmotic pressure draws more water into the intercellular space. There is a preferential focal or global accumulation of fluid in the white matter since it has more extracellular space than gray matter. Such edema is readily detected by MRI and gross examination. Microscopically with HE staining, edema appears as pale areas with widespread separation of myelinated axons by clear vacuolated spaces (Fig. 1.25B). In chronic edema there is a reactive gemistocytic astrogliosis.

Cytotoxic (cellular) edema

Cytotoxic edema occurs when the energy-dependent sodium and potassium pumps in endothelial and glial cells are impaired. Intracellular accumulation of sodium ions leads to fluid retention resulting in intracellular swelling (Fig. 1.25A). This effect is first apparent in endothelial cells, then in astrocytes and subsequently in neurons and oligodendrocytes. The physical blood–brain barrier remains intact and hence cytotoxic edema has low protein content. This type of edema is seen in various toxic and metabolic disorders (discussed in Chapter 6). Furthermore, it occurs in combination with vasogenic edema in ischemia. Macroscopically, brain swelling appears generally less severe in cytotoxic edema than in vasogenic edema. Histologically, cytotoxic edema causes a *spongy state (status spongiosus)* with sharply defined vacuoles in the white matter due to intramyelinic edema (Fig. 1.25C). Cell swelling can also be seen as vacuoles within processes of perineuronal and perivascular astrocytes. Initially the status spongiosus is devoid of reactive changes; in chronic edema diffuse reactive astrogliosis becomes apparent.

Interstitial edema

Interstitial edema results from increased permeability of the desmosomal junctions between lining ependymal cells of the ventricular system. With increased intraventricular pressure the ependymal lining ruptures and CSF accumulates interstitially in the periventricular white matter. In contrast to vasogenic edema, interstitial

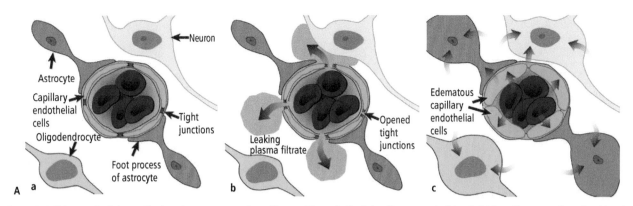

Fig. 1.25 Edema. A: Schematic drawing; a: normal capillary with endothelial cells connected by tight junctions creating the blood–brain barrier (BBB), supported by astrocytic endfeet processes; b: opening of the BBB with leakage of plasma into the interstitium (vasogenic edema); c: failure of ion/water pumps, water from blood enters the intracellular compartment (endothelial cells, astrocytes, neurons) with swelling of cells resulting in cytotoxic edema.

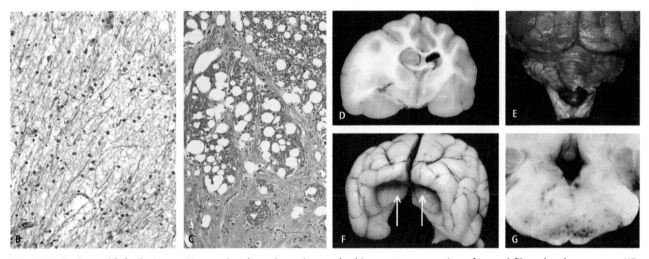

Fig. 1.25 B: Dog with brain tumor. Vasogenic edema in peritumoral white matter, separation of axonal fibers by clear spaces. HE. C: Calf with liver failure. Internal capsule. Spongy state with sharply delineated vacuoles. HE. D: Cat with brain tumor (meningioma extending in lateral ventricle). Massive edema particularly in white matter with swelling of the left hemisphere associated with the tumor. E: Dog with cranial trauma. Cerebellar coning with hemorrhagic necrosis of the herniated vermis and brainstem compression resulting from severe brain edema. F: Dog with brain tumor. Caudal view of occipital lobes, herniated cerebral cortex (arrows) underneath tentorium (tentorium has been removed). G: Dog with brain tumor and high intracranial pressure. Medulla oblongata. Multiple small hemorrhages (*Duret* hemorrhages).

edema has low protein content. Small pools of interstitial edema may coalesce leading to fluid-filled cavities of various sizes eventually leading to macroscopically visible cystic structures. In the spinal cord or brainstem such cavitations are called *syringomyelia* or *syringobulbia* respectively. In the brain, mostly connected to the lateral ventricles, they are called diverticula.

Effects of brain edema

Edema may cause focal or global CNS swelling usually associated with space-occupying masses such as abcesses, tumors or hemorrhages. Because the brain and spinal cord are closely confined by meninges and the rigid calvarium and vertebrae, brain or spinal cord swelling

causes increased intracranial or intraspinal pressure, respectively, with life-threatening secondary complications as described in Chapter 4. The brain is compressed against the skull resulting in flattening of gyri and narrowing of sulci. In transverse sections marked mechanical distension, particularly of the white matter, and variable compression of the ventricular system can be observed (Fig. 1.25D). Global swelling of the cerebral hemispheres causes compression of the brainstem, which is flattened and distorted with close apposition of rostral colliculi. The mesencephalic aqueduct is narrowed, and in the brainstem and cerebellum small target hemorrhages (*Duret hemorrhages*) due to stretching and necrosis of blood vessels may be present

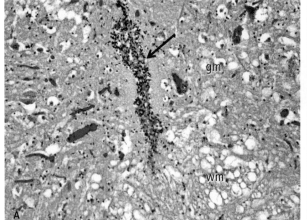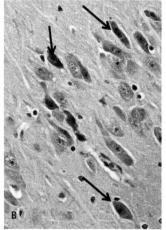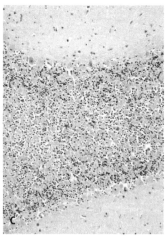

Fig. 1.26 Artifacts. A: Dog. Spinal cord. Advanced postmortem autolysis, marked vacuolation of gray (gm) and white (wm) matter, the structure of the central canal (large arrow) is largely disorganized with only the nuclei of the ependymal and subependymal cells indicating its presence. HE. B: Dog. cerebral cortex. Dark neurons (arrows) next to morphologically normal neurons. HE. C: Bovine. Cerebellar cortex. Extensive postmortem lysis of cerebellar granule cell layer, a common artifact in large animals. HE.

(Fig. 1.25G). The brain parenchyma expands caudally resulting in *cerebellar vermal herniation* (Fig. 1.25E) and herniation of the cerebral cortex underneath rigid structures (e.g. tentorium cerebelli: *transtentorial or subtentorial herniation* (Fig. 1.25F); falx cerebri: subfalcine herniation). Such herniation severely increases pressure in focal areas leading to small hemorrhages and ischemic necrosis following disruption of blood supply with a usually fatal outcome.

1.3.8 Artifacts, postmortem degeneration, pseudolesions and old age

Artifacts

Postmortem autolysis progresses quickly in nervous tissues leading to artifactual changes that may significantly interfere with detection and correct interpretation of lesions (especially for the untrained eye). In advanced autolysis, the CNS becomes mushy, macroscopic structures may become ill defined and cavities are caused by gas-forming bacteria.

The most common artifact of autolysis at the histological level is vacuolation (Fig. 1.26A). The latter can be especially prominent in the white matter. These vacuoles are irregular in shape and size and often not well delineated. Also rough handling of the tissues causes mechanical tearing and disruption of the tissue architecture with increased intercellular space, separation of neuronal layers and vacuolation. Inadequate processing (e.g. prolonged contact with 70% ethanol) causes significant vacuolation principally of the white matter. In the gray matter, there are excessively large clear spaces around neurons, blood vessels and glial

nuclei. Artifactual vacuolation has to be distinguished from pathological spongy state in the CNS as discussed in Chapter 6.

Purkinje cells undergo rapid perineuronal vacuolation, and granule cell depletion is also common after a prolonged interval before fixation (Fig. 1.26C). With advancing autolysis, neurons become pale and pink with a slightly foamy cytoplasm. Sometimes, oligodendroglial nuclei are uniformly surrounded by clear halos or opaque material, rendering the impression of a swollen cytoplasm. In advanced autolysis, the choroid plexus and ependyma become denuded of their epithelial-derived lining cells (Fig. 1.26A). A reliable sign of good tissue preservation is the presence of cilia on ependymal cells.

Inadequate fixation either in time or in fixative volume leads to blurring of structural detail in histological sections. Pale-basophilic staining, round structures (mucocytes, Buscaino bodies) may appear in significant numbers in the parenchyma as an artefact of formalin fixation, probably by reaction of myelin components with formalin.

A very common finding even in fresh, well fixed tissue are *dark neurons*. Their name derives from single or clusters of neurons anywhere in the CNS, which appear shrunken and strongly basophilic with corkscrew dendrites (Fig. 1.26B). Their significance has been hotly debated but they are most probably artifact due to tissue handling. Others interpret the uptake of the dye *fluorojade* as an early degenerative change in such neurons.

When such abnormalities are not associated with reactive changes (e.g. invasion of macrophages, gliosis,

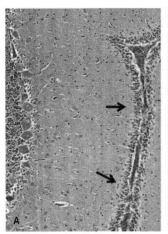 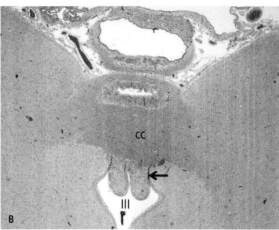 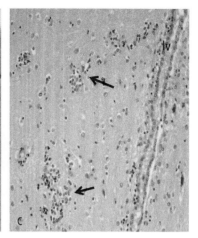

Fig. 1.27 Pseudolesions. A: Young dog. Cerebellum with an external granule cell layer (arrows). HE. B: Dog. Subcommissural organ (arrow) (cc, caudal commissure; III, third ventricle). C: Dog. Caudate nucleus. Clusters of primitive neuroectodermal cells (arrows) in the caudate nucleus in vicinity of lateral ventricle (lv). HE.

invasion of inflammatory cells, capillary proliferation) it is prudent to assume that they are artifacts unless they are found in optimally preserved and processed tissues.

Pseudolesions

Be aware of some normal microanatomical features suggesting a lesion:

- Very young animals may still have germinal cell layers notably subpially in the cerebellar cortex (*external granule cell layer*) (Fig. 1.27A). The density of glial cells in immature white matter is also much higher than in adult brains.
- The *circumventricular organs* (CVO). These small, highly specialized structures in the wall of the third and fourth ventricles contain numerous capillaries without a blood–brain barrier. Ependymal and neural cell processes contact the CVOs, which play a role in the coordination between neural and hormonal functions. The CVOs include the organum vasculosum, the subfornical organ, the subcommisural organ (Fig. 1.27B) and the area postrema in the fourth ventricle.
- Focal accumulations of *primitive undifferentiated glial and neuronal cell precursor cells* occur in the forebrain in subependymal and perivascular sites around the lateral ventricles (Fig. 1.27C). They are very prominent and dense in fetal and neonatal animals, also occurring in the thalamus and midbrain; they may again increase in numbers with old age.
- In the brainstem, neurons of certain nuclei such as the olivary and pontine nuclei uniformly lack the perinuclear Nissl substance; this is not to be confused with chromatolyis.
- In certain mammalian species normal secretory neurons of the hypothalamus and locus coeruleus contain cytoplasmic melanin.

- Eosinophilic intracytoplasmatic inclusion bodies occur occasionally in neurons (e.g. in the lateral geniculate body) in different species, notably cats (pseudo-Negri bodies).

Old age

Tissue changes associated with old age are quite consistent, and it is a quantitative problem whether to call them pathologic or simply physiologic attrition with age.

Old dogs often show a marked hydrocephalus and apparent shrinkage of the cerebrum (Fig. 1.28B) without ever having suffered from neurological signs during their lives. Although there is gliosis and increased numbers of glial cells around neurons (satellitosis) in the gray matter in old dogs with brain atrophy, it is not clear whether there is significant loss of neurons. Another conspicuous feature in old brains is a diffuse status spongiosus of the white matter (Fig. 1.28D), sometimes with fibrillary gliosis ("scar" tissue). This appears to be due to degeneration and loss of myelin associated with deposits of non-degraded ubiquitin–protein conjugates and complex galactolipids. A consistent finding in all species is the appearance of degenerated neurons and large spheroids in the accessory cuneate nucleus. The number of so-called subependymal and cortical glial nests in old brains seems to be increased compared with younger animals (in the rhinencephalic cortex, ventricular angles, caudate nucleus). A typical sign of old age is an accumulation of lipofuscin granules in the cytoplasm of neurons, in particular in the brainstem nuclei (Fig. 1.28C). Around blood vessels one often sees macrophages containing lipopigment. Senile plaques and congophilic angiopathy (Fig. 1.28F,G) have also been described in very old animals as discussed in Chapter 8 on degenerative disease. There is also a fibrotic thickening of the meninges and of the stroma of the choroid plexus.

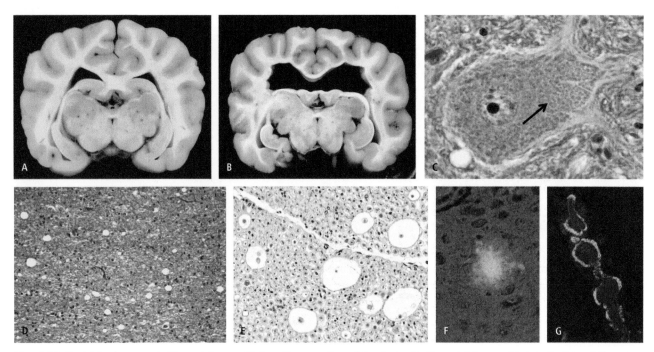

Fig. 1.28 Geriatric changes. A: Normal 2-year-old dog. Cross-section of forebrain. B: Normal 14-year-old dog. Section at the same level, marked thinning of the cerebral cortex and subcortical white matter with compensatory enlargement of the ventricles C: Old dog. Brainstem. Lipofuscin pigment accumulation (arrow) in a neuron. HE. D: Old dog. Cerebrum. Vacuolation and gliosis in the white matter. HE. E: Old dog. Spinal nerve roots. Ballooning of myelin sheaths. HE. F: Old dog. Cerebral cortex. Senile plaque (accumulation of beta amyloid). Thioflavine stain, UV fluorescence. G: Vascular amyloidosis. Thioflavine stain, UV fluorescence.

In old cats, we often see focal meningothelial proliferation/hyperplasia. In some species such as horses, there is mineralization and iron deposition in the walls of blood vessel walls mainly in the basal nuclei. In the PNS, old age is frequently characterized by extensive vacuolation of myelin sheaths particularly in nerve roots (Fig. 1.28E).

1.4 Recognizing major lesion patterns

Diagnostic neuropathology is based on the detection of lesions and their subsequent interpretation. In addition to being familiar with the basic reaction patterns as described in Section 1.3, two further essential requirements for a successful start in diagnostic neuropathology are: (a) being able to recognize the major gross and histological lesion patterns and (b) a working knowledge of the classification of neurological diseases including the major morphological hallmarks (lesion patterns) of each disease category.

1.4.1 The major lesion patterns

As we have seen in Section 1.3, the nervous system can only mount a relatively limited number of reactions to injury. It follows therefore that there are also only a

limited number of *basic* lesion types. Of course there are myriads of morphological variations of these basic lesion types but it is possible and necessary to recognize their most essential common features or patterns. At the macroscopic level we can recognize the following patterns: abnormal anatomy, space-occupying mass lesion, hemorrhage, malacia/necrosis, pallor/softening of the white matter. While even small hemorrhages can be seen with the naked eye, small foci of incipient malacia may require microscopic detection. Major microscopic patterns include, apart from malacia: spongy change, intracellular accumulation of abnormal material, hypercellularity, selective loss of neurons, axons or myelin. All these lesion patterns are briefly described below and illustrated in Fig. 1.29.

Deviation of normal anatomy

With some basic knowledge of neuroanatomy, abnormal anatomic disturbances are readily identified macroscopically as, for example, hydrocephalus or cerebellar hypoplasia. Deviation of the normal anatomy is most often a congenital malformation but can also be the result of some other acquired pathological process leading to atrophy of a certain region. Occasionally, part of the brain or cord, or sometimes the whole brain, is swollen

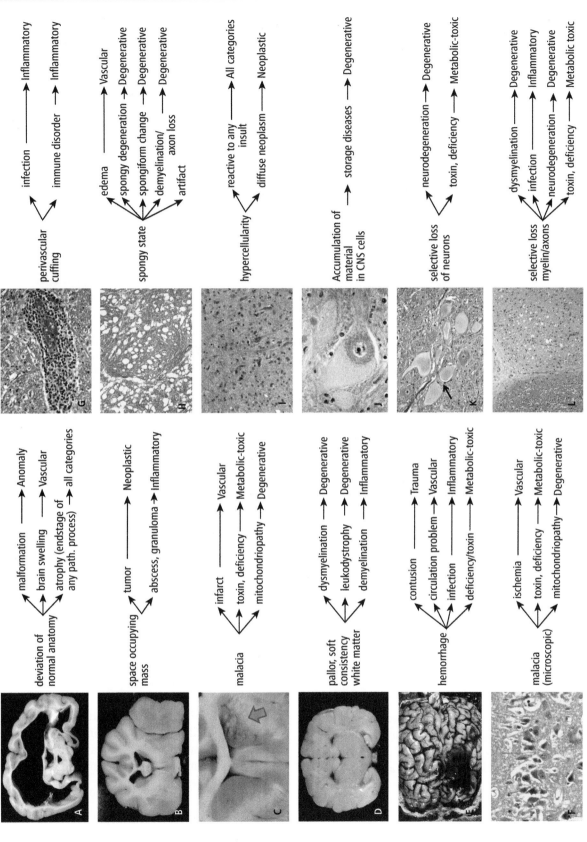

Fig. 1.29 Major lesion patterns and their interpretation. A: Major gross lesion patterns and their interpretation. B: Major histological lesion patterns and their interpretation.

due to mass lesions with cerebral edema. The resultant increased intracranial pressure can force areas of the brain underneath the tentorium cerebelli (*subtentorial herniation*) or the cerebellar vermis caudally through the foramen magnum (*cerebellar vermal herniation*). Also the cerebrocortical gyri are flattened and widened and the sulci compressed.

Space-occupying mass

Such a mass is usually easy to detect. Space-occupying mass lesions in small animals are generally due to primary or secondary tumors but can also be associated with excessive focal accumulation of inflammatory cells (abscess, granuloma) and result in a midline shift.

Malacia

Malacia is defined as grossly or microscopically detected softening and necrosis of the tissue resulting from destruction of most cells in the affected area leading to complete loss of the original architecture. Complete destruction with cavitation is easy to detect grossly, while acute lesions display a gelatinous consistency often with a change of color to gray or yellow. Histologically, malacic lesions are demarcated from normal tissue and appear paler or darker than their surroundings. The original architecture is lost, and the acutely affected tissue appears less compact, vacuolated and with widespread cell necrosis.

Pallor/softening of the white matter

Extensive lesions of the white matter are visible to the naked eye. The white matter is normally brilliantly white and in many areas is clearly demarcated from the gray matter. Following paucity/absence/loss of myelin the white matter becomes grayish, less distinguishable from the gray matter and may appear softened. Histologically on HE, loss of myelin is characterized by pale staining. Specific myelin stains are very useful to detect and define this lesion.

Hemorrhage

Accumulation of erythrocytes outside the blood vessels is usually grossly visible as red to dark brown in acute hemorrhage while orange/yellowish discoloration of the tissue is more indicative of chronicity. Hemorrhage results from damage to the blood vessels and is usually associated with malacia.

Perivascular cuffing

Accumulation of inflammatory cells around the blood vessels in the parenchyma is probably the easiest lesion to detect at the histological level. Such perivascular cell accumulations or cuffing can often be detected at low-power magnification and are highly characteristic for an inflammatory/infectious disorder but may also occur in a very limited extent in other disorders (e.g. hippocampal necrosis in cats).

Spongy state (status spongiosus)

This is a very common pattern resulting from many different types of injury and is also a common artifact. The tissue looks moth-eaten, there is an excessive number and size of clear spaces around neurons, glial cells and capillaries, and diffuse or distinct vacuoles in the neuropil and or specifically in gray and/or white matter. Such vacuolar change can be caused by postmortem artifact, (intra-myelinic) edema, loss of axons and/or myelin, or vacuolation of neurons, glial cells or their processes. A guide to the interpretation of this spongy state is extensively covered in Fig. 6.14.

Hypercellularity

This is apparent as focal or extensive areas with increased numbers or density of cells. Usually, in HE sections the cell nuclei are most prominently stained, thus we detect too many nuclei. This change is very common and there are several variations of this change.

- Infiltration and accumulation of inflammatory cells. Accumulation of large numbers of inflammatory cells in the leptomeninges and subarachnoid space can sometimes be detected on gross examination as a diffuse whitish or yellowish clouding of the meninges.
- Astrogliosis or microgliosis (proliferation of astroglial or microglial cells), a reactive change particularly of astrocytes or microglial cells, which can occur as a result of any kind of injury. Hypercellularity can thus be a feature of many disease categories.
- Proliferation of endothelial cells and increased density of microvessels or neovascularization in the affected area is a common reactive change in different types of injury.
- Diffuse neoplasia. While most tumors consist of compact expansile masses, in certain tumor types (e.g. astrocytomas), neoplastic cells may diffusely invade the tissue, leaving the original architecture of the tissue more or less undisturbed.

Accumulation of abnormal intracellular material or bodies

Such abnormal material can consist of inclusions, granules, foamy material or clear vacuoles and is relatively easy to detect in neurons because of their size. Such change can also be associated with swelling of cells and/or displacement of other cell components such as the nucleus.

Selective changes in neurons/axons/dendrites

Detection of this pattern requires careful histological examination and may be difficult without experience. The architecture of the tissue is changed, regularity is disrupted, the tissue appears less compact and there is loss of certain tissue elements. Recognition of these changes is greatly facilitated by knowing the normal microanatomy of the various areas of the CNS. This knowledge is acquired by making it routine to consciously register anatomical features while reading histological slides. Special histochemical or immunohistochemical stains for myelin and axons are very helpful to recognize selective change in the white matter. For example, such stains are required to distinguish between primary or secondary demyelinating lesions.

1.4.2 Lesion distribution pattern

As explained in later chapters, the anatomical distribution pattern of the lesions is of paramount importance in the differential diagnosis. Lesions which are either single (focal) or multiple (multifocal–disseminated) can already suggest different disease categories. Generally, bilateral involvement of specific anatomic areas is typical for metabolic–toxic and degenerative diseases. Particularly in the latter the lesions are mostly, but not always, symmetrical. Last but not least lesions may have a predilection for either gray or white matter. As we will see, the specific anatomical location of lesions may be highly diagnostic in many diseases.

1.4.3 Classification of neurological diseases

Recognition of the major patterns is a first important step in neuropathological diagnosis. The recognized patterns must then be placed in the appropriate disease category against a background of historical and clinical information. For diagnostic purposes, it makes sense to categorize diseases according to their common characteristics. To classify lesions, it is obviously best to consider disease mechanisms that are associated with specific morphological changes, and thus with certain patterns of lesions as described above. This is true to a certain extent, at least at the level of the large disease categories. However we prefer to use a classification system based not only on morphological criteria but which also includes assessment of clinical data, includ-

ing that obtained from MRI images. With this approach we can distinguish the following groups of diseases: vascular, inflammatory, traumatic, anomalous (malformation), metabolic–toxic, idiopathic, neoplastic, degenerative. The acronym **VITAMIN D** may be helpful as an initial memory aid for the neurologist as well as the pathologist.

While diseases in this scheme are classified according to traditional pathologic criteria, these categories not only have common morphological features (thus exhibiting one or more of the above lesion patterns) but also include some common clinical neurological denominators or at least trends with respect to breed, age, onset/course, involvement of other organ systems, focal or multifocal localization and CSF evaluation changes.

Vascular diseases

The main lesions of the CNS vasculature include vasculitis, hemorrhage and infarction. The latter results from focal vascular obstruction (e.g. septic or bland fibrin thrombi and emboli, fibrocartilage, atheroclerosis, intravascular lymphoma) or less commonly from global ischemia and consist of sharply demarcated areas of neuropil destruction termed malacia. Vascular diseases can occur in all age groups and provoke peracute, severe, often lateralizing neurological signs which remain stationary for some time and may gradually regress. Extraneural signs are found when the primary problem is located in the cardiovascular system, e.g. bacterial endocarditis. Cerebrospinal fluid is usually altered with protein increase, excess red blood cells (RBCs) and sometimes pleocytosis with macrophages.

Inflammatory diseases

The hallmark of this group is parenchymal invasion of blood-derived leucocytes around blood vessels (perivascular cuffing) and infiltrating into the parenchyma, as well as proliferation of endogenous microglia (hypercellularity), resulting in encephalitis, myelitis, meningitis, ependymitis, choroid plexitis and neuritis. Inflammatory lesions are most frequently associated with infections but also with immune-mediated disorders. Infectious diseases of the CNS can occur in any age group but are generally more frequent in young animals. They are usually of acute onset with rapid progression but a subacute–chronic course may occur. Infections can be restricted to the CNS but may also be associated with disseminated lesions in other organ systems. Inflammatory lesions are generally *multifocal, disseminated* or *diffuse*. Focal lesions may become space-occupying masses. Neurological signs may suggest multifocal involvement but one single localizing sign may predominate. Pleocytosis and protein increase in the CSF is typical of CNS inflammatory diseases.

Trauma

Cranial or spinal trauma results in mechanical disruption of tissue compounded by traumatic injury to blood vessels resulting in hemorrhage and usually malacia. Trauma leads to peracute neurological signs, which in the case of hemorrhage, may rapidly worsen. The neurological signs may improve in the days and weeks following trauma. In the case of endogenous spinal cord trauma (e.g. intervertrebral disc disease) a subacute to chronic intermittent course is frequently seen. Neurological signs are mostly focal. CSF sampling is contraindicated in cranial trauma due to concurrent edema and raised intracranial pressure. In spinal cord trauma various spectra of CSF changes may be found.

Anomalies or malformations

Abnormal development of the CNS *in utero* may lead to gross or more subtle malformations or anomalies of the normal anatomy, e.g. hydrocephalus, cyclopia, cerebellar hypoplasia or spina bifida. Most malformations occur as single point genetic mutations, and much less commonly as a result of intrauterine transplacental infections or intoxications. Malformations are usually clinically apparent at birth or within the first months of life. Usually, neurological signs are focal and remain stationary, although some compensation or progression may develop in time. Routine CSF evaluation fluid is unremarkable.

Metabolic–toxic diseases

Deficiencies and toxins can lead to acute destruction of nervous tissue in certain anatomically restricted sites in a *bilateral, usually symmetrical distribution pattern*. Tissue destruction is frequently severe with malacia, cavitation and hemorrhage. An additional common microscopic lesion is a spongy vacuolar change. In some conditions lesions are more discrete and therefore resemble degenerative diseases. Metabolic–toxic diseases are usually in groups of animals, and of rapid onset and progression reaching maximal clinical intensity within a short time. Surviving animals may gradually recover. Neurological signs reflect a particular localization but without lateralization. There are usually non-specific but marked changes in the CSF in both protein level and cell content. Metabolic encephalopathies resulting from primary extraneural organ failure (e.g. renal or hepatic) exhibit a fluctuating course and diffuse localization.

Idiopathic diseases

Idiopathic means of obscure or unknown cause. Because this designation is still applicable for many animal CNS diseases, idiopathic disorders comprise the single largest group of diseases, which in our opinion is no longer practical. Therefore we use the term idiopathic for a group of diseases with abnormal *functional* neurological signs but without morphologically detectable changes of the nervous tissue. Such syndromes or diseases are not covered in this book. Examples are epilepsy, myasthenia, narcolepsy and the scores of clinically ill defined "movement disorders". Such diseases often demonstrate clinically a paroxysmal (e.g. seizures) or fluctuating course. Routine CSF evaluation is unremarkable. It is important to note that in such cases on neuropathological examination no lesions are detected even though the animal may demonstrate severe neurological signs.

Neoplasia

Primary CNS tumors, pituitary tumors and metastatic tumors originating from surrounding tissues (e.g. nasal cavity) or from other organs all compromise the CNS by either destructive invasion or compression by tumor cell proliferation (hypercellularity). Such focal space-occupying lesions can result in a rise in intracranial pressure and secondary peritumoral edema. Tumors can also obstruct CSF flow with secondary distension of the ventricular system. Tumors mostly affect older animals. The clinical course is usually subacute to chronic but a sudden increase in intracranial pressure may lead to rapid progression. Neurological signs are focal and lateralizing. In metastatic brain tumors, signs may be multifocal and clinical evidence of the primary tumor may be found. CSF changes include mild to severe protein elevation, sometimes with exfoliation of tumor cells.

Degenerative diseases

These diseases are characterized by progressive degeneration of specific cell types in the nervous system in a *bilaterally symmetrical* and restricted anatomical localization. Common patterns are: selective change of neurons/myelin/axons with gliosis (hypercellularity), spongy state, pallor or loss of white matter and abnormal accumulation of material in neurons. Such lesions are attributed to specific gene defects. Most degenerative diseases occur in young animals in certain breeds. Sometimes they are of late onset. The course of the disease is slowly progressive. Most degenerative diseases are restricted to the CNS; however in lysosomal storage diseases there is also selective involvement of extraneural tissues. Selective involvement leads to focal neurological signs without lateralization. The CSF is usually normal.

1.4.4 General strategy

Gross lesions

Recognition of the major lesion patterns and the anatomically based lesion distribution is the important first step and will direct the neuropathological assessment towards specific disease categories. The latter are covered in the subsequent chapters of this book. It is important to use this systematic stepwise approach before assessing details. Fig. 1.29 shows examples of major lesion patterns. The first five images relate to recognizable changes at the macroscopic level: deviation from normal anatomy, space-occupying mass, hemorrhage, malacia and selective white matter changes. When such changes are seen, various diagnostic options are listed with their respective VITAMIN D category.

At the next level, microscopic lesions are generally more difficult to interpret for beginners with one exception: it is easy to recognize perivascular cuffing, the hallmark of inflammatory diseases. With further experience additional patterns can be recognized including, in increasing order of difficulty, microscopic malacic lesions, spongy change, intracellular accumulation of abnormal material, hypercellularity and selective lesions/loss of neurons, axons or myelin.

The major patterns may often occur in combinations, e.g. hemorrhage together with malacia or hypercellularity together with pallor of the white matter. It is important to realize that lesions are dynamic processes and their morphology can be modified with time.

Detecting changes and recognizing the major patterns are both major steps towards diagnosing neuropathological problems. In the following chapters these basic patterns will be further subdivided and detailed and their underlying mechanisms will be discussed. In approach, pattern recognition and understanding disease mechanisms is most effective in achieving a neuropathological diagnosis.

1.5 Neuropathology in the clinics: magnetic resonance imaging (MRI)

Johann Lang DECVDI, Department of Clinical Veterinary Medicine, Division of Clinical Radiology, Vetsuisse Faculty, Univ. Bern

In recent years, MRI has become an essential non-invasive diagnostic method in veterinary neurology. This technique allows visualization of the nervous system in sections, very much like in the macroscopic examination of brain slices. The interpretation of MRI images requires not only physical and neuroanatomical but also neuropathological knowledge. Thus this is an area where diagnostic imaging and diagnostic pathology increasingly overlap. In fact, neuropathologists are often consulted to help in the interpretation of images and, conversely, the MRI findings have become an integral part of the documentation of neurological cases submitted to necropsy. Therefore neuropathologists should become familiar with the principles of MR image interpretation.

1.5.1 Basic MRI physics

MRI generates sectional images of the body by exploiting the nuclear magnetic resonance of atomic nuclei in the body. The most commonly used (and most abundant) atom in this respect is hydrogen.

According to the quantum theory, hydrogen nuclei act like rotating gyroscopes, which have a dipole moment about their rotational axis, the so-called nuclear spin. In MRI, the rotational axis of the nuclear spin, which has a random and disorganized orientation at rest, is polarized by a strong magnetic field and consequently hydrogen nuclei of the body align along this field. This may occur in two directions: either parallel or anti-parallel to the direction of the magnetic field, where they rotate along their axis in a frequency that is defined by the strength of the magnetic field and the proton in question (precession). Then, a short radio frequency pulse is emitted by a coil, which is placed around the body part of interest. The hydrogen nuclei with the same frequency as the emitted radiopulse will absorb the energy (resonance frequency or "Larmor frequency") and as result the nuclear spin changes its orientation in the magnetic field (resonance). When the radio wave pulse is turned off resonating protons return to their original low-energy (equilibrium) state, a process called relaxation, and the released energy can be registered by a receiver coil. An image can be produced because relaxation rates of hydrogen protons vary depending on their chemical binding in a given tissue and the water content of the latter. Therefore, with the additional help of paramagnetic contrast media, MRI is able to detect subtle differences between soft tissues. In the nervous system, this method allows the direct and anatomically exact reproduction of gray and white matter, the ventricular system with the CSF, the spinal cord, the spinal nerves, the intervertebral discs and the surrounding fat. Only the resolution of bony structures and bone/air interfaces is poor.

Two relaxation components are differentiated: the so-called T1 (or longitudinal) and the T2 (or transverse) relaxations. The length of T1 relaxation (T1 relaxation time) lies in the range of seconds for fluids but is much shorter for soft tissues (tenths of seconds). The T2 relaxation time, like the T1 relaxation time, has a great influence on the signal intensity of a given tissue and image contrast. In T2-weighted (T2W) images, brain tissue has a short T2 relaxation time, whereas CSF has a long T2 relaxation time which is displayed as high signal intensity structure (white).

1.5.2 Principles of interpretation

Practical examples are shown in Fig. 1.30, Fig. 1.31 and Fig. 1.32. Please note that radiologists use the perspective of the examiner standing in front of the animal. The right side of the image corresponds with the left side of the animal.

The standard image planes in an MRI examination are oriented in a transverse, sagittal and dorsal direction. However, any other sections are also possible. As these slices have a certain thickness, MRI renders a two-dimensional image containing all the information within these tissue slabs. By using a variety of so called sequences, the different components of the tissue can be seen in different ways. In the brain, the basic examination usually includes T1W (read as T1-weighted) images, T2W images and FLAIR (fluid attenuated inversion recovery) images for the suppression of the signal from free fluid such as the CSF.

T1W images are basically used for differentiating fat from water and carry excellent anatomical information. Tissues with short T1 relaxation times such as fat or tissues that accumulate contrast agents have high signal intensity and appear bright, substances with a long T1 such as CSF have low signal intensity. As the white matter in the brain contains more fat than the cortex (due to its myelin content) and has therefore a shorter T1 relaxation time, the T1W image provides good gray–white matter contrast and hence an excellent anatomical picture of the brain. Due to the usually increased water content causing prolongation of the T1 relaxation time, most pathological changes appear as hypointense structures compared to normal tissue.

In T2W images, brain tissue has a comparatively shorter T2 relaxation time and lower signal intensity than CSF, which has high signal intensity in this sequence, resulting in good portrayal of the ventricular system. The contrast of the white to gray matter is reversed compared to T1W sequences: the gray matter is more hyperintense than the white matter on T2W images. T2W are sensitive for pathologies since they emphasize change of water content as it occurs in most pathologies including tumors, edema and inflammation. Increased water content causes a prolongation of the T2 relaxation times and therefore lesions are more hyperintense on T2W images than normal tissues. Furthermore, iron-containing structures such as the basal nuclei and nuclei in the brainstem and cerebellum are hyperintense in T2W images compared to the surrounding brain tissue.

Special sequences and images using contrast agents can selectively increase the contrast between different tissue components and diseased versus normal areas. In the brain, the single most important sequence is the FLAIR (fluid attenuated inversion recovery) sequence which selectively suppresses the signal from free fluid such as the CSF but not of brain edema facilitating the detection of lesions in the subarachnoid space and in the brain parenchyma close to the ventricular system.

The diagnostic yield of a MRI investigation can be enhanced with the injection of paramagnetic contrast agents such as gadolinium. Paramagnetic substances accelerate energy exchange of spins in the vicinity of the contrast agent thus shortening the T1 relaxation time of the hydrogen protons and leading to increased signal intensity. Since the contrast agent does not penetrate the intact blood–brain barrier (BBB) of normal brain, only structures without BBB will be hyperintense after application of contrast media. Examples are the pituitary gland or the highly vascularized choroid plexus. In pathological tissue with absence or disturbance of the BBB, lesions will show high signal intensity and increase the contrast to normal tissue thus enhancing the sensitivity of an MR examination. The degree and pattern of contrast uptake also varies between different types of abnormalities therefore increasing also the specificity of the examination. See MRI Atlas.

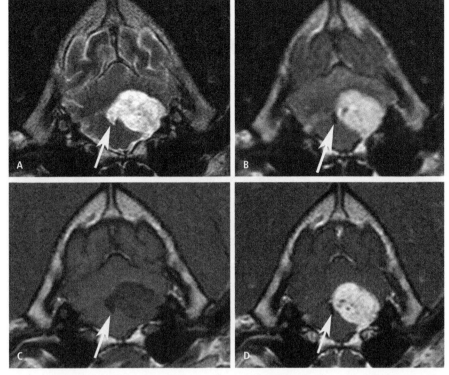

Fig. 1.30 Male, 8-year-old crossbreed dog with clinical signs of central vestibular disease. MRI (High Field Open Magnet from Philips, 1 Tesla) including transverse T2W (A), FLAIR (B), T1W pre- (C) and post-contrast (D) images of the posterior fossa. Diagnosis was choroid plexus papilloma. There is a 1.5 × 2 cm extra-axial lesion in the left cerebellopontine angle causing mild right-sided deviation of the medulla. The lesion has broad-based contact with the left petrosal bone, which is clearly delineated and has normal signal intensity (SI). The lesion shows high SI in FLAIR and T2W images, and low SI in the pre-contrast T1 sequence, and there is severe contrast uptake of the lesion. Note the small triangular area dorsal to the medulla and continuous with the lesion (arrows) representing the compressed fourth ventricle. It displays the SI of fluid with T2W hyper-, T1W hypo-, FLAIR hypointensity, and there is no contrast enhancement. In the post-contrast series, fine hypointense and sharply delineated tubular structures can be seen coursing through the lesion. The meninges surrounding this lesion appear normal.

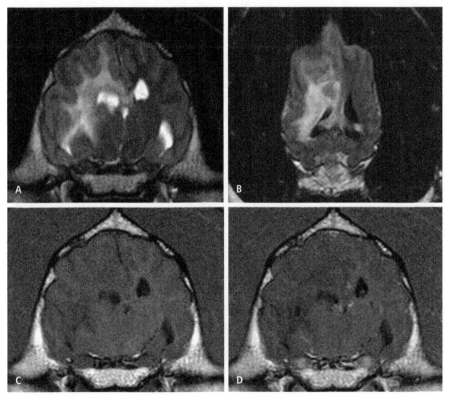

Fig. 1.31 Male, 7-year-old Flatcoated Retriever with reduced consciousness. MRI (High Field Open Magnet from Philips, 1 Tesla) including transverse T2W (A), dorsal FLAIR (B), transverse T1W pre- (C) and post-contrast (D) images of a severe vasogenic brain edema, located in the white matter. It is hyperintense in T2W and FLAIR images with high contrast to the dark ventricles in the FLAIR studies. Typically, edema is hypointense in T1W images and shows no contrast uptake. Space occupying mass in right frontal lobe visible in dorsal FLAIR image.

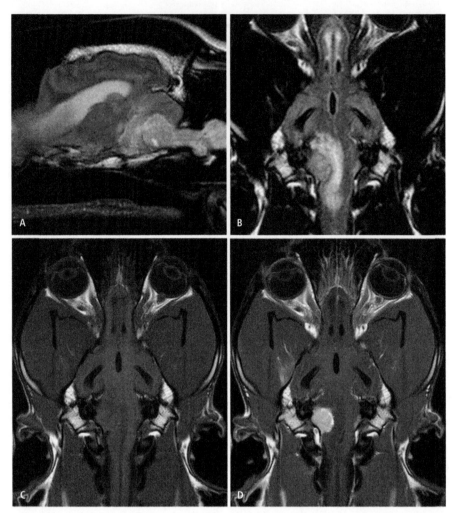

Fig. 1.32 Male, 11-year-old Magyar Vizsla dog with suspected right-sided brainstem lesion. MRI (High Field Open Magnet from Philips, 1 Tesla) including sagittal T2W (A) , dorsal FLAIR (B), dorsal T1W pre- (C) and post-contrast (D) images of the brain. Diagnosis was meningioma. The paramedian sagittal T2 sequence reveals dilated right lateral ventricle with high SI, and also ill defined high SI in the brainstem, cerebellum and spinal cord. In the center, there is arounded focal lesion delineated by a hyperintense rim. In the dorsal FLAIR, the CSF in the ventricular system is suppressed, the perifocal edema presents hyperintense, and the well delineated extra-axial lesion slightly hypointense compared to the edema. There is also hyperintense periventricular edema in the olfactory bulb bilaterally. In the pre-contrast T1 image, lesion and edema present mildly hypointense compared to the brain, and there is massive homogeneous contrast enhancement of the broad-based tumor.

Further reading

Neuropathology general

Bolon B, Butt MT. Fundamental Neuropathology for Pathologists and Toxicologists. Hoboken, NJ: Wiley, 2011.

DeLahunta A, Glass E. Veterinary Neuroanatomy and Clinical Neurology, 3rd ed. St. Louis, MO: Saunders/Elsevier, 2009.

Grant Maxie M. (ed) Jubb, Kennedy, and Palmer's Pathology of Domestic Animals, 5th ed. Edinburgh, New York: Elsevier Saunders, 2007.

Gray F, Poirier J, De Girolami U. Escourolle and Poirier's Manual of Basic Neuropathology, 4th ed. Philadelphia, PA: Butterworth-Heinemann, 2003.

Love S, Louis DN, Ellison DW. (eds) Greenfield's Neuropathology, 8th ed. London: Hodder Arnold, 2008.

McGavin MD. Pathologic Basis of Veterinary Disease, 4th ed. St. Louis, MO: Mosby Elsevier, 2007.

Mayhew J. Large Animal Neurology, 2nd ed. Chichester, UK: Wiley-Blackwell 2008.

Perry A, Brat DJ. Practical Surgical Neuropathology: A Diagnostic Approach. Philadelphia, PA: Churchill Livingstone/Elsevier, 2010.

Summers B, Cummings JF, deLahunta A. Veterinary Neuropathology. St. Louis, MO: Mosby, 1995.

http://www.vet.cornell.edu/oed/neuropathology/index.asp

Neurology/functional neuroanatomy

DeLahunta A, Glass E. Veterinary Neuroanatomy and Clinical Neurology, 3rd ed. St. Louis, MO: Saunders/Elsevier, 2009.

Platt, SR, Olby NJ. BSAVA Manual of Canine and Feline Neurology, 3rd ed. Quedgeley, UK: British Small Animal Veterinary Association, 2004.

Lorenz MD, Coates JR, Kent M. Handbook of Veterinary Neurology, 5th ed. St. Louis, MO: Elsevier Saunders, 2012.

http://www.ivis.org/special_books/Braund/toc.asp

Neuroanatomy

Canine brain transections. http://vanat.cvm.umn.edu/brainsect/

Brain biodiversity bank. Michigan State University. https://www.msu.edu/user/brains/

Brain maps org. http://brain-maps.org/index.php?p=timeline

Comparative brain collections. http://brainmuseum.org/

DeLahunta A, Glass E. Veterinary Neuroanatomy and Clinical Neurology, 3rd ed. St. Louis, MO: Saunders/Elsevier, 2009.

Jenkins TW. Functional Mammalian Neuroanatomy: with emphasis on dog and cat, including an atlas of the central nervous system of the dog, 2nd ed. Philadelphia, PA: Lea & Febiger, 1978.

Kim RKS, Liu CN, Moffitt RL. A Stereotaxic Atlas of the Dog's Brain. Springfield, Il: Charles C Thomas, 1960.

Leigh EJ, Mackillop E, Robertson ID, Hudson LC. Clinical anatomy of the canine brain using magnetic resonance imaging. Vet Radiol Ultrasound 2008;49:113–121.

Singer M. The Brain of the Dog in Section. Philadelphia, PA: WB Saunders Company, 1962.

Techniques for PNS and muscle

Shelton GD. Routine and specialized laboratory testing for the diagnosis of neuromuscular diseases in dogs and cats. Vet Clin Pathol 2010;39:278–295.

Basic tissue reaction patterns

Facecchia K, Fochesato LA, Ray SD, Stohs SJ, Pandey S. Oxidative toxicity in neurodegenerative diseases: role of mitochondrial dysfunction and therapeutic strategies. J Toxicol 2011; 683728. Epub 2011 Jul 14.

Stetler RA, Gan Y, Zhang W, Liou AK, Gao Y, Cao G, Chen J. Heat shock proteins: cellular and molecular mechanisms in the central nervous system. Prog Neurobiol 2010;92:184–211.

Sofroniew MV, Vinters HV. Astrocytes: biology and pathology. Acta Neuropathol 2010;119:7–35.

Czeh M, Gressens P, Kaindl AM. The yin and yang of microglia. Dev Neurosci 2011;33:199–209.

Edema

Lencean SM. Brain edema – a new classification. Medical Hypotheses 2003;61:106–109.

Kimelberg HK. Water homeostasis in the brain: basic concepts. Neuroscience 2004;129:851–860.

Artifacts, pseudolesions, old age

Borràs D, Ferrer I, Pumarola M. Age-related changes in the brain of the dog. Vet Pathol 1999;36:202–211.

Bukovics P, Pál J, Gallyas F. Aldehyde fixation is not necessary for the formation of "dark" neurons. Acta Neuropathol 2008;116:463–464.

Garman RH. Histology of the central nervous system. Toxicol Pathol 2011;39:22–35.

Head E. Neurobiology of the aging dog. Age (Dordr) 2011;33:485–496.

Kherani ZS, Auer RN. Pharmacologic analysis of the mechanism of dark neuron production in cerebral cortex. Acta Neuropathol 2008;116:447–452.

Pugliese M, Carrasco JL, Gomez-Anson B, Andrade C, Zamora A, Rodríguez MJ, Mascort J, Mahy N. Magnetic resonance imaging of cerebral involutional changes in dogs as markers of aging: an innovative tool adapted from a human visual rating scale. Vet J 2010;186:166–171.

Sisó S, Jeffrey M, González L. Sensory circumventricular organs in health and disease. Acta Neuropathol 2010;120:689–705.

Magnetic resonance imaging

Gavin PR, Bagley RS. Practical Small Animal MRI. Ames, IO: Wiley-Blackwell, 2009.

Elliott I, Skerritt G. Handbook of Small Animal MRI. Oxford, UK: Wiley-Blackwell, 2010.

This book is accompanied by a companion website which is maintained by
the Division of Diagnostic Imaging, Dept of Clinical Veterinary Medicine,
Vetsuisse Faculty, University of Bern, Switzerland:

www.wiley.com/go/vandevelde/veterinaryneuropathology

2

Vascular disorders

In this group of diseases there is a disturbance of blood circulation in the CNS. The lesions in these diseases include ischemic damage to the nervous tissue resulting from a deficient blood supply and hemorrhage when blood vessels are injured. Vascular disorders are considered to be relatively rare in domestic animals as compared to humans but are being recognized with increasing frequency as a result of advances in veterinary diagnostic imaging.

2.1 Pathophysiology of ischemia

Because the CNS has a high glucose and oxygen demand (a third of the total energy generated by the body) and a very limited storage capacity, it is dependent on a high and permanent supply of oxygen and glucose by arterial blood. Cerebral arterial blood flow remains relatively constant despite significant changes in blood pressure. It is maintained by the constriction and dilation of small cerebral arteries and arterioles depending on whether the systemic blood pressure rises or falls. This type of "autoregulation" protects the brain from ischemia as long as the cerebral blood flow is not reduced by more than 60%. However, when the ischemic threshold is exceeded, the supply of oxygen and glucose and also the removal of potentially toxic metabolites are insufficient and cellular damage occurs.

Global ischemia occurs following either severe loss of blood or decrease of blood pressure (e.g. cardiorespiratory arrest, heart disease, narcotic drug overdose), whereas local ischemia results from vascular occlusion (infarct). Neurons, which are totally dependent on oxidative glycolysis, are particularly vulnerable and therefore the first cell type to be affected by ischemia, followed by oligodendrocytes, astrocytes, microglia and endothelial cells. Lack of oxygen, even for a few minutes, leads to irreversible neuronal damage. Circulatory or respiratory disorders, as well as some toxins influencing the oxygen content of the blood, affect the neurons in a characteristic way. The change is called *acidophilic neuronal necrosis*. These cells show a sharply delineated shrunken cell body with a bright eosinophilic, homogeneous cytoplasm ("red and dead neurons") and pyknotic nuclei (see Chapter 1.3.1). These irreversible changes are induced after a few minutes of ischemia and become microscopically visible approximately 8 hours after the insult. The pathogenesis of this change is complex and not completely understood. The accepted mechanism involves excitotoxicity as described in Chapter 1.3.1.

Immediately adjacent to areas of complete ischemia with irreversible tissue necrosis is a rim of tissue in which the cerebral blood flow is only partially compromised. This rim is called the *penumbra*, in which the damage may be reversible.

A second wave of neuronal injury occurs during reperfusion. Restored blood flow allows for influx of blood-borne leukocytes and oxygen resulting in synthesis of reactive oxygen species and nitric oxide, edema and hemorrhage, further exacerbating cell damage.

2.2 General strategy for diagnosing vascular lesions

- The typical clinical presentation is an animal of any age with a history of peracute/acute onset of neurological signs suggesting a focal lesion which generally do not progress in severity. If the animal survives, signs may abate with time. Focal vascular insults may be clinically silent and hence detected as an incidental finding on MRI or on the neuropathological examination.
- Vascular lesions are often detected on gross examination while sectioning the brain. In the spinal cord they may be easily overlooked unless there is a clear clinical/imaging localization. If a spinal localization is suggested by the history, systematic sectioning of all segments may be required.

Veterinary Neuropathology: Essentials of Theory and Practice, First Edition. Marc Vandevelde, Robert J. Higgins, and Anna Oevermann.
© 2012 John Wiley & Sons, Ltd. Published 2012 by John Wiley & Sons, Ltd.

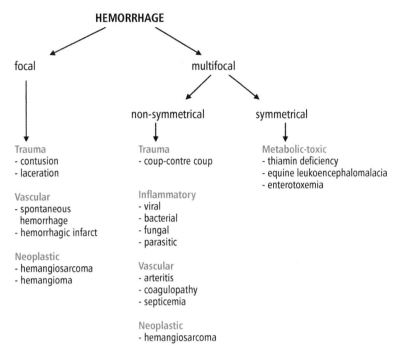

Fig. 2.1 Differential diagnosis of hemorrhage.

- The prevailing lesion patterns are gross or microscopic well demarcated areas of malacia and/or hemorrhage.
- In most cases, these lesions are focal, but depending on the etiology (e.g. vasculitis, systemic hypertension, global ischemia due to low blood pressure) they may be multifocal or (rarely) diffuse. Consult Fig. 6.1 for the differential diagnosis of malacia.
- For hemorrhagic lesions see Fig. 2.1 on the differential diagnosis of hemorrhage.
- The finding of focal or non-symmetrical multifocal malacic or hemorrhagic lesions quickly points to a circulatory problem. The next step is to determine the underlying primary disease. Optimally solid clinical or necropsy data may pinpoint a defined circulatory problem (e.g. cardiac disease) but this data is often lacking. Searching for the cause of the problem in brain sections focuses then on finding vascular lesions or obstructions. Unfortunately these are often not found and in many cases the vascular etiology remains presumptive.

2.3 Common vascular lesions

2.3.1 Vascular lesions of the brain

Ischemic brain infarct

Infarcts may occur as a result of vascular obstruction either due to local cerebrovascular disease causing vascular thrombosis or due to embolization of a process in a distant organ (**thromboembolism**). Emboli arising from cardiac diseases, e.g. from chronic endocarditis of the mitral valve or from mitral valve insufficiency, are an important cause of vascular obstruction. Metastatic **tumor emboli** may occasionally obstruct major blood vessels. Rarely, vascular lesions resulting from (accidental) **intracarotid injections** have been described in the horse. Vascular obstruction may also be caused by a primary lesion of the cerebral blood vessel wall. Inflammatory lesions of vessels occur in the frame of infectious/immune diseases and are covered in the section on inflammation (Chapter 3). Vascular degeneration resulting from toxins is discussed in the section on toxic–metabolic diseases (Chapter 6). Primary vascular diseases such as *atherosclerosis*, *arteriosclerosis* and *arteriolosclerosis* as it occurs in humans are very rarely observed in domestic animals, possibly due to their relatively low incidence of hypertensive disease. Predisposing factors for brain infarction in animals are hypothyroidism or hyperadrenocorticism, diabetes mellitus, hyperlipemia, hypercoagulative state and hypertension.

Focal ischemia leads to the formation of infarcts, a circumscribed area of malacia. The localization of an infarct depends on the arterial system involved. In all species the brain receives blood from the basilar artery. In dogs, as in man, the brain circulation is additionally

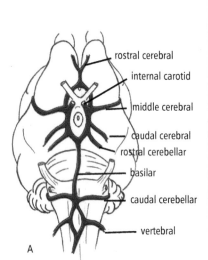
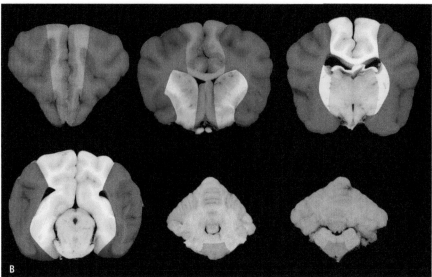

Fig. 2.2 A: Anatomy of large arteries in the canine brain. B: Schematic representation of arterial perfusion areas of the canine brain. Red: middle cerebral arteries. Violet: rostral cerebral arteries. Yellow: caudal cerebral arteries. Green: striate arteries. Blue: perforating arteries. Gray: rostral cerebellar arteries. Orange: caudal cerebellar arteries. Brown: vertebral arteries.

supported by the internal carotid artery; in cats and sheep it is supported by the maxillary artery. A special anatomical feature in ruminants, pigs and cats is the rete mirabile, a mass of convoluted blood vessels in the area of the sella turcica. In the dog, the brain is supplied by five pairs of large arteries (Fig. 2.2A). These branch off the arterial cerebral circle, a ring-shaped structure at the base of the brain formed by the bifurcating basilar artery, the internal carotid arteries and communicating arteries between them. The five main arterial systems are: the rostral, middle and caudal cerebral arteries as well as the caudal and rostral cerebellar arteries. All these run dorsally along the surface of the brain and give off superficial and deep perforating arteries to supply the deep structures of the brain. Fig 2.2B shows the perfusion areas of the major arteries. Cerebral infarcts are less common in dogs than in humans, presumably because of the presence of numerous vascular anastomoses and lower prevalence of vascular and hypertensive diseases. When a main artery is obstructed, a *territorial infarct* ensues; obstruction of the smaller perforating arteries leads to *lacunar infarcts*. *Watershed infarcts* occur as a result of global cerebral ischemia that is accentuated at the boundary between the territories of two major cerebral arteries. The predilection site for ischemic infarction in that case is the internal capsule and surrounding area (terminal perfusion area of the rostral and middle cerebral arteries or middle and caudal cerebral arteries). In dogs, infarcts are most often found in the cerebellum and forebrain.

In the vast majority of cases, infarcts are solitary lesions. Ischemic infarcts occur extremely rarely in multiple locations simultaneously. Occasionally, we have observed ischemic infarcts of different ages within the same canine brain. Recurrence has also been observed in clinical MRI studies and pathological studies show infarcts of different stages to be common in aging pigs.

Macroscopically ischemic infarcts appear mostly as single, well circumscribed areas of discoloration (tan) and softening (malacia) predominantly of the gray matter but sometimes extending into the surrounding white matter (Fig. 2.3A,B). See MRI Atlas. Although white matter is considered less vulnerable than gray matter to ischemic injury, isolated white matter infarcts (predominantly in the centrum semiovale) may occur in rare instances. Similar lesions may be seen in absence of gray matter lesions following carbon monoxide intoxication (see Chapter 6.2.5).

In acute lesions there is often edema surrounding the infarcted area. In HE sections, during the acute stage the infarcted area is pale compared to the normal brain and sharply demarcated (Fig. 2.3C). On higher magnification, acidophilic neurons and swollen axons are observed (Fig. 2.3D). Astrocytes may have swollen nuclei. The necrotic tissue is soon invaded by large numbers of macrophages removing the dead tissue (Fig. 2.4A). In the penumbra there is vascular proliferation and astrogliosis. In surviving animals, infarcts usually become cavities that are lined and traversed by dense astroglial scar

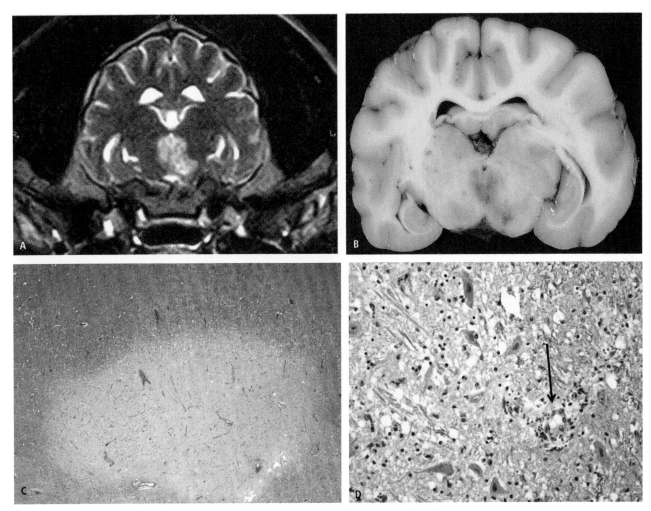

Fig. 2.3 Dog. Anemic infarct. A: MRI (T2W sequence) showing a well demarcated hyperintense lesion representing a lacunar infarct involving a perforating artery of the rostral midbrain. B: Same animal as in A, well demarcated area of brownish discoloration on both sides of the third ventricle extending into the substantia nigra of the right side. C: On HE the infarcted area appears well demarcated and pale. D: Higher magnification reveals acidophilic neurons, spongy state and prominent capillaries with hypertrophic endothelium (arrow).

tissue (Fig. 2.4B). In many cases of suspected cerebral infarction the vascular obstruction is not found on histological examination.

Ischemic encephalopathy

Global ischemia leads to widespread, bilaterally symmetrical neuronal death in selectively vulnerable neuronal populations (in human medicine referred to as **ischemic encephalopathy**). Generally, the brain is not uniformly involved, but due to the vascular anatomy and varying vulnerability of neuronal subtypes, neuronal necrosis appears first in the cerebral cortex (in the so-called watershed zones), where the hippocampus appears to be the most sensitive part, followed by the cerebellar

cortex (Purkinje cells), the basal nuclei and thalamic nuclei ("selective vulnerability"). Widespread ischemic damage with a bilateral distribution in the most vulnerable areas can be seen e.g. following **anesthesia accidents** and **cardiac arrest**, furthermore in **neonatal maladjustment syndrome**, severe **anemia**, **hypotension** and **hypovolemic shock**. However, in animals dying immediately or within hours following the ischemic insult, which is very often the case, there is not sufficient time for microscopic lesions to develop and the brain may appear normal. Depending on duration and intensity of ischemia, the neuropathology varies from a few necrotic neurons (only visible with the microscope) to pseudolaminar necrosis of the cerebral cortex (polioencephalomalacia) to global infarction of the brain, which

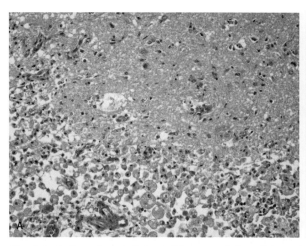
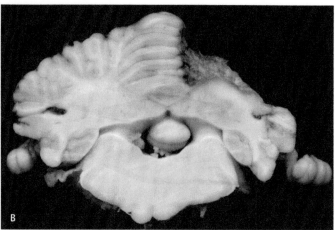

Fig. 2.4 A: Dog. Anemic infarct. After several days, infarcted areas become infiltrated with gitter cells. Note the sharp demarcation between the infarcted and unaffected tissue. HE. B: Dog. Chronic cerebellar infarct in a dog involving the perfusion area of the right rostral cerebellar artery. The right cerebellar hemisphere is largely replaced by a cystic area (now collapsed), note sharp demarcation from the unaffected tissue.

can be appreciated macroscopically. Ischemic encephalopathy has to be differentiated from metabolic toxic encephalomalacias which in the absence of adequate anamnestic information may be quite difficult. Consult Fig. 6.1.

Feline ischemic encephalopathy

This condition is well known in the US in adult cats with acute forebrain signs, which may resolve in time. In **feline ischemic encephalopathy** there is unilateral extensive infarction of the cerebral cortex and hippocampus sometimes including the deeper structures. In

surviving animals, there is marked atrophy of one hemisphere. The underlying cause is parasitic migration of *Cuterebra* larvae (see also Chapter 3.3.8). Presumably, toxic effects of the parasite induce vascular spasms leading to ischemia.

Hemorrhagic brain infarcts

These may occur following thrombosis of veins (Fig. 2.5A,B). Obstruction of large extracerebral veins, for example the dural venous sinus as in humans, has been very rarely documented in animals. More common is vascular damage with increased leakage of erythrocytes

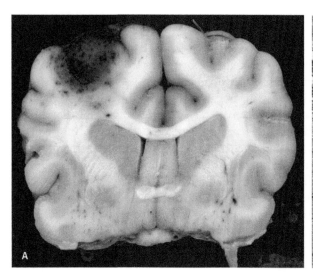
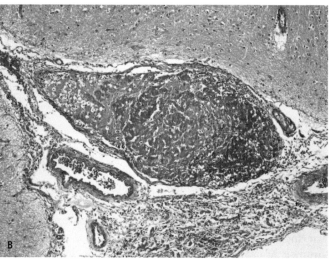

Fig. 2.5 A: Dog. Left parietal cortex. Hemorrhagic infarct associated with brain swelling and midline shift. B: This infarct was caused by venous thrombosis that was associated with a metastatic carcinoma. HE.

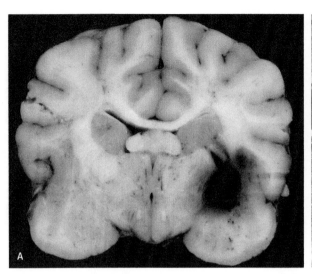 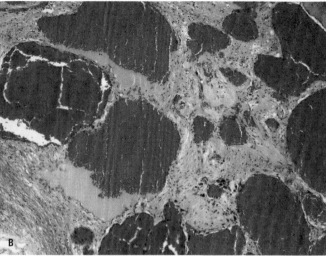

Fig. 2.6 A: Dog. Spontaneous hemorrhage in area of globus pallidus dissecting the internal capsule. B: Dog. Cerebral hemangioma associated with spontaneous cerebral hemorrhage showing plexiform arrangement of numerous cross-sections of well differentiated and thin-walled vessels. HE.

when reperfusion occurs in focal ischemia. This leads to ring hemorrhages which may coalesce to form larger hemorrhagic lesions. Hemorrhagic cerebral infarcts must initially be differentiated from traumatic lesions (frequently meningeal contact, meningeal hemorrhage, possibly "contre-coup" lesions in other locations) or from embolic encephalitis following septicemia (multiple, less circumscribed hemorrhages) (see Fig. 2.1). For septic encephalitis and trauma see chapters 3 and 4.

Hemorrhage/hematoma

Hemorrhage (Fig. 2.6A) is a common major lesion pattern and can be caused by trauma, toxic–metabolic, infectious/inflammatory vascular injury (e.g. septicemia or vascular tumors). Consult Fig. 2.1 for differential diagnosis. In contrast to humans, in which spontaneous brain hemorrhage (hemorrhagic stroke) is a relatively frequent cause of neurological dysfunction, spontaneous rupture of blood vessels is rare in domestic animals since the underlying combination of vascular changes and primary hypertension as in humans is lacking. In animals, large space-occupying hematomas can be caused by preexisting vascular pathologies such as vascular tumors (**cavernous hemangiomas**) and rarely malformations (**vascular hamartomas** or **aneurysms**). However, it is often difficult to find evidence of such vascular lesions amidst massive hemorrhage in histological sections (Fig. 2.6B). In these cases, hematomas are generally focal, mostly rounded solitary lesions. See MRI Atlas. Multiple hemorrhages

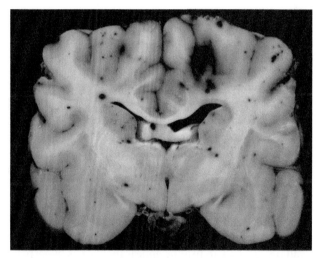

Fig. 2.7 Dog with septicemia. Cross-section of forebrain. Multifocal and randomly distributed hemorrhages of varying size in the gray and white matter.

indicate coagulation disorders induced by an imbalance between coagulation and fibrinolysis (e.g. disseminated intravascular coagulation), toxins (e.g. dicumarol intoxication), vasculitis (Fig. 2.7), trauma or metastatic vascular tumors.

If the animal survives the initial vascular insult, the hematoma becomes infiltrated by macrophages, which metabolize hemoglobin in various stages from the phagocytosed erythrocytes to hemosiderin. The latter becomes visible in HE sections from about 3 days following hemorrhage and may persist throughout life.

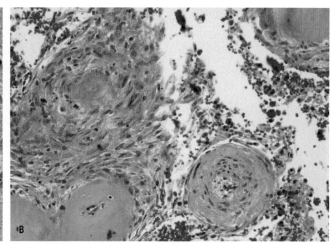

Fig. 2.8 Cat. Feline hypertensive encephalopathy A: Hyaline changes and thickening of arteriolar walls, secondary proteinaceous exudation, edema and gliosis in the surrounding brain parenchyma. HE. B: Subarachnoidal arteries showing hyperplastic changes with massive thickening of the wall due to adventitial fibroblast proliferation and subendothelial deposition of hyaline material. HE.

Feline hypertensive encephalopathy

Neurological signs compatible with hypertensive encephalopathy as it occurs in humans have been described in cats in association with systemic hypertension and renal failure. Hypertensive encephalopathy develops with an abrupt and prolonged increase of systemic blood pressure that overwhelms the autoregulatory mechanisms of the brain. Neuropathologically, it is characterized by hypertensive vascular changes in arteries and arterioles (Fig. 2.8). These may present as hyalinosis of the vessel wall (thickening due to leakage of eosinophilic material and its deposition in the vessel wall resulting in an hyaline appearance) or as hyperplastic arteriolosclerosis (thickening of the vessel wall due to concentric hyperplasia of spindloid cells). Secondary changes include severe vasogenic edema, hemorrhages in the parenchyma and subarachnoid space that may be significant, and ischemic necrosis with influx of phagocytes.

2.3.2 Vascular lesions of the spinal cord

The spinal cord is supplied by two dorsal (dorsal spinal arteries) and one ventral (ventral spinal artery) superficially located arteries formed by anastomosing branches of the dorsal and ventral radicular arteries and extending over much of the length of the cord.

Perforating arteries arising from the dorsal and ventral spinal arteries supply specific areas of any given cord segment as depicted in Fig. 2.9A.

Fibrocartilagenous emboli (FCE)

Spinal cord infarcts resulting from **fibrocartilaginous embolism** are quite common in dogs and occur less frequently in other domestic animals. Animals with such spinal cord infarcts show peracute often lateralized spinal signs without pain. The fibrocartilaginous emboli are histochemically identical to nucleus pulposus of the intervertebral discs, hence it is postulated that they originate from this source. However, the precise mechanism by which the emboli access the spinal cord blood supply, particularly large-caliber arteries, from the nucleus pulposus is unclear. It has been proposed that nucleus pulposus material may penetrate into the vertebral vessels or into the venous sinus of the bone marrow of the vertebral body during trauma/exercise. From the latter it is claimed to enter arteries and veins by retrograde flow through arteriovenous anastomoses. In people the explanation is that Schmorl's nodules break off from the outer cartilaginous plate of the disc into the medulla of the vertebral body. Several other mechanisms have been proposed. Whatever the real mechanism and source of this fibrocartilagenous embolus is, occlusion of the arterial supply or venous drainage leads to characteristic patterns of ischemic necrosis. Spinal cord

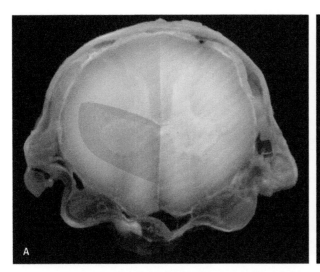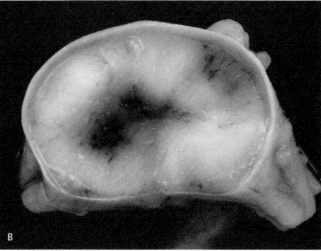

Fig. 2.9 A: Schematic representation of spinal cord perfusion areas (based on de Lahunta and Glass, Veterinary Neuroanatomy and Clinical Neurology, Saunders Elsevier 2009). Red: central (sulcal) branch of the ventral spinal artery. Blue: circumferential branches (arterial vasocorona) of the ventral radicular arteries. Green: circumferential branches (arterial vasocorona) of the dorsal spinal artery. B: Dog. Spinal cord infarction due to showering of the circumferential branches of the dorsal spinal artery and the central branch of the ventral spinal artery by fibrocartilagenous emboli. Relatively well demarcated areas of hemorrhage and malacia (brown discoloration) are present in the right dorsolateral funiculi and in the central gray matter.

arteries have numerous anastomoses and hence it is likely that in order to cause spinal cord infarction multiple vessels must be simultaneously occluded by a shower of fibrocartilageneous emboli. Depending on the size of the embolus, occlusion of the spinal artery or its central (sulcal) branches leads to necrosis of gray matter. In contrast, occlusion of the circumferential branches (arterial vasocorona) of the spinal and radicular arteries, which supply the white matter, leads to a restricted pattern of leukomyelomalacia. If both systems are involved in multiple showering then there is confluent, sharply defined myelomalacia. These resultant areas of polio- or leuko- or confluent myelomalacia can be seen macroscopically, especially when they have become cystic or hemorrhagic (Fig. 2.9B). Venous occlusion leads to hemorrhagic malacia. The emboli may involve several consecutive or multifocal segments and more rarely the brainstem and cerebellum. Histologically, temporal features are similar to those described in cerebral infarcts.

Fibrocartilagenous emboli are generally, but not always, found in both arteries and veins (Fig. 2.10). Because this material stains metachromatically it can be best detected by Giemsa, toluidine blue or alcian blue histochemical stains (Fig. 2.10D).

Sometimes no fibrocartilagenous emboli can be detected in myelomalacia but just thrombi or emboli composed of fibrin clots and degenerated blood cells.

Other causes of spinal cord infarction

Spinal cord infarction resulting from the same causes as in brain infarcts is very rare, presumably because the collateral circulation in the cord is well developed. It might occur as a complication in severe cases of **canine steroid-responsive meningitis arteritis** (SRMA, see Chapter 3), in which thrombi occlude major perforating arteries as a result of arterial wall necrosis.

Spinal cord hemorrhage

Spontaneous hemorrhage may result from vascular malformations or tumors as in the brain. **Hematomyelia** has also been rarely seen in dogs with SRMA when the inflammatory process leads to rupture of a large artery. Extensive subarachnoid hemorrhage of the brain and spinal cord following myelography has been described in dogs. The pathogenesis is not clear: hemorrhage may be the result of traumatic injury of a vessel during lumbar puncture or of an idiosyncratic response to the contrast medium. **Post-anesthetic hemorrhagic myelopathy**, with acute diffuse hemorrhagic myelomalacia in many segments of the cord, occurs in horses undergoing surgery in dorsal recumbency. The mechanism is not understood.

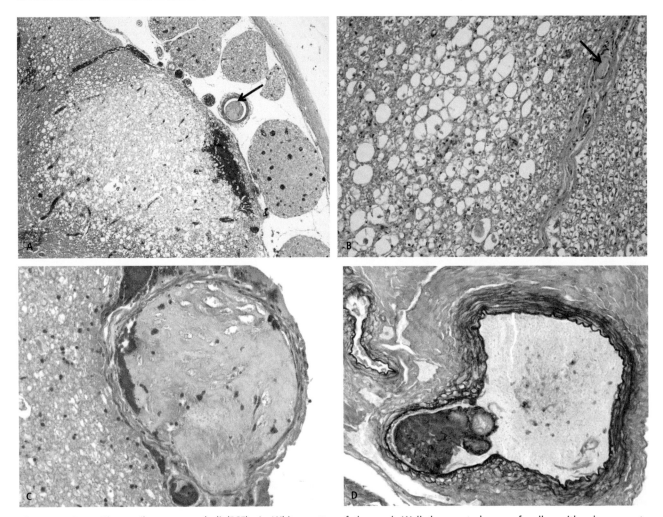

Fig. 2.10 Dog. Fibrocartilagenous emboli (FCE). A: White matter of the cord. Well demarcated area of pallor with edema, acute necrosis and hemorrhage. Embolus occludes the dorsal radicular artery (arrow). HE. B: Infarcted area with edema, dilation of myelin sheaths, fibrocartilagenous embolus (arrow). HE. C: A large fibrocartilagenous embolus almost completely occludes a subarachnoidal vein. HE. D: Fibrocartilagenous emboli stain bright blue with alcian-blue stain.

2.3.3 Ischemia in the peripheral nervous system and muscles

Distal aortic thrombosis

This is a relatively common disorder in cats associated with hypertrophic cardiomyopathy and occurs rarely in dogs. These cats show a sudden onset of paraparesis to paraplegia with painful hard muscles and lacking a femoral pulse. The aortic thrombosis leads to acute ischemic necrosis of the tibial and peroneal nerves and of the muscles of the hindlimbs. The spinal cord is spared.

Further reading

Cerebral infarcts

Garosi LS. Cerebrovascular disease in dogs and cats. Vet Clin North Am Small Anim Pract 2010;40:65–79.

Garosi LS, McConnell JF. Ischaemic stroke in dogs and humans: a comparative review. J Small Anim Pract 2005;46:521–529.

Wessmann A, Chandler K, Garosi L. Ischaemic and haemorrhagic stroke in the dog. Vet J 2009;180:290–303.

Hemorrhage

Martin-Vaquero P, Moore SA, Wolk KE, Oglesbee MJ. Cerebral vascular hamartoma in a geriatric cat. J Feline Med Surg 2011; 13:286–290.

Packer RA, Bergman RL, Coates JR, Essman SC, Weis K, O'Brien DP, Johnson GC. Intracranial subarachnoid hemorrhage following lumbar myelography in two dogs. Vet Radiol Ultrasound 2007;48:323–327.

Hypertensive encephalopathy

Brown CA, Munday JS, Mathur S, Brown SA. Hypertensive encephalopathy in cats with reduced renal function. Vet Pathol 2005;42: 642–649.

Littman MP. Spontaneous systemic hypertension in 24 cats. J Vet Intern Med 1994;8:79–86.

Fibrocartilagenous emboli

De Risio L, Platt SR. Fibrocartilaginous embolic myelopathy in small animals. Vet Clin North Am Small Anim Pract 2010;40:859–869.

Aortic thrombosis

Smith SA, Tobias AH, Jacob KA, Fine DM, Grumbles PL. Arterial thromboembolism in cats: acute crisis in 127 cases (1992–2001) and long-term management with low-dose aspirin in 24 cases. J Vet Intern Med 2003;17:73–83.

This book is accompanied by a companion website which is maintained by the Division of Diagnostic Imaging, Dept of Clinical Veterinary Medicine, Vetsuisse Faculty, University of Bern, Switzerland.
www.wiley.com/go/vandevelde/veterinaryneuropathology

3

Inflammatory diseases

The term inflammation is currently often used in a broad sense covering a wide range of reactive processes resulting from tissue injury. In this chapter we focus on inflammatory diseases in the traditional sense of the word, i.e. lesions characterized by strong participation of the immune system. Morphological evidence of such an immune reaction consists of accumulation of inflammatory cells in the meninges, around the blood vessels and in the parenchyma. Most of these lesions are associated with infectious diseases but some result from derangement of the immune system.

3.1 Pathophysiology of inflammation

3.1.1 Entry and effect of infectious agents in the nervous system

Hematogenous spread from other infected organs is common in bacterial infections with infected thromboemboli becoming lodged in small blood vessels in the CNS. Viruses can enter the CNS from the blood through endothelial cell infection or penetration of the blood–brain barrier within circulating infected mononuclear cells. A few areas of the CNS (choroid plexus, circumventricular organs) have fenestrated capillaries where agents may access the brain directly. Some infectious agents, such as herpes viruses and the *Listeria* bacterium, can also enter the peripheral nerves to get into the CNS by traveling within axons. The agent is then carried transsynaptically by axonal transport from one neuronal pool to the next. Infectious agents can also spread through the CSF. This is common in bacterial infections, once the agents have entered the cerebrospinal fluid compartment.

Many agents, especially viruses such as rabies virus, have an affinity for neurons often with specific tropism for certain neuronal populations. The process of viral replication may kill the neurons by apoptosis or necrosis leading to serious neurological signs. An extreme example is the severe cerebrocortical necrosis in herpes virus infections. Bacteria and fungi and some viruses (e.g. equine herpes virus) damage endothelial cells with disturbance of blood vessel permeability with resulting brain edema and/or hemorrhage. Some agents may target the cells of the white matter causing myelin destruction.

3.1.2 Immune reaction of the host against the infectious agent in the CNS

The innate immune system

Similar to other tissues, the CNS also possesses an innate immune system represented by pattern recognition receptors (PRRs) such as Toll-like receptors (TLRs) that are capable of recognizing certain molecular structures on pathogens or altered tissue constituents. PRRs are strongly expressed on microglial cells and also on astrocytes. Recognition of pathogens by these receptors elicits an immediate reaction with secretion of toxic molecules and swift recruitment of other cells such as neutrophils, macrophages and natural killer cells. An example of such an innate immune reaction is the formation of micro-abscesses in listeriosis.

The adaptive immune response

Compared to other organs, the CNS seems poorly equipped to participate in the adaptive immune response. A significant residential lymphocyte population, and lymphatic drainage system are lacking. A blood–brain barrier (BBB) effectively shields the CNS from the blood and, normal CNS cells, with the exception of microglia, do not express antigen presenting (MHC) molecules on their surface. Still, antigen can drain from the CSF to the cervical lymph nodes or, in the case of viruses replicating in endothelial cells, may be expressed at the luminal surface of the blood vessels in the nervous system, thus becoming recognizable by circulating lymphocytes. Activated T cells spontaneously cross the BBB and may accumulate when they

Veterinary Neuropathology: Essentials of Theory and Practice, First Edition. Marc Vandevelde, Robert J. Higgins, and Anna Oevermann.
© 2012 John Wiley & Sons, Ltd. Published 2012 by John Wiley & Sons, Ltd.

recognize their antigen presented by microglial cells. The replication of agents in the CNS and changes directly induced by them leads to a range of complex reactive events.

Invasion of immune cells in the nervous system

A range of molecules has been recognized to play a crucial regulatory role in CNS inflammation. These include, among others, *adhesion molecules*, *metallo-proteinases*, *chemokines* and *cytokines*. All these molecules can be constitutively expressed by CNS cells, albeit usually at low levels. Most play an important role in CNS development and homeostasis. Some are inducible by certain stimuli and all can be upregulated by a wide range of noxious events. Because of their potency, even in very small quantities, it is not surprising that the expression of these molecules is tightly regulated at several levels. This regulation is extremely complex. These molecules frequently act by binding to their corresponding receptors mediating signal transduction with upregulation of the cell's machinery, for example increased transcription activity. Frequently they are produced as precursor molecules that need to be cleaved into their active form by specific enzymes which in turn are regulated by still other factors. Some are regulated by specific inhibitors secreted by the CNS tissue.

Entry of inflammatory cells into the CNS across the blood–brain barrier is an important first step in reaction to injury. *Integrins*, transmembranous molecules regulating communication between the extracellular compartment and the cytoplasm, and *adhesion molecules*, expressed by endothelial cells, play an important role in leukocyte trafficking across the blood–brain barrier. *Matrix metallo-proteinases* (MMPs) are enzymes which can degrade the extracellular matrix in this way disrupting the blood–brain barrier for entry of leukocytes into the CNS parenchyma. The MMPs are present in an inactive form, which must be cleaved by other enzymes in order become effective. They are additionally regulated by *tissue inhibitors of metallo-proteinases* (TIMPs) illustrating the complex control mechanisms for such potent compounds. MMPs are, for example, upregulated in canine distemper virus infection along with the invasion of inflammatory cells through the blood vessel walls.

Cellular migration and *chemotaxis* (the process by which inflammatory cells are attracted to the brain) is further modified by *chemokines* and their receptors expressed by glial cells in the CNS. Both can be upregulated by various inflammatory mediators. Each chemokine has its specific receptor but multiple receptor usage is also possible, again providing a means for complex regulation.

An important class of inflammatory mediators, which play a role in the regulation of the inflammatory response are the *cytokines*. This is a large group of compounds with such widely diverging activities that their lumping together in one class of molecules is rather arbitrary. Cytokines can promote inflammation, others are anti-inflammatory. Some cytokines such as *tumor necrosis factor alpha* (TNF alpha) and *interleukin-1* (IL-1) are involved in tissue damage by triggering the release of toxic molecules from macrophages. However, cytokines not only enhance or induce tissue damage but are also involved in repair and neuroprotection depending on timing of the pathological process, amount of mediator produced and interaction with other molecules. An example for cytokine activity is the release of IL-8 in the spinal fluid of dogs with steroid-responsive meningitis arteritis which leads to invasion of inflammatory cells into the CSF compartment. In canine distemper infection there is an upregulation of pro-inflammatory cytokines, whereas anti-inflammatory cytokines remain at base level explaining the long-lasting nature of the disease.

All the complex molecular interactions described above finally lead to infiltration of inflammatory cells across the BBB.

3.1.3 Morphological aspects of the immune response

The major morphological hallmark of inflammation is accumulation of inflammatory cells around blood vessels or *perivascular cuffing*. The infiltrating inflammatory cells also invade the perivascular parenchyma and the CSF spaces.

The imported specifically sensitized immune cells quickly expand upon interaction with their target (antigens of the infectious agent) , and many additional cells are recruited from the blood into the CNS. Following the cellular immune response (cytotoxic and helper T cells), a humoral immune response is initiated as B cells are recruited and develop into immunoglobulin-producing plasma cells. This leads to the intrathecal production of antibodies against the infectious agent, which can be detected in the cerebrospinal fluid in the live animal.

In the wake of the inflammatory response, with the presence of numerous highly active molecules, the local residential cells are stimulated to participate. Proliferation of glial cells can be diffuse but is often nodular along with the location of the infectious agent. These *glial nodules* consist of a mixture of invaded inflammatory cells, microglial cells/macrophages and astrocytes. The nodules are particularly prominent in neurotropic viral infections. Macrophages are usually strongly upregulated in bacterial and fungal infections with the formation of granulomas. As in other types of tissue injury, endothelial cells can proliferate with formation of capillary sprouts. Capillary proliferation is often a prominent feature in protozoal infections.

Generally, the intrathecal immune response should lead to clearance of the infection and recovery. Indeed, this is frequently observed in immunohistochemical studies of infections, such as tick-borne encephalitis virus, which is usually rapidly eliminated. Also the bacterial load in encephalitis caused by *Listeria mono-cytogenes* decreases sharply during the course of the disease. However, the extent to which an animal will recover depends on the infectious load in the CNS. When the immune response evolves very early and rapidly, spread of the agent within the CNS is limited and animals may only suffer from mild and transient signs. If not, large or multiple areas of the CNS become infected eliciting widespread inflammation. In that case the immune response directed against intra-cellular agents can also induce significant damage to the tissue when cells are killed together with the agent. Immunopathologic complications can result in severe tissue damage with encephalomalacia or demyelina-tion. For example extensive tissue destruction associated with suppurative inflammation is common in listeriosis.

In some infections, invasion and proliferation of inflammatory cells is so intense that large space-occupying inflammatory lesions are formed. This is the case in granulomatous encephalitis or brain abscesses arising from bacterial and fungal infections. Space-occupying lesions in the CNS cause compression of the surrounding tissues, formation of edema and rise in intracranial pressure, similar to neoplasms. Inflammatory changes in the CSF compartment can cause obstruction of CSF flow with development of hydrocephalus. This happens frequently in feline infectious peritonitis (FIP) or bacterial CNS infections in neonatal food animals because the inflammation occurs within the CSF pathways.

3.2 General strategy for diagnosis of inflammatory lesions

The typical presentation is an animal at any age with acute multifocal neurological signs, which usually progress quite rapidly. Morphologically, the prevailing major pattern is perivascular cuffing. Additional major patterns which can be encountered are hemorrhage, malacia, space-occupying lesion, hypercellularity and loss of myelin. Thus there is a very large number of additional morphological features to be analyzed requiring a systematic approach outlined in Fig. 3.1.

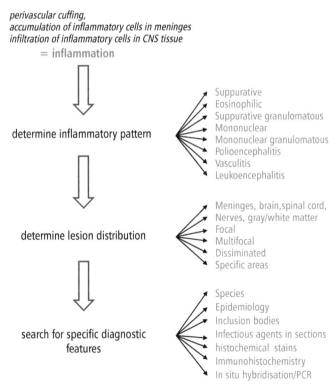

Fig. 3.1 General strategy for diagnosis of inflammatory disorders.

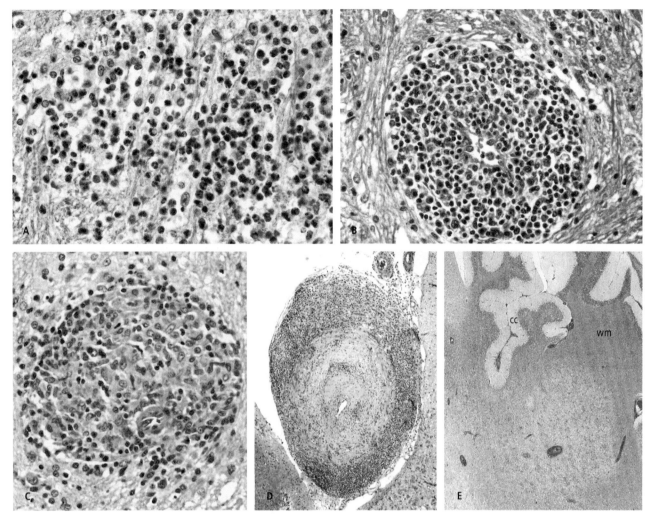

Fig. 3.2 Examples of major inflammatory reaction patterns A: Bacterial sepsis. Bovine. Cerebral white matter. Suppurative inflammation. Focal infiltration with neutrophils. HE. B: Bovine. Brainstem. Sporadic bovine encephalitis. Perivascular cuffing with mononuclear infiltrates of lymphocytes, plasma cells and macrophages. HE. C: Dog. Cerebral white matter. Granulomatous meningoencephalitis. Eccentric angiocentric perivascular cuffing with histiocytes and some lymphocytes. HE. D: Arteritis. Cat. Basilar meninges. Large artery with intense accumulation of inflammatory cells within and around the arterial wall. HE. E: Necrotizing leukoencephalitis. Dog cerebellum. Intense focal inflammation in the white matter (wm) (cc, cerebellar cortex). HE.

3.2.1 Recognizing major inflammatory reaction patterns

The invading inflammatory cells are reacting to the presence of an infectious agent and/or altered (and sometimes normal) tissue constituents. Depending on the particular disease there are a number of different basic reaction patterns which we can distinguish morphologically. In addition to the type of reactive pattern we can also quickly distinguish some obvious trends for an inflammatory process to specifically target certain tissue compartments: gray matter, white matter or blood vessels.

Thus recognizing these patterns helps us to direct the further examination and diagnosis. However, while spe-

cific groups of organisms have a clear tendency to induce specific patterns, there are no absolute rules! More than one pattern may occur in the same lesion. The next step is to determine the prevailing inflammatory pattern. The major patterns are briefly described here below and some basic morphological features are illustrated in Fig. 3.2.

Suppurative inflammation

In this type of inflammatory response polymorphonuclear leukocytes are the predominating cell type (Fig. 3.2A). In suppurative processes, influx of inflammatory cells may be so intense that it is macroscopically visible as clouding of the meninges. Large focal accumulations of polymorphonuclear cells lead to formation of an *abscess.* In the subacute and chronic stage of initially suppurative inflammation mononuclear cells with lymphocytes, histiocytes and plasma cells also participate and gradually increase in number, leading to a pyogranulomatous pattern.

Non-suppurative (mononuclear) inflammation

Here mononuclear cells (lymphocytes, plasma cells, monocytes) dominate the infiltrates (Fig. 3.2B). In viral infections, this type of infiltration is usually accompanied by specific involvement of certain cell populations: neurons (neurotropic), endothelial cells (endotheliotropic), white matter (demyelinating) leading to additional typical patterns discussed below.

Eosinophilic inflammation

This is a relatively rare type of inflammation. Significant numbers of eosinophils in an inflammatory infiltrate are immediately apparent in histological sections. They are commonly associated with parasitic and also fungal infections.

Granulomatous inflammation

Granulomatous inflammation generally occurs with intracellular infectious agents, parasites and foreign bodies, but also in a modified pattern in immune-mediated disorders (e.g. GME). The characteristic feature in this pattern is a marked accumulation/proliferation of activated histiocytic cells/macrophages (epithelioid macrophages) in the inflammatory infiltrates (Fig. 3.2C). The latter often invade the perivascular tissue with formation of large, often macroscopically visible space-occupying lesions: *granulomas*. In some lesions multinucleated giant cells are formed. Granulomatous inflammation can be associated with suppurative or with non-suppurative infiltration of inflammatory cells. The former is also called pyogranulomatous inflammation and represents the chronic stage of initially suppurative lesions.

Polioencephalitis

This is a frequent variant of non-suppurative inflammation, particularly in viral infections that have an affinity for neurons. Therefore, the lesions are often exclusively localized or most severe in the gray matter (*polioencephalitis/poliomyelitis*). Depending on the agent, specific populations of nerve cells are targeted. Thus, the distribution pattern can indicate a specific etiology. In neurotropic infections one finds varying degrees of neuronal degeneration with neuronophagia, neuronal loss and gliosis.

Leukoencephalitis/demyelination

Some infectious diseases and immune disorders focus on the white matter (Fig. 3.2E). Destruction of the myelin sheaths with sparing of the axons is called primary demyelination. In the context of inflammatory diseases demyelination may be primary or secondary, in the latter case resulting from the inflammatory response in which axons are affected as well.

Vasculitis

Some inflammatory diseases are characterized by severe lesions of the veins and arteries as a result of infiltration with inflammatory cells within the blood vessel walls (Fig. 3.2D). Damage of the blood vessel wall causes leakage of plasma and blood cells with formation of perivascular hemorrhages and/or ischemic tissue damage.

A spectrum of diseases can be included within a major reaction pattern as shown in Table 3.1.

3.2.2 Determining the distribution pattern of the lesions

Inflammation may be focal but more often multiple areas of the CNS are affected with a multifocal (several separate lesions), disseminated (many small lesions) or diffuse (all areas affected) distribution pattern.

The anatomical distribution of the lesions is also very important. A specific infectious agent or immune response may target specific areas of the nervous system. This can be related to the mode of entry or, particularly in the case of viruses, to a tropism for certain cell types, such as for example motor neurons in the cord and brainstem. The latter will then lead to a distinct polioencephalomyelitis. Bacterial and fungal infections are generally less selective because in most cases they invade the brain hematogenously, frequently causing widespread infection in the CSF pathways or abscesses and granulomas. Immune-mediated diseases often have specific targets, e.g. the proximal portions of the motor nerves in polyneuritis or the meningeal arteries in SRMA. Thus assessment of the anatomical location of the lesions (CSF, gray or white matter, nerves, blood vessels, specific anatomical areas) is helpful for the diagnosis of inflammatory disorders.

3.2.3 Specific features

Since most infectious agents have a specific species spectrum and varying geographical incidences, the species as well as the local epidemiological situation have to be considered in the interpretation of pathological findings. Finally, demonstration of an agent allows a specific

Table 3.1 Interpretation of inflammatory patterns (FIP, feline infectious peritonitis; NE, necrotizing encephalitis; NME, necrotizing meningoencephalitis; SRMA, Steroid-responsive meningitis arteritis).

INFLAMMATORY PATTERN	ETIOLOGY	SPECIFIC DISEASES
Suppurative	Bacterial	Tuberculosis, embolic encephalitis, sellaturcica empyema (ruminants), meningo-ependymitis during septicemia (food animals, horses), listeriosis (ruminants); *Streptococcosis*, melioidosis
	Fungal, algal	Aspergillosis, candidiasis, mucormycosis, blastomycosis, coccidiodomycosis, protothecosis, cryptococcosis, encephalitozoonosis, cladosporiodiosis, fusariosis
	Non-infectious	SRMA (dog)
	Viral	Arbovirus, herpesvirus (in peracute stage)
Eosinophilic	Helmintic	*Angiostrongylus, Baylisascaris, Spirocerca lupi* (dog); *Cuterebra* (cat); *Strongylus, Angiostrongylus, Halicephalobus* (horse); *Setaria* (horse, sheep, goat); *Elaphostrongylus, Parelaphostrongylus* (sheep, goat); coenurosis, cystecercosis (ruminants)
	Protozoal	Equine protozoal myeloencephalitis, sarcosporidiosis (sheep), toxoplasmosis (dog, cat), neosporosis (dog), amebiasis (dog, bovine, equine)
	Non-infectious	Eosinophilic meningoencephalitis, eosonophilic granuloma (dog)
Suppurative–granulomatous	Bacterial	Tuberculosis, abscess
	Fungal, algal	Aspergillosis, candidiasis, mucormycosis, blastomycosis, coccidiodomycosis, protothecosis, cryptococcosis, encephalitozoonosis, cladosporiodiosis, fusariosis
	Viral	Feline infectious peritonitis
Non-suppurative	Viral	Neurotropic, endotheliotropic, demyelinating
	Bacterial	Listeriosis
	Protozoal	Equine protozoal myeloencephalitis, sarcosporidiosis (sheep), toxoplasmosis (dog, cat), neosporosis, (dog), amebiasis (dog, bovine, equine)
	Non-infectious	NE, NME (dog)
Polioencephalitis/-myelitis	Viral	Rabies, pseudorabies; spring-summer encephalitis, post vaccinal distemper (dog); feline poliomyelitis, Borna disease (cat, horse, sheep); West Nile virus (horse, cattle, sheep, dog, cat); Western, Venezuelan and Eastern equine encephalitis, Japanese encephalitis virus, Hendra virus (horse); bovine herpes 5, bovine paramyxovirus; louping ill (sheep); teschovirus, rubola virus, encephalomyocarditis virus, vomiting and wasting disease, swine vesicular disease (pig)
	Non-infectious	Greyhound encephalitis
Non-suppurative–granulomatous	Viral	Visna, caprine arthritis encephalitis, equine infectious anemia
	Non-infectious	GME, NE, NME (dog); cauda equina neuritis

(Continued)

Table 3.1 (*Continued*)

INFLAMMATORY PATTERN	ETIOLOGY	SPECIFIC DISEASES
Vasculitis	Fungal	Aspergillosis, mucormycosis
	Bacterial	Rocky mountain spotted fever (dog), thrombotic meningoencephalitis (bovine), embolic encephalitis
	Viral	Canine hepatitis, FIP, equine herpes virus 1, malignant catarrhal fever (bovine), classical swine fever, African swine fever
	Chlamydial	Sporadic bovine encephalitis
	Protozoal	Equine trypanosomiasis
	Non-infectious	SRMA (dog)
Leukoencephalitis/ demyelination	Viral	Canine distemper, feline immunodeficiency virus, feline leukemia virus myelopathy, visna, border disease
	Non-infectious	Polyneuritis, allergic encephalitis, NE

etiological diagnosis. Using histochemical stains such as a Gram, GMS (Grocott's silver–methenamine) and Periodic Acid Schiff (PAS), bacteria and fungi are easier to detect. In the case of viral infections, the detection of inclusion bodies may be helpful. Specific immunohistochemical (ICH) staining or in situ hybridization (ISH) techniques, both of which work very well in paraffin sections, are available for a wide range of agents. Quite often, however, no infectious agents can be found and we are left with a morphological diagnosis and some speculation as to the etiology. In the immune-mediated diseases, the nature and distribution of the lesions is usually quite typical, allowing a specific morphological diagnosis.

3.3 Common CNS infections

3.3.1 Neurotropic viral infections

The typical neuropathological pattern in this group is a non-suppurative polioencephalitis/poliomyelitis with neuronal destruction, perivascular mononuclear cuffing and glial nodules (neuronophagia). In particularly aggressive infections (as occurs for example in West Nile Virus infection), widespread neuronal necrosis may elicit a transient invasion of neutrophils in the peracute stage of the disease.

Rabies

Rabies is caused by a *lyssavirus* of the family *rhabdoviridae*, which is pathogenic for all mammals and occurs around the world. When a polioencephalomyelitis, particularly of the brainstem, is detected on histological examination this disease has always to be included in the differential diagnosis regardless of the species. No correlation may exist between the severity of clinical symptoms and the intensity of the inflammatory response. There is a polioencephalitis with perivascular mononuclear cuffs and glial nodules, which is most obvious in the brainstem but may be very discrete (Fig. 3.3A). In horses, spinal cord involvement may be the main feature. Suspicion of rabies can be confirmed by finding typical cytoplasmic inclusion bodies in the neurons of the hippocampus and in the Purkinje cells of the cerebellum (*Negri bodies*) (Fig. 3.3B). Rabies antigen can be easily demonstrated with IHC in paraffin sections (Fig. 3.3C).

Herpes virus infections

Neurotropic herpes viruses belong to the α-herpes viruses. The infection with *suid herpes virus 1*, also called *pseudorabies virus* (*PRV*), occurs in swine in many areas of the world and may infect a wide variety of mammals and birds. Horses, primates and humans are resistant to infection. Most frequently, the virus spreads to ruminants housed in the same premises or to dogs and cats by ingestion of contaminated raw pork meat. **Pseudorabies** or **Aujeszky's disease** in sows leads to abortion and mummified fetuses; in piglets the mortality rate is high. In young pigs the encephalitis is located mainly in the cortex, most severe in the rhinencephalic parts and decreasing from rostral to caudal. There is extensive neuronal degeneration and polioencephalomalacia (Fig. 3.3D) with, in the peracute stage of the disease, invasion of neutrophils.

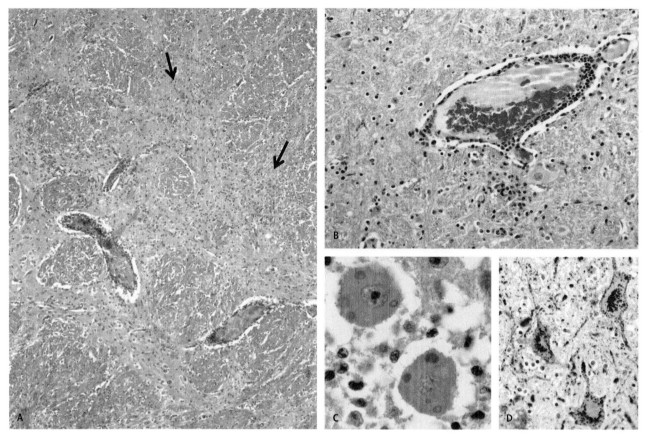

Fig. 3.3 A–D: Rabies. A. Sheep. Level of basal nuclei and capsula interna. Perivas cular cuffing and gliosis (arrows) in grey matter. B Dog.Discrete inflammatory lesions in brainstem with perivascular mononuclear cuffing and small microlial nodules (arrows), HE. C: Bovine. Cerebellum. Rabies viral inclusion bodies (Negri bodies) in cytoplasm of neurons, HE. D: Cat. Brainstem. Intense concentration of rabies virus antigen in neurons. Immunohistochemistry.

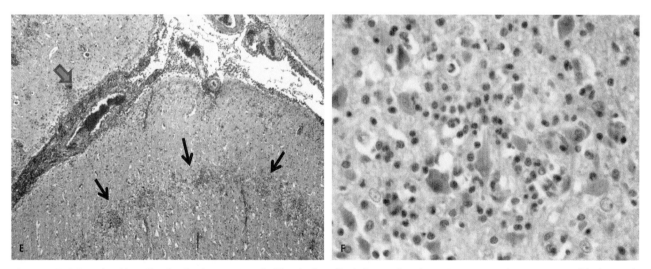

Fig. 3.3 E–F. Pseudorabies. Pig. Cerebral cortex. Band of focal microgliosis (arrows) and massive mononuclear meningitis (thick arrow). HE. F. same area as E, higher magnification. Degenerating neurons and diffuse infiltration with inflammatory cells including neutrophils.

Pruritus with violent scratching and automutilation of the head, and death within 2 days is the typical clinical history in dogs and cats. The lesions in small animals consist of mononuclear perivascular cuffs, neuronal necrosis and gliosis with large clear astrocytic nuclei with a hyperchromatic nuclear membrane. Neuronal and glial nuclei may contain eosinophilic inclusions. Lesions are mostly localized in the brainstem but there is also inflammation of the spinal and trigeminal ganglia.

Canine herpes virus encephalitis has only been reported in North America in very young puppies below the age of 6 weeks with widespread necrotizing polioencephalitis of the brainstem and cerebellar cortex. Primates, rabbits and hedgehogs are susceptible to human *herpes simplex* virus and show similar lesions of acute cerebrocortical necrosis of neurons as in humans. *Equine herpes virus 1* targets blood vessels (see below). **Bovine herpes encephalitis** is caused by *bovine herpes type 1 and type 5* viruses and presents as a polioencephalomyelitis in calves and occasionally adult animals with intense involvement of the cerebral cortex. Type 5 is much more neurovirulent than type 1 and is an important infection in developing countries, notably South America.

Arthropod-borne encephalitides (arboviruses)

These comprise a large group of agents from various viral families (*Togaviridae, Bunyaviridae, Flaviviridae, Reoviridae*) causing epidemics in various parts of the world in humans (with at least 80 different arbovirus-induced diseases known) as well as in domestic and wild animals. They are transmitted by arthropods such as ticks and mosquitoes, and because of global ecological changes their geographic distribution can shift dramatically. The most notorious example in this respect is the recent massive **West Nile virus encephalitis** epidemic in North America, and smaller outbreaks in several European and African countries, affecting humans, horses, birds, cattle, sheep and occasionally small animals. Further important arbovirus infections are the equine encephalitides in America (**Western, Venezuelan and Eastern equine encephalitis; WEE, VEE, EEE**) infecting horses and birds, and rarely other domestic animal species such as dogs. Others include **Japanese encephalitis** in Australasia infecting domestic pigs (the main reservoir) and horses, **louping ill** in sheep and **Russian spring–summer encephalitis (tick-borne encephalitis)** in dogs, horses and occasionally other domestic animals in Europe.

Arthropod-borne infections induce a polioencephalitis always with neuronal damage, mostly mononuclear inflammation and gliosis. In infections with a peracute lethal course (frequent in West Nile virus infection and equine encephalitides), neutrophils invade areas of neuronal destruction. The distribution of the lesions varies according to the agent. For example, in tick-borne encephalitis in dogs there is a characteristic pathology of the cerebellar cortex with necrosis and loss of Purkinje cells, which are replaced by glial cells forming so-called "glial shrubbery" (Fig. 3.4A). There is mononuclear perivascular cuffing and often remarkable glial cell proliferation and neuronophagia in the brainstem. Hemorrhage may occur, and some neutrophils can be found in the glial nodules and the perivascular cuffs. Meningitis usually is present. West Nile virus mostly targets the brainstem and spinal cord, and the equine encephalitis viruses the cerebral cortex (Fig. 3.4B). A

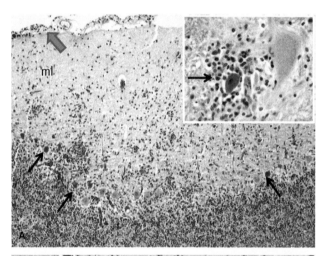

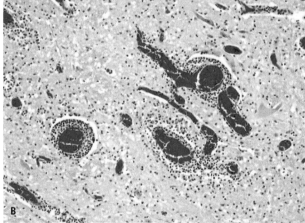

Fig. 3.4 Arbovirus infections. A: Dog. Tick-borne encephalitis. Cerebellum. Intensive microgliosis in Purkinje cell and molecular layers (ml) of the cerebellum, degenerating Purkinje cells with intense eosinophilia (several depicted by arrows), but minimal inflammatory infiltrate in meninges. HE. Inset: Neuronophagia in brainstem (arrow) next to normal neuron. HE. B: Horse. West Nile virus infection. Spinal cord. Massive perivascular mononuclear cuffing in gray matter and focal microgliosis. HE.

final diagnosis in all these infections requires immuno-histochemical and PCR identification of the agent.

Paramyxovirus infections

European sporadic bovine encephalitis with a subacute to chronic course occurs in adult cattle in central Europe and perhaps in other areas as well. A *paramyxovirus* was isolated from a few cases in the 1970s but was not further characterized. It is a disseminated non-suppurative polioencephalomyelitis of variable extent from slight to severe, with lympho-histio-plasmocytic meningitis and perivascular cuffs, gliosis as well as neuronal necrosis and neuronophagia (Fig. 3.5A). The lesions are most severe in the brainstem. In some cases marked destruction of the Purkinje cells in the cerebellar cortex, leading to cerebellar atrophy (Fig. 3.5B), or of the neurons in the hippocampus, with hippocampal sclerosis, are a predominant finding.

Post-vaccinal distemper has been reported in many areas of the world associated with vaccination with canine distemper virus (CDV) strains attenuated in canine cell lines presumably retaining some virulent potential. Thus the lesions are caused by the vaccine virus. Typically severe and lethal neural signs occur within 2 weeks following vaccination. The lesions consist of a non-suppurative polioencephalitis often with necrosis of the pontine nuclei. Large numbers of inclusion bodies are found. CDV can be readily demonstrated with IHC. Enhanced neuronotropism and polioencephalitis may also occur during natural infection with certain canine distemper virus lineages. See MRI Atlas.

A *porcine paramyxovirus* (*rubulavirus*, "blue eye diseases") causes a combination of pneumonitis and encephalitis, the latter especially in young piglets.

Henipaviruses are zoonotic agents causing respiratory and CNS disease in humans, horses (*hendra virus*) and pigs (*nipah virus*).

Borna virus infection

Horses, sheep, cats are spontaneously affected by **Borna disease** ("*staggering disease*") and it may rarely affect cattle and dogs in several European countries. In horses, sheep and cattle the disease is subacute to chronic and is characterized by a quite characteristic, very aggressive polioencephalitis inducing severe lesions in the hippocampus and cerebral cortex, with thick mononuclear cuffs, neuronal necrosis and loss as well as gliosis with fibrillary astrocytes (sclerosis). The so called *Joest–Degen* inclusion bodies may be present in the nucleus and rarely in the cytoplasm of large neurons of the hippocampus, but often remain undetected (Fig. 3.6). In cats

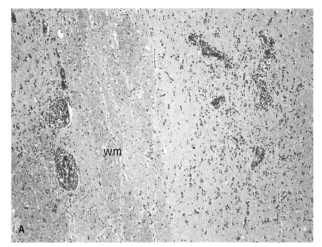

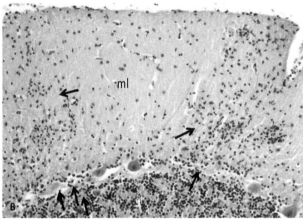

Fig. 3.5 European sporadic bovine encephalitis. Cow. A: Brainstem. Mononuclear cell perivascular cuffing and glial nodules restricted to gray matter (wm, unaffected white matter). HE. B: Cerebellum. Neuronophagia with loss of Purkinje cells in the cerebellum and marked microgliosis in molecular layer (ml, molecular layer; gl, granule cell layer). HE.

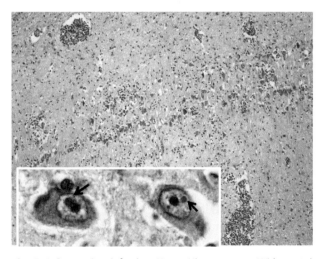

Fig. 3.6 Borna virus infection. Horse. Hippocampus. Widespread neuronal loss and microgliosis in the pyramidal cell layer with prominent perivascular cuffs of lymphocytes. HE. Inset: Two neurons each containing an intranuclear inclusion body (arrow). HE.

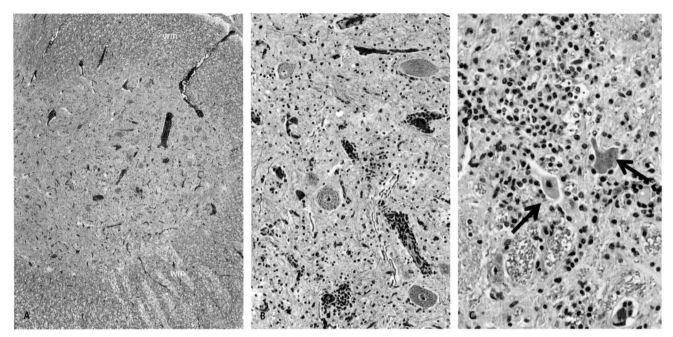

Fig. 3.7 Teschovirus infection. Pig. A: Spinal cord. Poliomyelitis, with inflammatory infiltrates restricted to the ventral horn, white matter (wm) is free of lesions. HE. B: Spinal cord. Perivascular mononuclear cuffing and microglial nodules in ventral horn. HE. C: brainstem. Microlial nodule with degenerating neurons (arrows) in brainstem. HE.

the lesions are more restricted to the brainstem. Recent studies indicate a Borna virus as the etiology of **psittacine proventricular dilatation syndrome (PPDS)**, also called **macaw wasting disease**, characterized by polyganglioneuritis, encephalitis, myocarditis and adrenalitis.

Neurotropic viral infections in pigs

This species appears to be particularly prone to viral CNS infections. In addition to the already described entities, many other viral agents cause CNS inflammation in pigs. Various porcine *teschovirus* strains (belonging to the *picornaviridae*) with varying degrees of neurovirulence are known around the world. In particular **teschen disease** is highly virulent with a high mortality rate. Lower brainstem, cerebellum and in particular ventral horns of the spinal cord are most severely affected, which is reflected by the clinical symptoms. The most striking feature is neuronal necrosis with glial nodules and neuronophagia. **Talfan disease** represents the clinically milder form of porcine poliomyelitis, which occurs sporadically but may be endemic in certain farms (Fig. 3.7).

Additional agents such as **vomiting and wasting disease** virus (also called hemagglutinating encephalomyelitis virus; coronaviridae), **swine vesicular disease** virus and **encephalomyocarditis** virus (both belonging to the picornaviridae) are known to cause nonsuppurative encephalitis mostly in piglets.

Feline polioencephalomyelitis

In cats and large felids in zoological gardens in North America and Europe a rare polioencephalomyelitis of variable severity occurs. The course of **feline polioencephalomyelitis** is rather protracted. The lesions can be mild and consist of disseminated, mononuclear perivascular cuffing and some gliosis with participation of microglial cells. In the spinal cord, there can be considerable neuronal loss and sclerosis. Despite very extensive isolation studies in large felids, the cause remains unknown, it has been speculated that this disease may represent a form of *Borna virus* infection.

3.3.2 Viral granulomatous inflammation

The prevailing pattern in these diseases is strong participation of macrophages in the inflammatory infiltrate possibly with formation of granulomas.

Lentivirus infection of small ruminants

Lentiviruses belong to the *retroviridae* and cause typically a granulomatous leukoencephalitis. The designa-

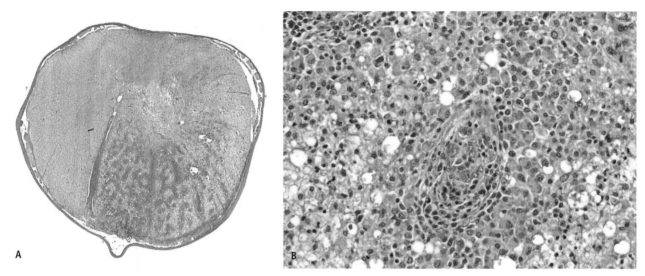

Fig. 3.8 Caprine arthritis encephalitis (CAE). Goat. Spinal cord. A: Granulomatous myelitis with numerous large perivascular cuffs, white matter necrosis and unilateral swelling of the cord (courtesy of Dr. L. Cork, Stanford University CA). HE. B: Extensive tissue necrosis with perivascular cuffing and dense granulomatous infiltrates. HE.

tion lentivirus points to the very long incubation time. **Caprine arthritis encephalitis (CAE)** virus causes severe arthritis mainly in the carpal joints and mastitis in adult goats in most industrialized countries. In goat kids up to 6 months of age, the virus can cause a severe multifocal granulomatous meningoencephalomyelitis, especially in the brainstem, spinal cord and cerebral white matter. Massive perivascular cuffs containing numerous macrophages are associated with significant destruction of the nervous tissue (Fig. 3.8A,B). In sheep and rarely in goats two manifestations of *maedi-visna virus* infection are known: **maedi,** a proliferative lymphohistiocytic pneumonitis, and **visna,** an encephalomyelitis. The disease was endemic in Iceland, but has been eradicated. In most other sheep-raising countries, except Australia and New Zealand, both *maedi* and *visna* are still observed sporadically. Both forms rarely occur together in the same animal. Maedi-visna infection in sheep also induces a granulomatous inflammation, particularly around the ventricles and in the spinal cord white matter; it can also cause primary demyelination as described in Section 3.3.4.

Equine infectious anemia virus

This *retrovirus* which occurs around the world has only a low neurotropism but occasionally can cause a severe neurological disease characterized by intense periventricular granulomatous inflammation with multinucleated giant cells and malacia of the white matter.

Feline infectious peritonitis

There are several clinical manifestations of **feline infectious peritonitis (FIP)**, a systemic disease caused by *feline coronavirus,* which is ubiquitous around the world especially where cat populations are dense. Neurological complications may accompany other extraneural signs but, often, only neurological signs are noted. The lesions in the CNS are probably to a large degree induced by virus–antibody complexes which get trapped in post-capillary venules, inducing violent inflammation following complement fixation. The dilated ventricles are sometimes filled with grayish–blue exudate, and the ependyma is thickened and glassy. Ependymal lesions in the mesencephalic aqueduct and fourth ventricle lead to obstructive hydrocephalus (Fig. 3.9A). Histologically the meninges, choroid plexus, ependyma and subependymal parenchyma are transformed into pyogranulomatous masses (Fig. 3.9) also containing many plasma cells. The subependymal lesion may extend deep into the parenchyma. The number of neutrophils varies from case to case. Vasculitis of the immune-complex type is frequently found in subependymal sites, the meninges and choroid plexus (Fig. 3.9D). Formation of connective tissue is conspicuous, sometimes with formation of fibrotic granulomas space occupying. See MRI Atlas.

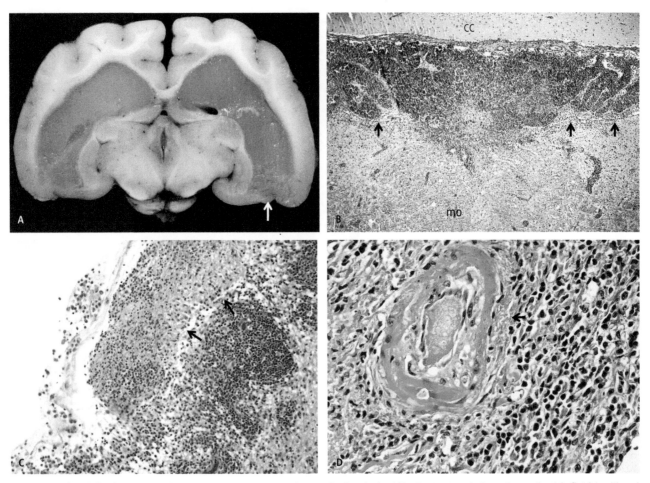

Fig. 3.9 Feline infectious peritonitis. Cat. A: Transverse section at the level of midbrain. Accumulation of protein-rich fluid in dilated ventricles, malacia of periventricular tissue particularly around temporal horn of lateral ventricle (arrow). B: Fourth ventricle. Intense granulomatous and lymphocytic chorioiditis, ependymitis and extension into the IV ventricle (arrows); destructive inflammation has replaced the medulla under the fourth ventricle (cc, cerebellar cortex; mo, medulla oblongata). HE. C: Mesencephalic aqueduct. Pyogranulomatous inflammation with destruction of the ependymal lining (arrows) with massive perivascular mononuclear cuffing. HE. D: Brainstem. Meningitis with acute fibrinoid necrosis of the vascular wall (arrow) with an intense infiltration of inflammatory cells in the subarachnoidal space. HE.

3.3.3 Viral vasculitis

In this group of viral infections, the pattern of non-suppurative inflammation is associated with significant damage to the blood vessel walls. This may lead to hemorrhage and/or ischemic changes.

Classical swine fever

Classical swine fever (hog cholera) *virus*, a *pestivirus*, is closely related to bovine virus diarrhea/mucosal disease (BVD/MD) virus and occurs in most swine-raising countries around the world. As BVD/MD in cattle, *classical swine fever virus* in swine is teratogenic (see Chapter 5) but in young and adult pigs it may also cause a disseminated vasculitis with perivascular, mostly lymphocytic infiltration of the vascular adventitia. As all the blood vessels throughout the body are the target tissue of the disease, the lesions may occur in any location of the CNS, white and gray matter. Hemorrhages and microglial nodules accompany the vascular changes. Similar lesions are found in African swine fever, an asfivirus, which is endemic in sub-Saharan Africa with occasional outbreaks in European countries.

"Fox encephalitis", hepatitis contagiosa canis

Contagious hepatitis or **Rubarth's disease** in dogs is caused by *canine adenovirus type 1*, which has a world-wide distribution. The targets are the blood vessels, and severe endothelial damage leads to hemorrhages, necrosis and edema throughout the body. The liver becomes necrotic, and a pathognomonic sign at necropsy is a thickened wall of the gall bladder due to edema. The

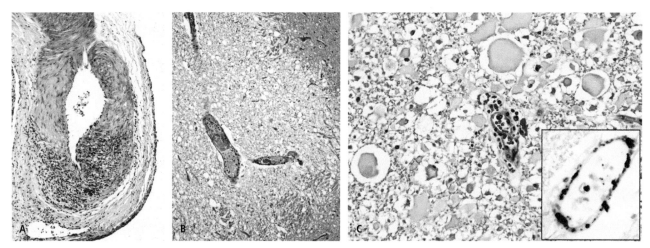

Fig. 3.10 Viral vasculitis. A: Cow with malignant catarrhal fever. Rete mirabile of the carotid artery. Mononuclear arteritis, focal invasion with inflammatory cells in the arterial wall. HE. B: Horse with equine herpes virus (EHV) infection. Brain. Sharply delineated infarct in the brain with vascular trombosis. C: Same case. Spinal cord. EHV-induced vasculitis and perivascular leukomyelomalacia with axonal necrosis, axonal spheroids and macrophage infiltrates. HE. Inset: EHV antigen in endothelial cells, IHC.

CNS vessels may be affected too, and the animals show nervous symptoms. The ensuing encephalitis is always inconspicuous. It is a mononuclear vasculitis, with rarely more than a single layer of mononuclear cells and hemorrhages. Large baso- or amphophilic homogeneous inclusion bodies are found in the swollen nuclei of endothelial cells.

Equine herpes myelitis

Equine herpes myelitis is caused by *equine herpes virus (EHV) type 1 (α-herpes virus)*, which is ubiquitous in horse populations around the world. This currently re-emerging disease is thought to occur more frequently in mares in areas which experienced abortion storms. Rapidly progressing weakness and ataxia are often accompanied by cauda equina signs. Macroscopically, one finds multifocal petechial or ecchymotic hemorrhages in white and gray matter of brain and spinal cord. The brain may contain multiple, random foci of yellowish-gray malacia. Microscopically there is primary vasculitis with endothelial cell necrosis and secondary thrombosis, edema, polymorphonuclear cell infiltration and hemorrhages. Primary vasculitis results in secondary ischemia with perivascular malacia often with axonal spheroids particularly in the spinal cord. There can be multinucleate syncytial cell formation (Fig. 3.10B,C).

Malignant catarrhal fever

Malignant catarrhal fever (MCF) is due to an infection with *ovine herpes virus 2 (OHV-2), alcelaphine herpes virus 1 (AHV-1)* or *caprine herpes virus 2 (CpHV-2)*, which occurs in cattle and cervids that have contact with sheep, goats or wild ruminants, the reservoirs for the virus. The disease is acute to subacute, with fever, nasal discharge, mucosal ulcerations and characteristic corneal opacity. CNS lesions are best seen in the arteries of the *rete mirabile*, a dense network of blood vessels surrounding the pituitary gland. It is a necrotizing and mononuclear vasculitis with a variable amount of neutrophils, the pathogenesis of which is not clear (Fig. 3.10A). The inflammatory vascular cuffs in the parenchyma of the CNS are mostly mild but are often accompanied by hemorrhage and leakage of plasma. Occasionally these typical vascular lesions are accompanied by a dissiminated polioencephalitis.

3.3.4 Viral leukoencephalitis

The lesion pattern in this group is non-suppurative inflammation with destruction of the white matter. The inflammatory component may be minimal in the initial stages of the infection or may be lacking altogether. In this case we are not really dealing with an inflammatory disease but with virus-induced myelin degeneration similar to certain hereditary diseases covered in Chapter 8.

Canine distemper virus (CDV)

The etiology of this worldwide disease of canids and other species is a *morbillivirus* belonging to the *paramyxoviridae*. Neurological signs in **nervous canine distemper** occur with or without preceding systemic disease consisting of gastrointestinal and respiratory

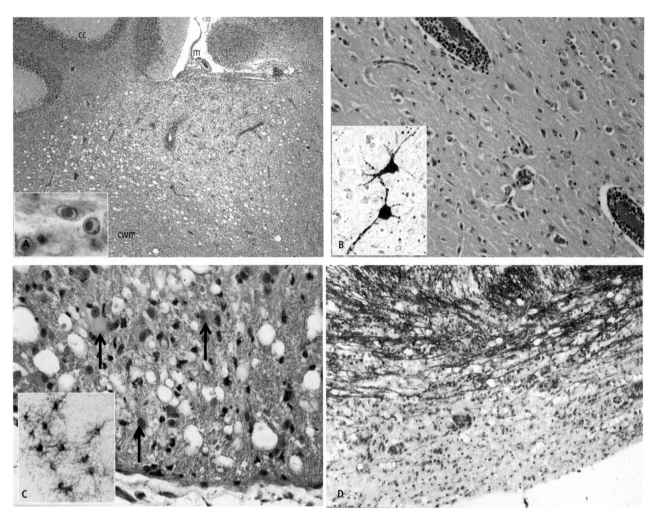

Fig. 3.11 Canine distemper virus (CDV) infection. Dog. A: Cerebellar white matter. Demyelinated plaque with intense inflammation (cc, cerebral cortex; cwm, cerebellar white matter; m, meningeal space). HE. Inset: Intranuclear viral inclusion bodies in astrocytes. HE. B: Cerebral cortex. Polioencephalitis with perivascular cuffs and mild microgliosis. Inset: Neurons containing CDV antigen. IHC. C: Medulla. Acute demyelination with spongy state of white matter and swollen gemistocytic astrocytes (arrows). HE. Inset: Microglial cells containing CDV antigen revealed by immunohistochemistry. D: Medulla. Demyelinating lesion with intact myelin stained blue. Luxol fast blue-cresyl Echt violet.

signs. There are multifocal to disseminated lesions in the gray and in the white matter. The highly characteristic and unique lesion in this disease is primary demyelination. In HE sections, primary demyelination impresses as multifocal areas of pale staining and vacuolation in the white matter (Fig. 3.11A,C), most prominently in the cerebellar folia and around the fourth ventricle, optic tracts and spinal cord, often bordering the CSF spaces. The myelin sheaths have disappeared, while the axons are still present. These foci of demyelination are best visible with special myelin stains (Fig. 3.11D) The lesions are accompanied by vascular proliferation, swelling of endothelial nuclei, gliosis and macrophages, which often contain myelin debris, and intranuclear and

intracytoplasmic eosinophilic inclusion bodies in astrocytes (Fig. 3.11A inset). In the subacute and chronic stage of the disease, perivascular cuffs (Fig. 3.11A) occur often with progression of demyelination to frank necrosis. In the gray matter of the cerebral cortex and the brainstem characteristic lesions are often located submeningeally. They consist of perivascular cuffing, vascular proliferation with swelling of endothelial nuclei, and gliosis with intracytoplasmic and intranuclear inclusion bodies in neurons (Fig. 3.11B). Neurons may show degenerative changes. In very young puppies there is polioencephalitis with secondary encephalomalacia. In a very rare variant of nervous distemper, so-called **old dog encephalitis**, there is diffuse and equally severe involvement of both gray and white matter with extensive tissue destruction and intense inflammation in the forebrain with sparing of the cerebellum and brainstem. See MRI Atlas.

Maedi-visna

In addition to the granulomatous inflammation described above (Section 3.3.2), in **maedi-visna** there are also areas of primary demyelination which look very much like those in CDV infection before intense inflammation becomes apparent. In advanced inflammatory lesions demyelination progresses to malacia.

The periventricular white matter, rostral cerebellar peduncles and thoracic cord are predilection sites. Sometimes there are only spinal cord lesions. Spinal foci often are visible macroscopically as brownish, wedge-shaped unilateral swellings.

Feline immunodeficiency virus

Reports on the neuropathology of this worldwide infection are somewhat inconsistent. Microglial cells appear to be a primary target of the infection. Early reactive changes in experimental infection are infiltration of lymphocytes in epineurium of the nerves, meninges and choroid plexus. Later there is marked perivascular cuffing, especially in the white matter, and gliosis. In advanced stages there is also pallor or vacuolation of the white matter and demyelination. These lesions can be found in the brain as well as in the spinal cord.

Feline leukemia virus associated myelopathy

As a relatively rare complication of chronic feline leukemia virus (FeLV) infection, cats may develop lesions of the spinal cord white matter, particularly the ventromedial and dorsolateral columns with demyelination but also axonal damage. These lesions are associated with infection of endothelial, glial and neuronal cells. There is no inflammation.

Dysmyelination due to intrauterine infections

Dysmyelination is a defect of myelin formation (see Chapter 8). Some forms of faulty myelinogensis are caused by *intrauterine affects* on the fetus (infections, intoxications). **Congenital tremor type A** in pigs, caused by *classical swine fever virus*, is associated with weak myelination in the white matter of the spinal cord and also mild status spongiosus. Hypomyelinogenesis may also be caused by intrauterine infection with bovine viral diarrhea virus (BVDV) in calves and *border disease virus (BDV; flaviviridae)* in lambs, which both have a worldwide distribution. The affected lambs have a generalized body tremor and abnormal "curly" fleece (hairy

shaker disease). Histologically there is hypomyelinogenesis in the white matter throughout the CNS. If an animal is kept alive long enough, the symptoms – underweight, tremors, abnormal fleece – may gradually disappear within 3–4 months. The myelin defect is related to hypothyroidism resulting from *BDV infection* in the pituitary gland. A further example is a **myelinopathy in Cretan puppies** described to be associated with leukoencephalitis due to *canine parvovirus type 2* infection.

3.3.5 Bacterial infections

The inflammatory infiltrate in bacterial infections nearly always contains varying amounts of polymorphonuclear cells. In chronic infections and infections with intracellular bacteria a non-suppurative inflammatory pattern with perivascular mononuclear cuffing and/or a granulomatous pattern is also seen. Thromboembolic encephalitis is frequently associated with vasculitis.

Tuberculosis

All species are susceptible to *Mycobacterium tuberculosis*. Both human and bovine **tuberculosis (TB)** have been markedly reduced around the world, although in some areas it is considered to be a re-emerging disease. Rarely cases are seen in zoo animals including monkeys. An infected animal shows the typical changes of TB in all organs, including the CNS. The meninges are thickened and whitish, and encapsulated pyogranulomas might be present anywhere in the CNS. A typical feature are the Langhans' giant cells, large cells with a ring of multiple, marginally located nuclei. Bacteria can be demonstrated with acid-fast stains within epithelioid macrophages and giant cells.

Streptococcal sepsis in piglets

Streptococcal chorio-meningo-ependymitis is caused by *Streptococcus suis serotype 2* and can occur in an outbreak like fashion in all swine-producing countries. As well as inducing bronchopneumonia and arthritis, the agent has an affinity for the CNS. The same bacterium can also cause a CNS infection in humans, which is currently considered to be a re-emerging zoonosis. Piglets up to 3 weeks of age, but sometimes also older animals, show severe neurological symptoms. Most animals die in the acute stage of the disease but a protracted course is also observed. At necropsy a massive ventricular dilation is observed; meninges, ependyma and choroid plexi are thickened and the ventricles are filled with suppurative exudate. Histologically there is a purulent chorio-meningo ependymitis with erosion of the ependymal lining and neuropil. This change is also present in the central canal of the cord. In the subacute stage the inflammatory infiltrate contains increasing numbers of mononuclear cells.

Bacterial meningitis and ventriculitis in large animals

This disease in juvenile animals is caused by **bacterial sepsis** with suppuration in many organ systems. Frequently isolated bacteria in calves are *E. coli*, *Salmonella* and *Pasteurella spp*, in foals *Salmonella spp* and *Actinobacillus equuli*, in small ruminants also *Staphylococcus pyogenes* and in swine *Hemophilus par-*

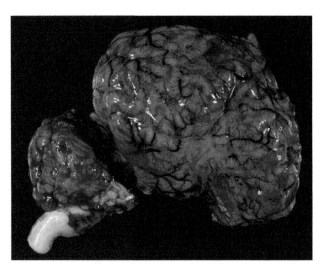

Fig. 3.12 Acute suppurative bacterial meningitis. Calf. Congestion and whitish-yellow clouding of the meninges due to accumulation of predominantly polymorphonuclear inflammatory cells.

asuis. In addition to purulent meningitis with clouding of the meninges (Fig. 3.12) there is also suppuration of the choroid plexus and ependyma with accumulation of pus in the ventricles. As a result of the ependymitis, the subependymal parenchyma is destroyed and replaced by large abscesses. A thick granulomatous and fibrous capsule around such abscesses indicates chronicity of the process.

Embolic purulent encephalitis in dogs and cats

In small animals, bacterial infections can affect the CNS in septicemic patients or when bacterial thromboemboli, arising for example from valvular endocarditis, get lodged in the cerebral circulation with spread of the bacteria in the parenchyma. Macroscopically, in **embolic bacterial encephalitis** foci of hemorrhagic malacia of different sizes are found throughout the brain, particularly in the gray matter (Fig. 3.13A). Histologically the hemorrhages are associated with necrotic vessels surrounded by sheets of neutrophils (Fig. 3.13B). There is formation of multiple small abscesses throughout the brain and sometimes severe ischemic necrosis of the parenchyma in affected areas.

Abscess

Many bacterial agents are known to cause brain abscesses, e.g. *Diplococci (Pneumococci)*, *Arcanobacterium pyogenes*, *Pasteurella* spp., *Pseudomonas aeruginosa* and *Mycoplasma* spp.) Agents may enter the CNS hematogenously and lead to a multifocal embolic purulent

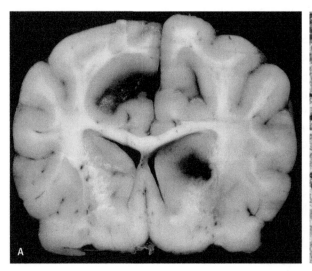
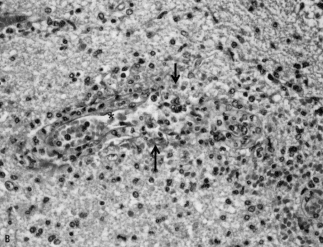

Fig. 3.13 Embolic bacterial encephalitis. Dog. A: Transverse section at level of basal nuclei. Hemorrhagic and acutely malacic lesions in cortex, caudate nucleus and internal capsule. B: Cerebral cortex. Invasion of inflammatory cells in the wall of a vein with subsequent necrosis (arrows) and perivascular hemorrhage. HE.

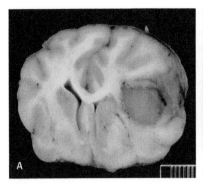
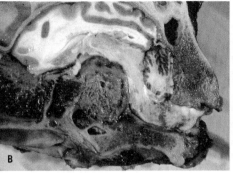
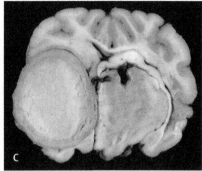

Fig. 3.14 Brain abscess. A: Dog. Transverse section at level of basal nuclei. B: Pig. Sagittal section of the head. Abscess in the sella turcica with marked dorsal compression of the thalamus. C: Deer. Cross-section at level of thalamus. Well encapsulated intradural extra-axial abscess with marked right shift (courtesy of Dr. R. Lecouteur).

meningoencephalitis, initially small foci becoming abscesses. Primary brain abscesses can arise as a consequence of trauma, or by direct extension from the sinuses. **Otogenic abscesses** occur in various species, in particular swine, sheep and rabbits, and rarely in dogs and cats. See MRI Atlas.

The infectious process starts in the middle and inner ear with vestibular symptoms. It progresses along the eighth cranial nerve and reaches the basolateral meninges of the medulla oblongata and from there spreads into the parenchyma where it forms unilateral abscesses, often of considerable size. Migrating grass seeds have also been described as a cause of **foreign body brain abscesses**. In the brain, an abscess has the same characteristics as in other organs: a purulent mass with a necrotizing center surrounded by a rim of macrophages and lymphocytes and a fibrous capsule on the outside (in chronic cases) (Fig. 3.15). Particularly in food animals (e.g. as a consequence of tail biting in swine or taildocking in sheep), **spinal abscesses** occur with compression and sometimes invasion of the spinal cord. In dogs, bacterial infection (most frequently staphylococci and streptococci, and *Brucella canis* in endemic areas) of the spine may start as an infection of the intervertebral disc, which than spreads to the adjacent bone leading to **discospondylitis**.

Empyema of the sella turcica

In food animals, the tissues in the *sella turcica*, a shallow groove of the sphenoid bone in which the pituitary gland is located, may become infected presumably because the surrounding *rete mirabile caroticum* with its many convoluted vessels easily traps bacterial emboli. The dura mater forms a strong barrier between the sella turcica and the adjacent basal meninges and brain, so

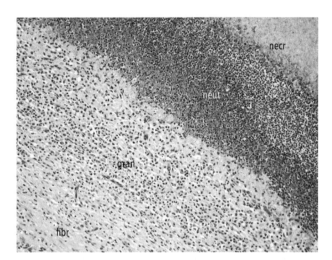

Fig. 3.15 Abscess. Dog. Cerebrum. Histological structure of an organized abscess: necrotic center (necr) surrounded by partially degenerated neutrophils (neut), a granulomatous wall (gran) formed by macrophages and an outer fibrous capsule (fibr). HE.

that the infection often remains local, encapsulated in the sella turcica without spreading further (Fig. 3.14B). In other animals, however, abscessation of the adjacent brain tissue and trigeminal nerves occurs.

Thrombotic meningoencephalitis in cattle (TME)

The agent, *Histophilus somni*, is a Gram-negative coccobacillus and a normal inhabitant of the respiratory flora, but may cause respiratory and reproductive disease around the world, particularly in North American cattle feedlots. It can also lead to acute vasculitis, which primarily affects the CNS. Initially, the animals show high temperature, rapidly falling to normal or subfebrile levels. After severe neurological signs and coma the animals die within a few to 48 hours. Macroscopically, in **thrombotic meningoencephalitis** multifocal, fairly well demarcated hemorrhages on surfaces and cut sections of brain and spinal cord are seen. The vascular lesions result from interaction of the bacterial lipooligosaccharides with platelets and endothelial cells. Histologically the hemorrhages are infiltrated with neutrophils; ensuing necrosis is due to vascular thrombosis and necrosis. Foci of Gram-negative bacteria may be seen.

Listeriosis

Listeria monocytogenes, a Gram-positive and facultatively intracellular bacterium, causes encephalitis of the brainstem (**listeric rhombencephalitis**) in ruminants (cattle, goats and sheep); it is one of the most common neurological diseases in these species around the world and an important zoonotic infection. Silage has been suspected to be the carrier of the pathogen. The infection spreads through cranial nerves from the oral cavity to the medulla oblongata and is thus often more marked on one side. Invasion of the bacteria leads to focal suppuration with microabscesses sometimes aligned along fiber tracts (Fig. 3.16A,C). Using immunohistochemistry, bacteria can be seen in axons, neurons and microabscesses (Fig. 3.16D,E). Infection and suppuration induce areas of malacia with prominently swollen axons (Fig. 3.16B). Simultaneously a strong cell-mediated immune response is mounted with a mononuclear meningitis, often most severe over the cerebellum, and large

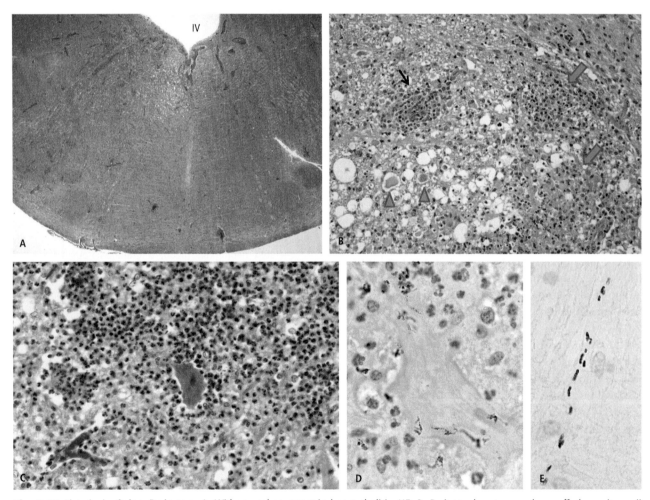

Fig. 3.16 Listeriosis. Ovine. Brainstem. A: Widespread asymmetrical encephalitis. HE. B: Perivascular mononuclear cuffs (arrow), small granulomas (large arrows) and area of malacia with vacuolation and axonal spheroids (arrow heads). HE. C: Suppurative encephalitis with microabscesses in acute lesion. HE. D: *Listeria* sp. bacteria in a neuron, immunohistochemistry. E: *Listeria* sp. bacteria inside axons in medulla oblongata, IHC.

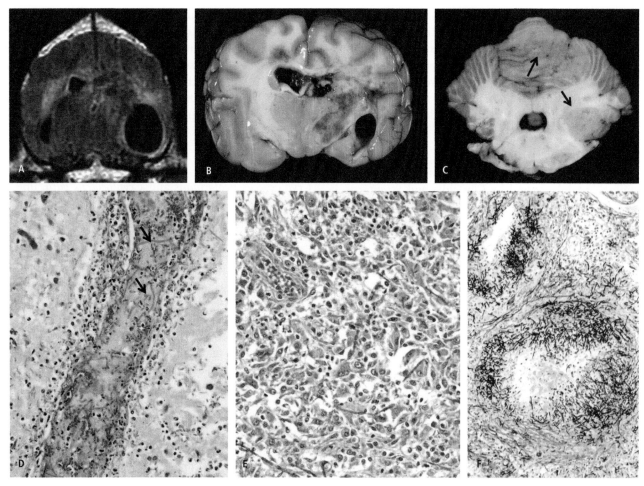

Fig. 3.17 Fungal encephalitis. A: Dog. *Chladiophora bantianum* infection. Cerebrum. Transverse MRI (FLAIR sequence) with multifocal hyperintense lesions in brain. B: Gross image of same lesion as in A, multiple severe granulomatous necrotizing lesions. C: Dog. Aspergillosis. Cerebellum. Two granulomas (arrows). D: Horse. Aspergillosis. Cortex. Fungal hyphae are present within the lumen and invade vessel wall (arrows). HE. E: Dog. *Chladiophora bantianum*. Cerebrum. Granulomatous encephalitis with numerous pigmented hyphae. HE. F: Dog. Aspergillosis. Brainstem. Predilection for invasion of vessel walls by fungal hyphae. GMS.

mononuclear perivascular cuffs (Fig. 3.16B). In the chronic stage, the neutrophils in the microabscesses are gradually replaced with macrophages and astrogliosis becomes prominent. The infection may spread from the brainstem to other rostral areas of the CNS. See MRI Atlas.

Melioidosis

Melioidosis, which occurs in tropical and sub-tropical areas, is caused by *Burkholderia pseudomallei*, a Gram-negative facultatively intracellular bacterium. It causes a multisystemic disease in humans, and all domestic animals, particularly ruminants and horses. The neuropathology is somewhat similar to listeriosis with a combination of suppuration and a cell-mediated mononuclear meningoencephalitis.

Miscellaneous bacterial infections

Ehrlichiosis, caused by *Ehrlichia canis*, occurs in many countries with warm climate around the world. It is a multisystemic infection in dogs including a non-suppurative meningoencephalitis mainly in the ventral portions of the brainstem and periventricular tissue. *Rickettsia* infections of the CNS have been reported in different species in several areas of the world. **Rocky Mountain spotted fever** in dogs in North America is caused by *Rickettsia rickettsii* and is associated with a disseminated suppurative vasculitis. **Salmon poisoning** (*Neorickettsia helminthoeca*) in dogs and foxes on the American Pacific coast is characterized by cerebellar meningitis. A chlamydia (*Chlamydophila pecorum*) is the cause of **sporadic bovine encephalitis** (also called Buss disease) in North America and some European countries, which is characterized by polyserositis and disseminated mononuclear–suppurative inflammation with vasculitis and necrotizing lesions throughout the neuraxis. **Neuroborreliosis** (*Borrelia burgdorferi*) has been associated with suppurative–granulomatous meningoradiculitis in horses. Similar lesions have been found in *Bartonella* spp infection in dogs.

Bacterial myositis

Bacterial infections of the muscle tissue occur in large animals mainly caused by Clostridia and Streptococci sp. There are varying degrees of myofiber necrosis, hemorrhages and infiltration with inflammatory cells.

3.3.6 Mycotic and algal infections

The initial neuropathological pattern is suppurative inflammation. There is frequently vasculitis and significant parenchymal destruction. Protracted lesions exhibit a marked granulomatous inflammatory pattern.

Aspergillosis, mucormycosis

The most common agents of mycotic CNS diseases are *Aspergillus*, *Mucorales* and *Candida* spp, which occur around the world. Any animal species is susceptible to mycotic infection, but cattle are the most important hosts with a variety of organs involved, including the CNS. Even aborted fetuses have been found with **mycotic encephalitis**. In horses, CNS **aspergillosis** may originate from guttural pouch mycosis. The histologic lesion is a necrotizing purulent meningoencephalitis with vascular necrosis and often thrombosis and perivascular accumulation of neutrophils (Fig. 3.17D,F). The fungal hyphae may be seen already in the HE stain in inflamma-

tory foci, vascular lumina and necrotic walls as well as the intravascular thrombi (Fig. 3.17D). If the lesions strongly suggest of a mycotic infection but no fungal hyphae are found a special silver stain like GMS (Fig. 3.17F) or PAS may be useful. In chronic lesions a granulomatous reaction prevails with formation of granulomas (Fig. 3.17C,E) often containing multinucleated giant cells. See MRI Atlas.

Cryptococcosis

Cryptococcus neoformans and *Cryptococcus gatii*, ubiquitous yeasts, mostly affect dogs and cats and occasionally horses, generally in areas with a hot humid climate. Clinically the symptoms of **cryptococcosis** indicate involvement of various organ systems. CNS symptoms are due to a marked suppurative meningitis and submeningeal encephalitis, sometimes with ependymitis and plexus chorioiditis and involvement of the subependymal parenchyma. Occasionally, tumor-like granulomas are formed (Fig. 3.18A). In the necrotic suppurative masses and cavities formed by vastly expanded Virchow-Robin spaces, called *pseudocysts*, cryptococcal organisms are found in large quantities (Fig. 3.18B,C). The organism is round and has a clear halo. This halo is the polysaccharide capsule, which can be specifically stained with mucicarmine (Fig. 3.18B).

Encephalitozoonosis

Encephalitozoonosis is mostly found in rabbits, but other species (dog, wild carnivores) around the world can be affected. The current name of the agent is *Encephalitozoon cuniculi*, but in the older literature the term of *Nosema* and *nosematosis* may also be encountered. The organism is now considered to be

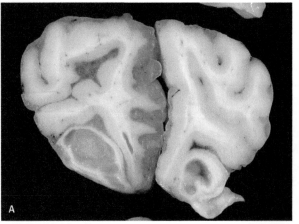
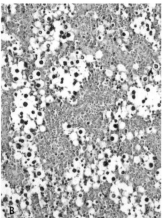
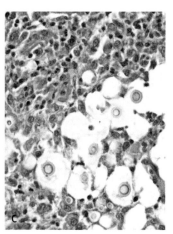

Fig. 3.18 Cryptococcosis. Dog. Frontal lobe. A: Transverse section of frontal lobes. Massive accumulation of gelatinous material in the meninges with a large, left-sided space-occupying mass within the olfactory peduncle. B: Histologically there are numerous *Cryptococcus neoformans* organisms embedded in a chronic granulomatous inflammatory response. Mucicarmine stain. C: High magnification showing granulomatous inflammation and characteristic yeasts with an outer clear capsule. HE.

fungal (belonging to the microsporidia). Granulomas of various sizes throughout the brain are the main constituent of the CNS lesions. Nodules consisting of epithelioid histiocytes, so-called "hepatoid" foci because they look like liver tissue, are characteristic. The organisms are very difficult to find, because they do not stain with HE. "Empty" spaces may be seen in the inflammatory foci or the adjacent tissue at low magnification; at higher magnification these contain loosely arranged oblong parasites, which stain positively with Ziehl-Nielson and Gramstain.

Other mycotic infections

These include **blastomycosis, coccidiodomycosis** and **histoplasmosis** as common infections in endemic areas. Further reported entities include **cladosporiodiosis, fusariosis** and sporadic cases of infection with, for example, *Ochroconis* and *Cladophialophora* sp. Such systemic infections with multiple organ involvement occur mostly in small animals in endemic areas; in the CNS they all cause pyogranulomatous lesions in which the agents can be detected.

Algal infections

Prototheca spp. are algal agents, which cause systemic infection with colitis, ocular and CNS involvement, mainly in dogs in tropical and subtropical areas around the world. There are disseminated necrotic–inflammatory lesions in the brain and spinal cord containing prothecal cells, which are easily recognized on HE-, PAS- and GMS-stained sections.

3.3.7 Protozoal infections

These infections often elicit a non-suppurative inflammation pattern very much like viral infections. They can also induce a suppurative pattern associated with severe tissue necrosis. The inflammatory infiltrate sometimes contains significant numbers of eosinophils.

Toxoplasmosis, neosporosis

Toxoplasma gondii replicates in the gut of cats but rarely causes disease in this species. *Toxoplasma gondii* and *Neospora caninum* cause identical CNS lesions in dogs. **Toxoplasmosis** and **neosporosis** occur worldwide and can be distinguished from each other by serological testing, immunohistochemistry and most reliably by polymerase chain reaction (PCR). The typical presentation is one of rapidly progressive myositis, with weakness progressing to paralysis in young puppies. Histological examination reveals destructive myositis (Fig. 3.19C) and multifocal lesions throughout the CNS and peripheral nerves. These CNS lesions consist of perivascular mononuclear cuffing, gliosis and often marked capillary proliferation (Fig. 3.19D). The lesions are similar to those of viral encephalitides. Characteristic parasitic cysts composed of tightly packed bradyzoites surrounded by a conspicuous wall (Fig. 3.19D inset) or the presence of tachyzoites within a parasitophorous vacuole confirm the histological diagnosis. In older animals, pure CNS involvement may occur with highly destructive lesions. In histological sections of the latter cases, a granulomatous and necrotizing encephalitis is present usually without special anatomical predilection. However, in a peculiar form of canine protozoal encephalitis the cerebellar cortex is specifically affected with macroscopically visible cerebellar atrophy (Fig. 3.19A). Foci of necrosis are accompanied by thick mononuclear perivascular cuffs, marked gliosis mixed with inflammatory mononuclear cells, neutrophils and eosinophils (Fig. 3.19E). There is also vascular proliferation and connective tissue formation. In cats, encephalomyelitis caused by *Toxoplasma gondii* (and related organisms) is very rare. A peculiar **segmental protozoal myelitis** has been reported in this species. See MRI Atlas.

Sarcosporidia, sarcocystis

Very often reactionless protozoal cysts, intensely basophilic, are found particularly in the cerebral cortex of ruminants. They apparently do not cause clinical disease in most animals. **Equine protozoal encephalomyelitis** caused by *Sarcocystis neurona* and, much less commonly, *Sarcocystis hughesi* occurs in North America. The lesions are more marked in the spinal cord (Fig. 3.19B) than the brain and are characterized by necrotizing inflammation in both gray and white matter with mononuclear perivascular cuffs and infiltration of the parenchyma with neutrophils, eosinophils and occasional giant cells. The sarcocystis organisms can be demonstrated in neurons, mononuclear cells and vascular endothelial cells. This CNS infection may also occur in the dog. In sheep, **protozoal encephalomyelitis** is caused by *Sarcocystis tenella*.

Amoebic infections

Amoebiasis been described in several animal species and occurs worldwide albeit rarely. Identified causes include *Acanthomoeba* in sheep and dogs, *Naegleria* species in cattle and horses and *Balamuthia sp* in dogs and primates. CNS infection in humans is known as primary amebic meningoencephalitis. The lesions consist of a focal and severe necrotizing pyogranulomatous meningitis and encephalitis (Fig. 3.20A). Amebae, which resemble large macrophages and stain with PAS, can be found in the lesions (Fig. 3.20B). A

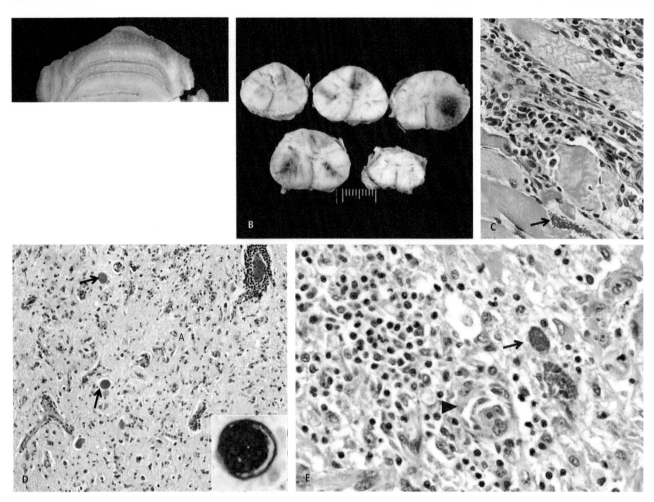

Fig. 3.19 Protozoal infections. A. Dog. Transverse section of cerebellum and brainstem. Severe necrosis of the cerebellar cortex due to *Neospora canis* encephalitis. B: Horse. Equine protozoal myelitis. Spinal cord. Multifocal granulomatous myelitis with hemorrhages due to *Sarcocystis neurona*. C: Dog. Skeletal muscle. Necrotizing non-suppurative myositis with *Neospora canis* organisms (arrow). HE. D: Dog. Cerebral cortex. *Neospora*-induced non-suppurative encephalitis with perivascular mononuclear cell cuffing, diffuse microgliosis, numerous protozoal cysts (arrows). HE. Inset: Protozoal cyst IHC for *Neospora canis*. E: Dog. Brainstem. Acute necrotizing encephalitis due to Neospora with inflammatory cell infiltrates including macrophages, lymphocytes, eosinophils, gemistocytic astrocytes, protozoal organisms (arrow) and endothelial cell proliferation (arrowhead). HE.

specific diagnosis requires immunocytochemistry (Fig. 3.20C).

Miscellaneous protozoal infections

Trypanosomiasis associated with *Trypanosoma evansi* infection was reported to cause a severe multifocal hemorrhagic necrotizing encephalitis, particularly of the cerebral white matter, in Brazilian horses. **Leishmaniosis** in dogs occurs mostly in southern countries worldwide and has been found to cause epidural granulomas in the spine and granulomatous meningitis. Agents like *Babesia* and *Theileria* are considered to be potentially associated

with CNS inflammation but the neuropathology of such infections has not been well defined.

3.3.8 Helminth infections

The inflammatory pattern is suppurative with variable numbers of eosinophils. Chronic lesions may develop a granulomatous component.

Nematodes

Migration of enteric nematode larvae into the CNS often occurs in aberrant hosts. *Ascaris* sp. invasion in the CNS is rare in small animals but can result in small, often clinically irrelevant, granulomas. Better known

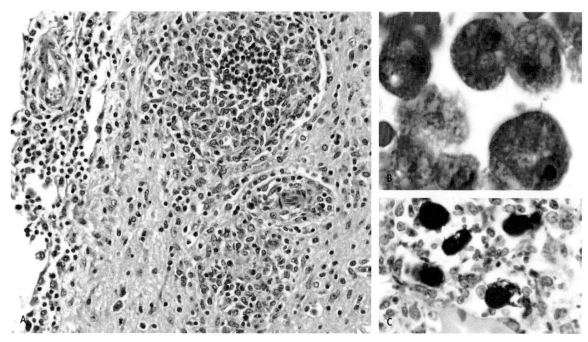

Fig. 3.20 Amebiasis, *Neagleari fowleri*. Bovine. A: Cerebral cortex. Pyogranulomatous meningoencephalitis. HE. B: Histologically the ameba resemble macrophages with foamy cytoplasm and a large eccentric nucleus. HE. C: Positive immunoreactivity of *Naegleria fowleri* in lesions. (Courtesy of Dr H. Kinde, CAHFS, San Bernadino, CA).

are **verminous encephalitis** caused by *Strongylus* sp, in the brain of horses (see MRI Atlas), *Elaphostrongylus* (in Europe) and *Parelaphostrongylus* (in North America), especially in the spinal cord of wild and domestic small ruminants. *Baylisascaris procyonis* infection has been described in North American dogs exposed to raccoons. *Angiostrongylus vasorum* and *Angiostrongylus cantonensis* have also been reported to induce neurological complications in dogs and foals respectively. *Halicephalobus gingivalis* (synonym *Halicephalobus deletrix, Micronema deletrix*) can induce a granulomatous encephalomyelitis in horses.

Migrating parasites induce areas of malacia mostly in the white matter with prominently swollen axons and various degrees of hemorrhage (Fig. 3.21B,C). These malacic/hemorrhagic lesions are round or elongated depending on whether they are cross- or longitudinally sectioned (Fig. 3.21C). The migration tracks induce reactive changes including vascular proliferation, invasion of macrophages and perivascular cuffing, containing varying amounts of eosinophils. Sometimes, histological slides contain sections of the parasite but they often do not (Fig. 3.21D). It is thought that the parasites may leave the brain after death, even when immersed in fixative. Indeed parasites may be detected in the fixative following centrifugation. Similar lesions but with more hemorrhage, especially affecting the

spinal cord, are described in small ruminants and in horses (**Kumri**) in Asia, caused by the microfilaria of *Setaria* sp. Microfilaria occasionally are found in the blood vessels of different species including birds without obvious parenchymal lesions. In subtropical and tropical areas, *Spirocerca lupi* has been found to invade the spinal cord of dogs with formation of granulomas.

Coenurosis, echinococcosis, cysticercosis

Coenurus, Echinococcus and *Cysticercus* are the larvae of tapeworms of the family the Taeniidae; e.g. those of *Multiceps multiceps* (*Coenurus cerebralis*), *Echinococcus granulosus, Echinococcus multilocularis* and *Taenia solium* (*Cysticercus cellulosae*). They also migrate and reach various organs, in particular liver and CNS. In the target organ, they form single or multiple cysts of different size, sometimes very large, which clinically act as a space-occupying process. **Echinococcosis** is a problem in human medicine and affects also dogs and non-human primates. Most important in veterinary medicine is **coenurosis** in sheep caused by *Coenurus cerebralis*. A characteristic symptom is walking in circles, hence the name "circling disease". Coenurosis has practically disappeared in developed countries as a result of better surveillance and treatment. At necropsy the cysts can be seen bulging from the brain surface,

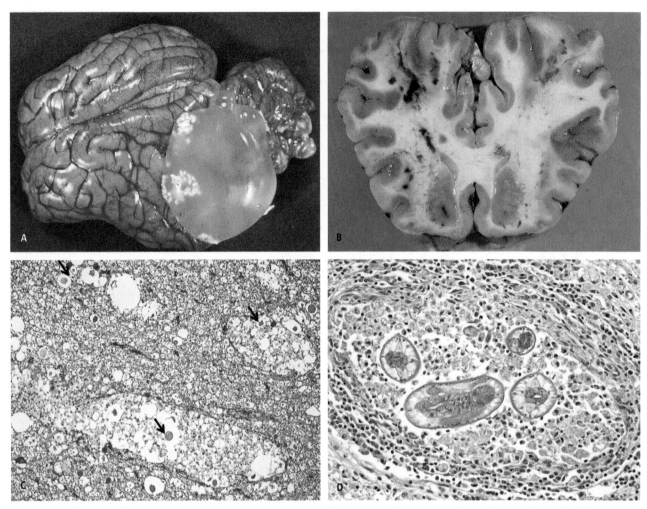

Fig. 3.21 Helminth infections. A: Sheep. *Coenurus* cyst in occipital lobe. Note clusters of white scolices in the wall of the cyst. B: Horse. Transverse section of frontal lobes. Verminous encephalitis caused by migrating aberrant strongyle larvae. Multiple hemorrhagic foci in the white matter. C: Goat. Spinal cord. *Elaphostrongylus* migration tracks in white matter with multiple areas of leukomyelomalacia containing swollen axons (arrows) and gitter cells. HE. D: Dog. Cerebellum. Several cross-sections of *Baylisascaris procyonis* larvae surrounded by an intense inflammatory reaction. HE.

filled with a clear fluid and with white granules fixed to the cyst walls (Fig. 3.21A). These granules are scolices of immature growing tapeworms, which are infectious. Compression, abscessation, granulomatous inflammation and hemorrhage may surround the cysts.

Cerebrospinal cuterebriasis

In cats in North America, the larvae of the *Cuterebra* fly may invade the CNS probably through the nasal cavity. Additionally to parasitic migration tracks similar to those in other helminth infections, there is extensive brain infarction, multifocal superficial cerebrocortical necrosis and widespread subependymal rarefaction. The cerebral lesions are also known as **feline ischemic encephalopathy**. The pathogenesis is not clear: putative larval toxins in the CSF inducing vasospasms and direct tissue damage have been proposed.

3.4 Non-infectious and immune-mediated inflammatory lesions

3.4.1 Definition

As with other organ systems, the nervous system can be targeted by the immune system leading to severe neurological disease. The prototype of immune-mediated CNS disease is **experimental allergic encephalitis (EAE)**, a multifocal demyelinating disease which can be induced by parenteral injections of CNS white matter resulting in an immune response against myelin antigens. EAE in small rodents is probably the most intensely studied animal model of T cell mediated autoimmune disease and has fostered an enormous body of knowledge on neuroimmunology. **Allergic encephalitis** also used to occur as a complication of rabies vaccination in people and animals but has largely disappeared since current rabies vaccines no longer contain brain tissue. One of the most important neurological diseases in humans resembling EAE is **multiple sclerosis (MS)**. MS is characterized by multifocal inflammatory demyelinating lesions, which are thought to result from autoimmunity against myelin. Interestingly, epidemiological studies have shown that an environmental factor (infection?) precipitates the disease. A spontaneous MS-like disease occurs in certain viral infections (e.g. **canine distemper**) in domestic animals.

The diseases reviewed in this section represent a rather heterogeneous group of lesions affecting either the meninges, the blood vessels, the brain/cord tissue or the peripheral nerves and muscles. Common to all these diseases is infiltration of inflammatory cells often associated with damage to the target tissue. They are assumed to be immune-mediated because all attempts to convincingly demonstrate infectious agents in such lesions or to isolate infectious agents from affected tissues have so far failed. Furthermore, many of these conditions are responsive to treatment with corticosteroids or other immunosuppressants. However, the underlying immunological mechanisms are only partially understood in a few of them. Cases are mostly sporadic and there may be a higher incidence in certain breeds or families. Most intriguing in this respect is the challenging and emerging group of canine non-infectious inflammatory encephalitides: granulomatous meningoencephalomyelitis (GME), necrotizing meningoencephalitis (NME) and necrotizing encephalitis (NE). The latter two conditions were initially called "breed-specific" (in Pugs and Yorkshire Terriers respectively).

3.4.2 Neurological diseases assumed to be immune-mediated

The most frequent pattern observed in this group of diseases is non-suppurative inflammation, often associated with variable degrees of granulomatous inflammation. In some diseases we find a suppurative or rarely an eosinophilic inflammation pattern.

Steroid-responsive meningitis arteritis

Steroid-responsive meningitis arteritis (SRMA) is a sporadic but not uncommon disease in dogs, which occurs more frequently in certain breeds (e.g. Boxer, Bernese Mountain Dog, Labrador Retriever) and may sometimes exhibit a familial pattern, e.g. in Boxers and Nova Scotia Duck Tolling Retrievers. In the latter genetic factors have been identified that seem to correlate with the disease. SRMA was first noticed in laboratory dog colonies (**Beagle pain syndrome**). The underlying mechanism is excessive IgA production probably as a result of immune dysregulation with a skewed Th2 response. Mostly young adult dogs are affected with acute relapsing fever, neutrophilia, neck pain and reluctance to move. In chronic cases, additional neurological signs with paresis and ataxia may be detected. The disease is glucocorticosteroid responsive but relapses can occur despite treatment.

Histologically there is suppurative inflammation of the meninges especially of the spinal cord. In subacute cases mononuclear infiltrates dominate and meningeal fibrosis becomes apparent. There is necrotizing arteritis (immune complex type) of the spinal arteries (Fig. 3.22A);

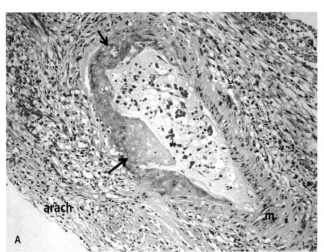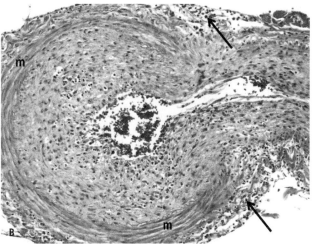

Fig. 3.22 Steroid-responsive meningitis arteritis (SRMA). A: Dog. Acute SRMA. Large spinal meningeal artery (partially thrombosed lumen); muscular layer (media, m) with focal acute fibrinoid necrosis (arrows), with intense inflammation in surrounding meninges (arach). HE. B: Dog. Chronic SRMA. Chronic stenosing arterial lesion. The original structure of the media (m) with concentrically arranged smooth muscle cells is intact. Between the media and the endothelium there is a massive layer of cell infiltration with sub-intimal fibrosis and stenosis of the vascular lumen. There is some non-suppurative inflammatory cell infiltrate in the meninges and perivascularly (arrows). HE.

sometimes there are meningeal hemorrhages or even hematomyelia. Chronic arterial changes are characterized by sub-intimal proliferation of spindle cells and stenosis (Fig. 3.22B). Sometimes there is extension of the inflammation to the cerebral meninges, choroid plexus and periventricular tissues.

Eosinophilic meningoencephalitis

Eosinophilic meningoencephalitis (EME) has been described in young male dogs, particularly Golden Retrievers and Rottweilers and rarely in cats; there are acute progressive neurological signs and CSF pleocytosis with many eosinophils. Pathologically there is an intensive meningitis and periventriculitis with eosinophils in part infiltrating in the underlying parenchyma. In one report, eosinophilic granulomas were described in Tervueren Shepherd Dogs. The cause is not known but an allergic mechanism is suspected. See MRI Atlas.

Canine granulomatous meningoencephalitis

Granulomatous meningoencephalitis (GME) is the current term for a disease probably first described in 1936 and still attracting a confusing and lengthy number of synonyms (e.g. *inflammatory reticulosis, lymphoreticulosis, neoplastic reticulosis*) reflecting changes only in immunological terminology. **Reticulosis** is a term that was introduced in human neuropathology by 1950, and then was essentially discarded by 1980 with the reclassification of reticulosis as a primary CNS B cell lymphoma. Surprisingly, use of the term reticulosis has persisted in dogs despite a lack of any similarities to the human lesion. GME has worldwide distribution, has no defined breed or gender specificity, and is characterized by a unique angiocentric granulomatous encephalitis consisting of a perivascular accumulation of macrophages often admixed with lymphocytes and plasma cells (Fig. 3.23). Focal excentric nodular accumulation/proliferation of histiocytic cells within the perivascular cuffs is characteristic in early lesions (Fig. 3.24). The perivascular cuffs may leave the Virchow-Robin space, invade the parenchyma and coalesce with neighboring cuffs eventually with destruction of the tissue. Currently, three major patterns of histologic lesion distribution in brain and spinal cord have been described: (1) the common disseminated form, in which the most intense lesions occur in the cranial cervical spinal cord, brainstem and midbrain, often with less severe extension rostrally into hemispheric white matter; (2) a disseminated form with angiocentric expansion forming multiple coalescing mass lesions of similar distribution; and (3) a focal form in which single discrete mass lesions occur in either the spinal cord, brainstem, midbrain, thalamus, optic nerves or cerebral hemispheres, without dissemination. It remains contentious whether the last is a neoplastic rather than an immunoproliferative process. Preliminary immunophenotyping studies on each of these disease patterns suggest that both disseminated forms exhibit similar phenotypic profiles. However, the focal form appears to be a neoplastic histiocytic

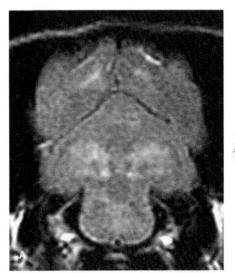
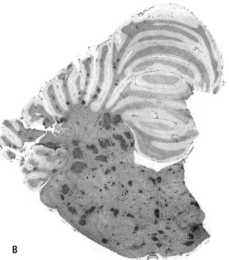

Fig. 3.23 Granulomatous meningoencephalitis (GME). Dog. A: Transverse MRI FLAIR sequence of cerebellum with multifocal hyperintense lesions. B: Same dog. Cross-section of cerebellum and medulla. Disseminated angiocentric granulomatous lesions revealed by immunohistochemistry for CD 18.

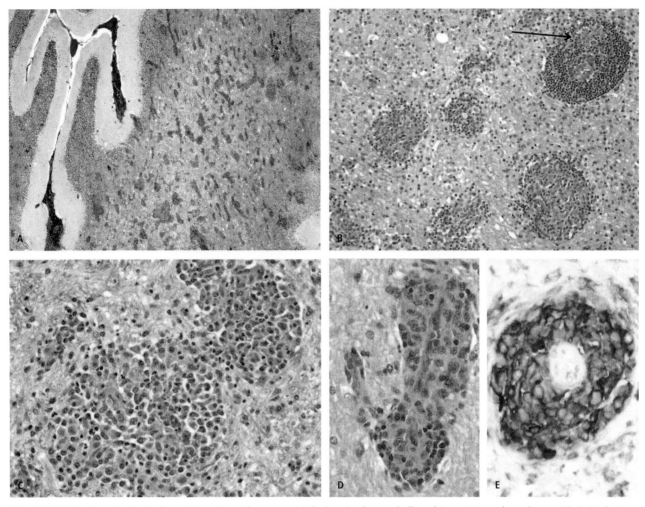

Fig. 3.24 GME. Dog. A: Cerebellum. Disseminated angiocentric lesions in the cerebellar white matter and meninges. HE. B: Brainstem. Perivascular cuffing around one vessel (arrow) of mostly lymphocytes but also an eccentric focus of macrophages. HE. C: Brainstem. Coalesence of expanding angiocentric cuffing by macrophages. HE. D: Brainstem. Eccentric perivascular cuffing with macrophages (histiocytes) in both longitudinal section and cross-section of affected vessels. HE. E: These macrophages are strongly immunoreactive with CD18. IHC.

dendritic cell phenotype. The pathogenesis of GME remains obscure though an autoimmune encephalitis induced by anti-GFAP antibodies in CSF, or a T cell mediated delayed hypersensitivity mechanism have been suggested. PCR-based screening for viral DNA (e.g., herpes, adeno- or parvoviruses) has been negative. See MRI Atlas.

Canine necrotizing meningoencephalitis

Necrotizing meningoencephalitis (NME) is a worldwide disease originally recognized in dogs in the US in the 1970s as a Pug dog, breed-specific disease, colloquially known as *"pug dog encephalitis"*. Since 1989, based on morphologically defined lesion patterns and histology, NME has been recognized in other small-breed dogs including Maltese, Chihuahua, Pekingese, Boston Terrier, Shih Tzu, Coton du Tulear and Papillon breeds. The pathogenesis and etiology remain obscure.

NME has both a characteristic anatomic distribution pattern and unique histological lesions not previously seen in other canine encephalitides of known etiology. Clinically the disease occurs in either gender but intriguingly so far only in small-breed dogs. Gross lesions occur as asymmetrical, multifocal bilateral areas of either acute encephalitis or chronic foci of malacia, necrosis and collapse of hemispheric gray and white matter decreasing in intensity rostrocaudally (Fig. 3.25). See MRI Atlas. Histologically there is a unique combination of focal meningitis and polio- and

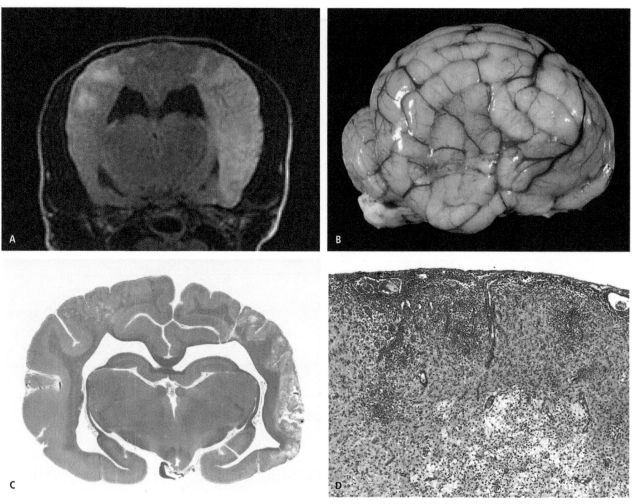

Fig. 3.25 Canine necrotizing meningoencephalitis (NME). Pug dog. A: Cerebrum.Transverse MRI FLAIR sequence showing massive acute hyperintensive bilateral lesions in cerebral cortex and subcortical white matter. B: Lateral view of the brain. Gross lesion in temporal lobe with multifocal areas of discoloration and underlying cortical necrosis. C: Histological section of the same dog at the same level as in B. Extensive destruction of cortex on right side and subcortical white matter on left side. D: Frontal lobe. Severe lymphocytic meningitis and polioencephalitis with necrotizing leukoencephalitis in underlying white matter. HE.

leukoencephalitis of adjacent white matter. The lesions are intensely inflammatory with meningitis and parenchymal histiocytic, microglial infiltrates accompanied by perivascular cuffing of lymphocytes and plasma cells (Fig. 3.25D). An acute non-suppurative encephalitis in the hippocampus, septal nuclei, and thalamus can coexist with chronic lesions. Usually, few inflammatory lesions are present in cerebellum, brainstem and spinal cord.

Canine necrotizing encephalitis

Necrotizing encephalitis (NE) was first described in 1993 in Yorkshire Terriers, and has been reported recently in the French Bulldog and Pomeranian. The pattern and histological type of the lesions are strikingly different from those of NME. Grossly the large focal asymmetric bilateral malacic necrotizing lesions are confined to hemispheric white matter (Fig. 3.26A,B) and the brainstem. See MRI Atlas. There is an intense histiocytic, microglial and macrophage cellular infiltrate with loss of white matter and thick perivascular lymphocytic cuffing (Fig. 3.26C). Other areas have acute exudation, severe edema, necrosis and eventual cyst formation, with a dramatic gemistocytic astrogliosis, histiocytes and gitter cells intermixed with thick perivascular lymphocytic cuffing (Fig. 3.26E, Fig. 3.27). Characteristically the overlying cortex and meninges are not involved. Multifocal intense inflammatory cell infiltrates of macrophages with dramatically thick perivascular lymphocytic cuffing are seen in the midbrain, brainstem and cerebellum. Thus, the classical lesions in NME and NE are distinctly different based on both dis-

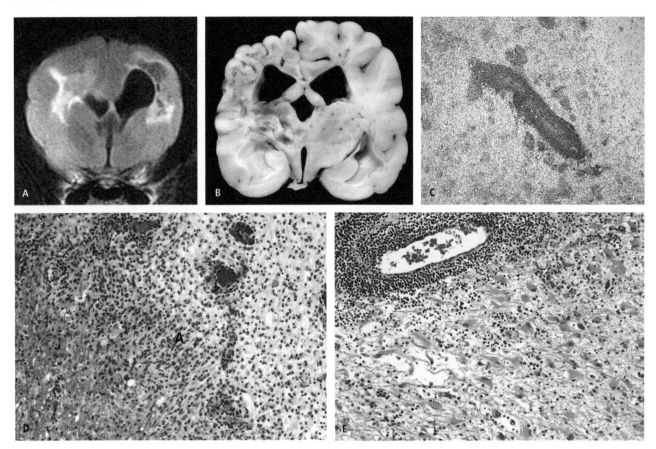

Fig. 3.26 Canine necrotizing encephalitis (NE). Dog. Yorkshire Terrier. A: Transverse MRI FLAIR image at level of basal ganglia. Hyperintense lesions in cerebral white matter. Destructive grey matter lesions on the right side. B: Similar case. Chronic lesion with cystic malacia and associated cerebral atrophy. C: Cerebrum. Destructive lesion with intense diffuse infiltration with inflammatory cells and several very prominent perivascular cuffs comprised mainly of lymphocytes. HE. D: NE. Dog. Yorkshire Terrier. Subcortical white matter. Severe diffuse infiltration with inflammatory cells in parenchyma at the edge of a malacic lesion. HE. E: "Burnt out" cystic lesion with distinctive proliferation of gemistocytic astrocytes and thick lymphocytic perivascular cuffing. HE.

tribution pattern and microscopic appearance. As with NME, limited immunophenotyping that has been restricted to paraffin-embedded specimens is consistent, but not diagnostically useful. Similarly to NME, neurological signs, results of CSF analysis and neuroimaging findings vary with intensity and location of lesions.

Whether these diseases (NME, NE) represent a much wider emergent spectrum of a single disease, or constitute a separate and unique disease manifestation, adds to the diagnostic dilemma presented by these encephalitides, and underlines an urgent need for a comprehensive review of existing information in order to establish working guidelines for classification and investigation of these entities.

Meningoencephalitis in Greyhounds

This appears to be a disease entity restricted to young Greyhounds in Ireland. Frequently, several pups within a litter are affected. There is a diffuse mononuclear encephalitis with severe gliosis predominantly in the cerebral cortex, caudate nucleus and periventricular gray matter of the brainstem but no evidence of neuronal targeting as in neurotropic viral infections. All efforts to detect infectious agents have been unsuccessful.

Acute polyneuritis

Acute polyneuritis or **polyradiculoneuritis** is considered to be an autoimmune disease of the PNS in dogs and cats, very rarely in other animal species. The cause in mostly not known. In North America hunting dogs bitten by raccoons may develop polyneuritis, in this case called **coon hound paralysis**. Presumably, antigens in raccoon saliva elicit an immune response which cross-reacts with PNS components. A similar disease in humans is also called **Guillain-Barré syndrome**. Clinically there is ascending paresis–paralysis of the limbs developing in a few days and areflexia with normal nociception. Recovery occurs within several weeks but relapses are possible. In the motor nerves, especially the proximal portions (spinal nerve roots), there are perivascular and interstitial lymphocytic infiltrations (Fig. 3.27), demyelination and axonal necrosis. In rare cases there may be prominent involvement of the cauda equina or cranial nerves.

Chronic hypertrophic polyneuritis

Chronic hypertrophic neuritis is a very rare condition in dogs with marked concentric proliferation of Schwann cells ("*onion bulbs*") associated with chronic mononuclear inflammation in cranial and spinal nerve roots occasionally leading to space-occupying lesions.

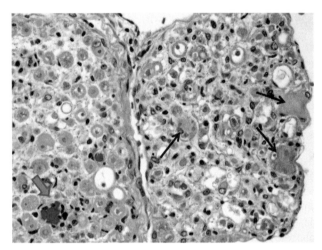

Fig. 3.27 Acute polyradiculoneuritis. Dog. Spinal nerve root. Diffuse lymphocytic infiltration (large arrow), several degenerating axons (arrows) within the fascicle. HE.

Sensory polyganglioneuritis

Sensory polyganglioneuritis is a rare disease in dogs of unknown etiology with severe mononuclear inflammation and axonal degeneration in the dorsal spinal root ganglia, trigeminal ganglia and associated nerves. There is also marked Wallerian degeneration of the dorsal columns.

Polyneuritis equi

Also called **cauda equina neuritis**, this is a rare sporadic disease in horses, of possibly autoimmune, perhaps post-infectious (e.g. herpes, adenovirus) origin. Mostly adult females are affected. The disease is chronic and progressive, with tail and sphincter paralysis and paresthesia/analgesia in the perineum. There is marked swelling of the cauda equina nerves with destructive inflammation of the nerves. The inflammation is often granulomatous with occasional multinucleated giant cells and massive fibrosis (Fig. 3.28). Occasionally there is involvement of the cranial nerves.

Autoimmune myositis

Autoimmune inflammation with destruction of muscle fibers has been described mostly in dogs and rarely in cats. Three distinct syndromes are recognized in skeletal muscles. In **polymyositis** all muscles of the body are affected with infiltration of T cells in the muscle tissue and variable degrees of tissue destruction. In **masticatory myositis** and **extraocular muscle myositis** only highly specific muscle groups are targeted by a severe destructive inflammatory process. Interestingly, specific autoantibodies against certain muscle components have been demonstrated and since specific breeds are more affected than others genetic factors appear to be

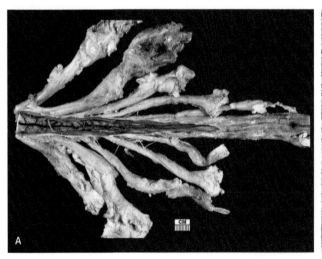

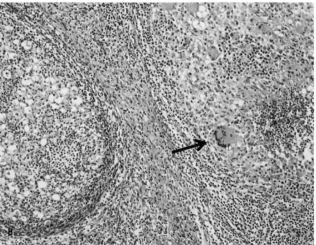

Fig. 3.28 Cauda equine neuritis. Horse. A: Massive enlargement of lumbosacral spinal nerves outside of the dura mater. B: Histologically there is a multifocal fibrosing, granulomatous and necrotizing polyneuritis sometimes with multinucleated giant cells (arrow). HE.

involved. This seems to be particularly true in Hungarian Vizlas.

Further reading

General

Greene C. Infectious Diseases of the Dog and Cat, 4th ed. St Louis, MO: Elsevier, 2012.

Wilson EH, Weninger W, Hunter CA. Trafficking of immune cells in the central nervous system. J Clin Invest 2010;120:1368–1379.

Neurotropic viral infections

Bukovsky C, Schmoll F, Revilla-Fernández S, Weissenböck H. Studies on the aetiology of non-suppurative encephalitis in pigs. Vet Rec 2007;161:552–558.

Cantile C, Del Piero F, Di Guardo G, Arispici M. Pathologic and immunohistochemical findings in naturally occuring West Nile virus infection in horses. Vet Pathol 2001;38:414–421.

Del Médico Zajac MP, Ladelfa MF, Kotsias F, Muylkens B, Thiry J, Thiry E, Romera SA. Biology of bovine herpesvirus 5. Vet J 2010;184:138–145.

Gosztonyi G. Natural and experimental Borna disease virus infections – neuropathology and pathogenetic considerations. APMIS Suppl 2008;124:53–57.

Kamata H, Inai K, Maeda K, Nishimura T, Arita S, Tsuda T, Sato M. Encephalomyelitis of cattle caused by Akabane virus in southern Japan in 2006. J Comp Pathol 2009;140:187–193.

Martella V, Blixenkrone-Møller M, Elia G, Lucente MS, Cirone F, Decaro N, Nielsen L, Bányai K, Carmichael LE, Buonavoglia C. Lights and shades on an historical vaccine canine distemper virus, the Rockborn strain. Vaccine 2011;29:1222–1227.

Staeheli P, Rinder M, Kaspers B. Avian bornavirus associated with fatal disease in psittacine birds. J Virol 2010;84:6269–6275.

Stein LT, Rech RR, Harrison L, Brown CC. Immunohistochemical study of rabies virus within the central nervous system of domestic and wildlife species. Vet Pathol 2010;47:630–633.

Theil D, Fatzer R, Schiller I, Caplazi P, Zurbriggen A, Vandevelde M. Neuropathological and aetiological studies of sporadic non-suppurative meningoencephalomyelitis of cattle. Vet Rec 1998;143: 244–249.

Weaver SC, Reisen WK Present and future arboviral threats. Antiviral Res 2010;85:328–345.

Yamada M, Kozakura R, Nakamura K, Yamamoto Y, Yoshii M, Kaku Y, Miyazaki A, Tsunemitsu H, Narita M. Pathological changes in pigs experimentally infected with porcine teschovirus. J Comp Pathol 2009;141:223–228.

Viral granulomatous infections

Benavides J, García-Pariente C, Fuertes M, Ferreras MC, García-Marín JF, Juste RA, Pérez V. Maedi-visna: the meningoencephalitis in naturally occurring cases. J Comp Pathol 2009;140:1–11.

Brown MA. Genetic determinants of pathogenesis by feline infectious peritonitis virus. Vet Immunol Immunopathol 2011;143:265–268.

Oaks JL, Long MT, Baszler TV. Leukoencephalitis associated with selective viral replication in the brain of a pony with experimental chronic equine infectious anemia virus infection. Vet Pathol 2004;41:527–532.

Poncelet L, Coppens A, Peeters D, Bianchi E, Grant CK, Kadhim H.Detection of antigenic heterogeneity in feline coronavirus nucleocapsid in feline pyogranulomatous meningoencephalitis. Vet Pathol 2008;45:140–153.

Viral vasculitis

Gilkerson JR, Barrett EJ. Equine herpesvirus neurological disease. Equine Vet J 2008;40:102–103.

Nelson DD, Davis WC, Brown WC, Li H, O'Toole D, Oaks JL. CD8(+)/perforin(+)/WC1(−) gammadelta T cells, not CD8(+) alphabeta T cells, infiltrate vasculitis lesions of American bison (*Bison bison*) with experimental sheep-associated malignant catarrhal fever. Vet Immunol Immunopathol 2010;136:284–291.

Demyelinating viral infections

Anderson CA, Higgins RJ, Smith ME, Osburn BI. Border disease. Virus-induced decrease in thyroid hormone levels with associated hypomyelination. Lab Invest 1987;57:168–175.

Benavides J, García-Pariente C, Fuertes M, Ferreras MC, García-Marín JF, Juste RA, Pérez V. Maedi-visna: the meningoencephalitis in naturally occurring cases. J Comp Pathol 2009; 140:1–11.

Carmichael KP, Bienzle D, McDonnell JJ. Feline leukemia virus-associated myelopathy in cats. Vet Pathol 2002;39:536–545.

Fletcher NF, Brayden DJ, Brankin B, Callanan JJ. Feline immunodeficiency virus infection: a valuable model to study HIV-1 associated encephalitis. Vet Immunol Immunopathol 2008;123:134–137.

Headley SA, Amude AM, Alfieri AF, Bracarense AP, Alfieri AA, Summers BA. Molecular detection of Canine distemper virus and the immunohistochemical characterization of the neurologic lesions in naturally occurring old dog encephalitis. J Vet Diagn Invest 2009;21:588–597.

Schaudien D, Polizopoulou Z, Koutinas A, Schwab S, Porombka D, Baumgärtner W, Herden C. Leukoencephalopathy associated with parvovirus infection in Cretan hound puppies. J Clin Microbiol 2010;48:3169–3175.

Vandevelde M, Zurbriggen A. Demyelination in canine distemper virus infection: a review. Acta Neuropathol 2005;109:56–68.

Bacterial infections

Barber RM, Li Q, Diniz PP, Porter BF, Breitschwerdt EB, Claiborne MK, Birkenheuer AJ, Levine JM, Levine GJ, Chandler K, Kenny P, Nghiem P, Wei S, Greene CE, Kent M, Platt SR, Greer K, Schatzberg SJ. Evaluation of brain tissue or cerebrospinal fluid with broadly reactive polymerase chain reaction for *Ehrlichia*, *Anaplasma*, spotted fever group *Rickettsia*, *Bartonella*, and *Borrelia* species in canine neurological diseases (109 cases). J Vet Intern Med 2010; 24:372–378.

Baums CG, Valentin-Weigand P. Surface-associated and secreted factors of *Streptococcus suis* in epidemiology, pathogenesis and vaccine development. Anim Health Res Rev 2009;10:65–83.

Beineke A, Bennecke K, Neis C, Schröder C, Waldmann KH, Baumgärtner W, Valentin-Weigand P, Baums CG. Comparative evaluation of virulence and pathology of *Streptococcus suis* serotypes 2 and 9 in experimentally infected growers. Vet Microbiol 2008;128:423–430.

Corbeil LB. *Histophilus somni* host-parasite relationships. Anim Health Res Rev 2007;8:151–160.

Fecteau G, George LW. Bacterial meningitis and encephalitis in ruminants. Vet Clin North Am Food Anim Pract 2004; 20:363–377.

Oevermann A, Di Palma S, Doherr MG, Abril C, Zurbriggen A, Vandevelde M. Neuropathogenesis of naturally occurring encephalitis caused by Listeria monocytogenes in ruminants. Brain Pathol 2010;20:378–390.

Fungal infections

Snowden KF, Lewis BC, Hoffman J, Mansell J. *Encephalitozoon cuniculi* infections in dogs: a case series. J Am Anim Hosp Assoc 2009;45: 225–231.

Stenner VJ, Mackay B, King T, Barrs VR, Irwin P, Abraham L, Swift N, Langer N, Bernays M, Hampson E, Martin P, Krockenberger MB, Bosward K, Latter M, Malik R. Prototheccosis in 17 Australian dogs and a review of the canine literature. Med Mycol 2007;45: 249–266.

Sykes JE, Sturges BK, Cannon MS, Gericota B, Higgins RJ, Trivedi SR, Dickinson PJ, Vernau KM, Meyer W, Wisner ER. Clinical signs, imaging features, neuropathology, and outcome in cats and dogs with central nervous system cryptococcosis from California. J Vet Intern Med 2010;24:1427–1438.

Protozoal infections

Alves L, Gorgas D, Vandevelde M, Gandini G, Henke D. Segmental meningomyelitis in 2 cats caused by *Toxoplasma gondii*. J Vet Intern Med 2011;25:148–152.

Caldow GL, Gidlow JR, Schock A. Clinical, pathological and epidemiological findings in three outbreaks of ovine protozoan myeloencephalitis. Vet Rec 2000;146:7–10.

Dubey JP, Chapman JL, Rosenthal BM, Mense M, Schueler RL. Clinical *Sarcocystis neurona, Sarcocystis canis, Toxoplasma gondii,* and *Neospora caninum* infections in dogs. Vet Parasitol 2006; 137:36–49.

Dubey JP, Lindsay DS, Saville WJ, Reed SM, Granstrom DE, Speer CA. A review of *Sarcocystis neurona* and equine protozoal myeloencephalitis (EPM). Vet Parasitol 2001;95:89–131.

Garosi L, Dawson A, Couturier J, Matiasek L, de Stefani A, Davies E, Jeffery N, Smith P. Necrotizing cerebellitis and cerebellar atrophy caused by *Neospora caninum* infection: magnetic resonance imaging and clinicopathologic findings in seven dogs. J Vet Intern Med 2010;24:571–578.

Rodrigues A, Fighera RA, Souza TM, Schild AL, Barros CS. Neuropathology of naturally occurring *Trypanosoma evansi* infection of horses. Vet Pathol 2009;46:251–258.

Helminth infections

Denk D, Matiasek K, Just FT, Hermanns W, Baiker K, Herbach N, Steinberg T, Fischer A. Disseminated angiostrongylosis with fatal cerebral haemorrhages in two dogs in Germany: a clinical case study. Vet Parasitol 2009;160:100–108.

Dvir E, Perl S, Loeb E, Shklar-Hirsch S, Chai O, Mazaki-Tovi M, Aroch I, Shamir MH. Spinal intramedullary aberrant *Spirocerca lupi* migration in 3 dogs. J Vet Intern Med 2007;21:860–864.

Wessmann A, Lu D, Lamb CR, Smyth B, Mantis P, Chandler K, Boag A, Cherubini GB, Cappello R. Brain and spinal cord haemorrhages associated with *Angiostrongylus vasorum* infection in four dogs. Vet Rec 2006;158:858–863.

Non-infectious and Immune-mediated inflammatory disorders

Aleman M, Katzman SA, Vaughan B, Hodges J, Crabbs TA, Christopher MM, Shelton GD, Higgins RJ. Antemortem diagnosis of polyneuritis equi. J Vet Intern Med 2009;23:665–668.

Anfinsen KP, Berendt M, Liste FJ, Haagensen TR, Indrebo A, Lingaas F, Stigen O, Alban L. A retrospective epidemiological study of clinical signs and familial predisposition associated with aseptic meningitis in the Norwegian population of Nova Scotia duck tolling retrievers born 1994–2003. Can J Vet Res 2008;72: 350–355.

Cuddon PA. Acquired canine peripheral neuropathies. Vet Clin North Am Small Anim Pract 2002;32:207–249.

Evans J, Levesque D, Shelton GD. Canine inflammatory myopathies: a clinicopathologic review of 200 cases. J Vet Intern Med 2004; 18:679–691.

Shelton GD. From dog to man: the broad spectrum of inflammatory myopathies. Neuromuscular Disorders 2007;17:663–670.

Shiel RE, Mooney CT, Brennan SF, Nolan CM, Callanan JJ. Clinical and clinicopathological features of non-suppurative meningoencephalitis in young greyhounds in Ireland. Vet Rec 2010;167: 333–337.

Talarico LR, Schatzberg SJ. Idiopathic granulomatous and necrotising inflammatory disorders of the canine central nervous system: a review and future perspectives. J Small Anim Pract 2010; 51: 138–149.

Tipold A, Schatzberg SJ. An update on steroid responsive meningitis-arteritis. J Small Anim Prac 2010;51:150–154.

Williams JH, Köster LS, Naidoo V, Odendaal L, Van Veenhuysen A, de Wit M, van Wilpe E. Review of idiopathic eosinophilic meningitis in dogs and cats, with a detailed description of two recent cases in dogs. J S Afr Vet Assoc 2008;79:194–204.

This book is accompanied by a companion website which is maintained by the Division of Diagnostic Imaging, Dept of Clinical Veterinary Medicine, Vetsuisse Faculty, University of Bern, Switzerland.
www.wiley.com/go/vandevelde/veterinaryneuropathology

4

Trauma

Traumatic lesions of the nervous system result from direct mechanical impact applied to the head, spine or peripheral nerves. In addition, during sudden acceleration or deceleration the skull and vertebral bone collide against the inert brain and spinal cord. Apart from direct mechanical disruption of the tissue (laceration), there is damage to the blood vessels leading to ischemia, hemorrhage and secondary changes. The space-occupying effect of the latter may cause additional injury of the gray and white matter because the CNS is located in the narrow confines of the skull and spine.

4.1 Pathophysiology of CNS trauma

Causes of brain trauma, commonly called traumatic brain injury (TBI), in animals include car accidents, falls, bites, kicks, gun shots and blows to the head. The extent of injury varies considerably with severity, speed and duration of the distortion. A special case is iatrogenic trauma associated with CSF puncture inadvertently penetrating the medulla.

4.1.1 Pathogenesis of brain trauma

Primary and secondary injury

The molecular pathogenesis of trauma is highly complex and only in part understood. Mechanical distortion of the tissue leads to lesions of the microvasculature with leakage of blood and plasma into the tissue. Following the immediate effect of sheer forces with disruption of neurons and other cells besides blood vessels (primary brain injury), a range of secondary events leads to additional damage within hours and days following the traumatic event. The secondary brain damage may significantly aggravate the initial traumatic injury and is frequently fatal. TBI induces disruption of cerebral blood flow autoregulation and an abrupt rise in catecholamines causing a rapid increase in blood pressure, which may cause life-threatening brain edema. These changes are compounded by the direct mechanical disruption of blood vessels resulting in ischemia and thus depletion of energy stores. Consequently, energy-dependent ion pumps break down with depolarization of membranes and excessive release of excitatory amino acids leading to exitotoxicity (see Chapter 1). When anti-oxidative defense mechanisms (e.g. superoxide dismutase) become depleted, oxygen radicals induce peroxidation of membranes of neural as well as vascular elements resulting in necrosis and can also initiate apoptosis. The altered tissue environment, e.g. with high levels of inflammatory mediators such as prostaglandin, can lead to vasospasm a few days after the trauma, aggravating the already compromised blood supply to the traumatized tissue. Membrane damage at the level of the blood–brain barrier leads to vasogenic and cytotoxic brain edema, within the confined space of the skull, further compromising tissue perfusion. Thus, much of the pathogenesis of TBI is basically due to ischemia. The destructive changes will eventually lead to an inflammatory reaction elicited by release of pro-inflammatory cytokines with initial influx of neutrophils followed by macrophages removing cell debris and blood.

Since only little free space is present within the rigid cranial vault, TBI-induced mass hemorrhage acts as a space-occupying lesion increasing intracranial pressure. The latter may further reduce cerebral perfusion leading to vascular leakage, ischemia and edema formation, increasing the intracranial pressure still more. This may eventually lead to significant brain swelling with midline shift and herniation of the occipital lobes underneath the tentorium cerebelli, resulting in lethal brainstem compression. The same mechanisms may result in caudal herniation of the cerebellum through the foramen magnum.

Mechanics of brain trauma

Traumatic lesions can occur immediately below the site of impact (*coup*), on the opposite side of impact

Veterinary Neuropathology: Essentials of Theory and Practice, First Edition. Marc Vandevelde, Robert J. Higgins, and Anna Oevermann.
© 2012 John Wiley & Sons, Ltd. Published 2012 by John Wiley & Sons, Ltd.

(*contre-coup*) or both as shown in Fig. 4.1. It is generally accepted that coup lesions are most severe and contre-coup lesions are small when a stationary (but mobile) head is hit by a moving object. In contrast, contre-coup lesions generally are more prominent than coup lesions when a moving head bounces against a stationary object. The pathomechanism of coup and contre-coup injuries is still under debate, but it is widely accepted that inertia of the brain is involved in the pathogenesis. The brain is suspended in the cerebrospinal fluid and therefore freely movable within the skull and thus subject to a range of different forces (e.g. linear and angular acceleration forces; shearing, rotational and tensile forces) in trauma. When the head is suddenly accelerated or decelerated

the inert brain is bounced against the inner surface of the calvarium or tentorium either on the side of impact or on the opposite side. Additionally, the physical properties of cerebrospinal fluid and tensile forces resulting in stretching of vessels and brain parenchyma (when the brain moves away from the skull) have been implicated in the development of contre-coup contusions. Thus, the distribution pattern of lesions is often complex involving not only superficial areas but also deep structures of the brain (Fig. 4.1D).

4.1.2 Pathogenesis of spinal cord trauma

Trauma to the spinal column may result in spinal cord injury following vertebral fractures, luxations, subluxa-

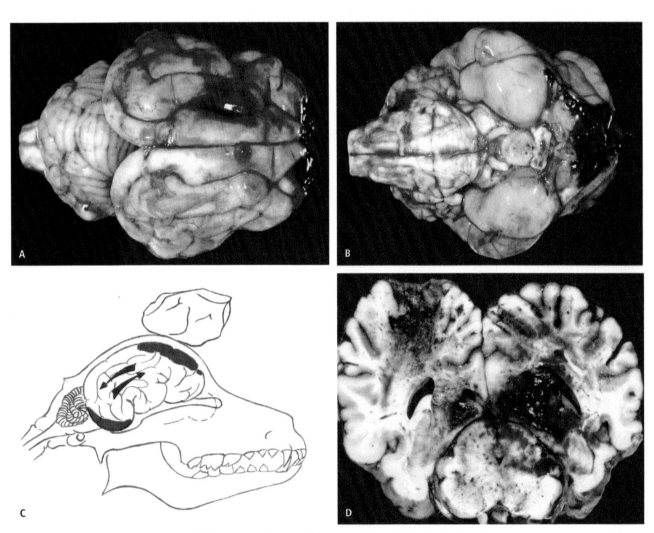

Fig. 4.1 Coup/contre-coup. A–B: Cat hit by car. A, dorsal and B, ventral view of the brain showing coup and contre-coup lesions. C: Simplified illustration of the coup/contre-coup mechanism during closed head trauma. Following impact the brain moves at a different speed to the skull because of its inertia and is bounced against the internal side of the skull resulting in contusion. The contusion may occur directly below (coup) or at the opposite side (contre-coup) of the impact. D: Horse. Severe closed head trauma (fell on obstacle in jumping competition) with a superficial wedge-shaped lesion in left hemisphere (probable coup) but also severe hemorrhagic lesions in the deep brain structures illustrating the frequently complex lesion distribution in cranial trauma.

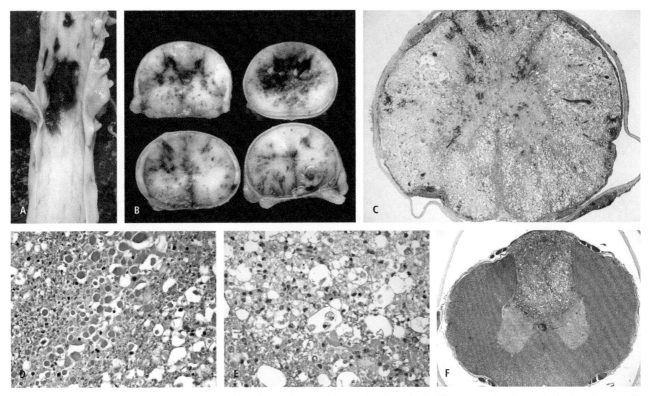

Fig. 4.2 Spinal cord contusion. A: Dog. Spinal cord. Focal area of hemorrhagic malacia (dura mater has been incised and opened). B: Dog. Cross-sections of spinal cord. Hemorrhagic myelomalacia more pronounced in center of the cord and gray matter. C: Transverse section. There are multiple hemorrhages more pronounced in gray matter with extensive myelomalacia. HE. D: Numerous swollen axons in the white matter in acute lesion. HE. E: Loss of tissue architecture with infiltration by macrophages. HE. F: Ascending hemorrhagic myelomalacia within the dorsal columns and central canal. HE.

tions and intervertebral disc herniations. Even without mechanical deformation of the spinal canal a sudden blow to the vertebral column may lead to severe cord lesions. In addition, traumatic lesions often lead to narrowing of the spinal canal exerting continuous pressure on the cord. Thus, basically two pathogenetic mechanisms have to be considered in cord trauma: contusion and compression. Often both mechanisms act synergistically. This is particularly true in intervertebral disc disease.

Contusion

Following impact, the cord, which is suspended and hence movable within in the spinal canal, collides with the bony wall of the spinal canal because of inertia resulting in *contusion*. At the site of impact there is damage to the microvasculature leading to intramedullary hemorrhage, which is typically more pronounced in the gray than in the white matter. This is because the gray matter is far more vascularized than the white matter. Secondary changes in the hours and days follow-

ing the traumatic event are based on the same mechanisms as described in brain trauma. As in the brain, hemorrhage is associated with acute ischemic necrosis of the tissue (Fig. 4.2). See MRI Atlas. The clinical consequences of hemorrhagic myelomalacia are frequently severe and have a bad prognosis. A peculiar secondary change in the cord is that the hemorrhage can extend over several segments from the site of impact thus producing *ascending* or *descending hemorrhagic myelomalacia* (Fig. 4.2F) often along the central canal and dorsal columns. The mechanism of this phenomenon is yet unknown, but vascular damage, hemorrhage, excitotoxicity, inflammatory mediators and reactive oxygen species likely contribute. In the worst of cases, it may involve many segments or even the whole cord.

Compression

Compression of the cord occurs when the spinal canal is narrowed, for example by a protruding intervertebral disc. The resulting pathology depends on the speed with

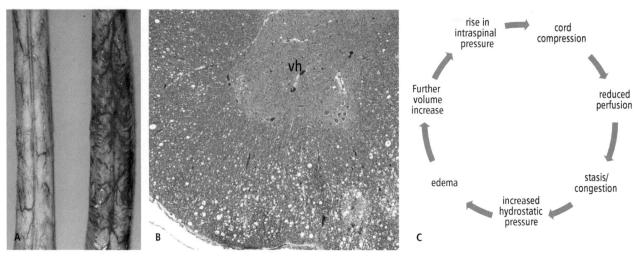

Fig. 4.3 Spinal cord compression. A: Wobbler syndrome. Horse. On the right side a compressed spinal cord segment with marked congestion and swelling compared to normal cord segment on the left. B: Acute Hansen's type I intervertebral disc herniation. Dog. Spinal cord. Marked spongy state of the white matter due to edema and swelling of myelin sheaths as well as axonal degeneration (vh, ventral horn). HE. C: Diagram of the events in the vicious closed cycle with the lesions induced by hemodynamic changes during compression.

which the compression develops. This is called the *dynamic factor*. Acute compressions that happen within seconds initially induce lesions very much like those described in spinal cord contusion. More often, we are dealing with compressive lesions that develop within hours, days or even weeks. Chronic ("chronic" as opposed to a sudden blow) compression in this case leads to hemodynamic changes depicted in Fig. 4.3. Important to understand the pathogenesis of chronic compression is that the cord is encased by the spinal canal, a rigid tunnel of bone, in which there is little spare space. Any pathological process, which occupies space will sooner or later compress the cord. This will then lead to perfusion failure, vascular stasis, leakage of plasma proteins and increased osmotic pressure in the tissue, leading to edema further increasing intraspinal pressure, thus establishing a vicious circle (Fig. 4.3C). For that reason, decompressive surgery is the treatment of choice in many cases.

On histological examination, the lesions are more obvious in the white matter. The involved cord segments show a marked spongy state of the white matter, which is most pronounced immediately adjacent to the compressive force. The spongy state is caused either by edema, visible as extensive vacuolation of the tissue with "empty" vacuoles and little evidence of lysis of cellular elements and reactive changes, or by destructive lesions, including demyelination and axonal disruption/swelling (Fig. 4.3B). Usually there is a mixture of both components. Depending on the severity and duration of com-

pression, the destructive component may be more or less pronounced. In severe lesions, we may find extensive necrosis of both gray and white matter. In compressive lesions of sudden onset, we find evidence for both contusion and compression.

Depending on the stage of the spinal cord injury, we find reactive changes such as invasion of neutrophils initially followed by macrophages, vascular proliferation and gliosis. In animals that survive for several days or more, Wallerian degeneration is present in the ascending and descending tracts of the cord. In fact, if the primary lesion has been overlooked, Wallerian degeneration indicates its presence. In chronic compressions, we often find loss of neurons and gliosis in the gray matter (see Fig. 4.8C) and we occasionally see enlargement of the central canal in the area of the lesion. The ependymal lining of the canal may rupture with leakage of spinal fluid in the tissue (*interstitial edema*) and formation of a fluid-filled cavity (*syringomyelia*).

In slowly progressive compression, e.g caused by tumors of the meninges or nerve roots, the cord can be remarkably attenuated with mild evidence of ongoing destruction but severe atrophy.

4.2 General strategy for diagnosis of traumatic CNS lesions

• The diagnosis of CNS trauma does not pose any problem when an animal is submitted with a clear history of a traumatic event or when other signs of mechanical injury are present such as skin abrasions, limb fractures etc. In domestic animals this is frequently not the case. Animals such as livestock on pastures or free-roaming pets are often not under close surveillance. A blunt trauma may not cause any externally visible mark. The only available history may be that neurological signs suddenly appeared.

- The predominant lesion pattern in trauma is hemorrhage often associated with malacia ("hemorrhagic malacia"). Thus when hemorrhagic lesions are seen, trauma can be suspected. However, there are many other causes of hemorrhage or hemorrhagic malacia. A differential diagnosis of hemorrhagic lesions in the CNS is presented in Fig. 2.1. Further information can be obtained in Fig. 6.1.
- Areas of dark brown, orange or yellowish discoloration are highly suggestive of an old hemorrhage, potentially due to trauma.
- Spinal cord injury of various causes discussed below is probably the most common cause of neurological disease in animals. A correct clinical localization in the spinal cord is often available. If not, whenever there is a history of paresis or paralysis in the hind limbs or all four limbs, the spinal cord (and spinal canal) should be examined as outlined in Chapter 1.
- Traumatic lesions in the cord and surrounding tissues are often visible with the naked eye and spinal cord can be sampled accordingly.
- In the absence of a clinical or external macroscopic localization, systematic sectioning of all segments may reveal a macroscopic change. If not, the presence of Wallerian degeneration in the routine histological sections indicates the presence of a focal lesion somewhere in the cord. If this primary lesion is not included in the original sections there may be an indication to trim in more spinal cord tissue.

4.3 Traumatic nervous system diseases

4.3.1 Trauma of the brain

Concussion

Concussion is the mildest form of head injury and is defined as temporary impairment of neurological function following rapid acceleration/deceleration during head trauma. Axonal injury may be involved in concussion. Mild lesions may be present on MRI, and hemorrhages and axonal/neuronal damage may be seen with light microscopy. This type of trauma is well known in human medicine, but data on animals are lacking.

Hemorrhage/hematoma

The common visible evidence of trauma is hemorrhage, which may occur diffusely or focally as mass hemorrhage (hematoma) that results from rupture of large blood vessels. The hemorrhage may be localized in the epidural or subdural space, but in animals occurs most commonly as extensive subarachnoid or intracerebral hemorrhages. The latter are observed in the cortex with contact to the leptomeninges, in the subcortical white matter or in the deeper structures (Fig. 4.4A,B).

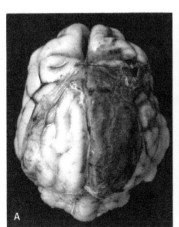
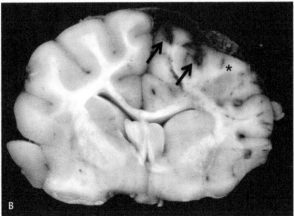
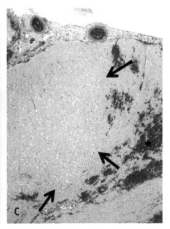

Fig. 4.4 Acute cerebral trauma. Dog, hit by car. A: Dorsal view on the brain. The right hemisphere is covered by a large subdural hematoma. B: Transverse section of the same brain. The subdural hematoma compresses the right parietal lobe. Contusive hemorrhages are found in the cortex and subcortical white matter (arrows). The cortex is swollen, and the boundary between white and gray matter blurred (asterisk) indicating edema and necrosis. C: Same case. Histologically, in this area focal hemorrhages (asterisk) border a large area of spongy state (arrows). The overlying subarachnoid space is infiltrated by macrophages. HE.

Frequently, hemorrhages are particularly extensive or even selectively localized in the gray matter because the latter is much more vascularized than the white matter.

Contusion, laceration

Contusions and lacerations result from blunt trauma to the head and consist of focal to extensive parenchymal/arachnoidal hemorrhages and tissue necrosis (Fig. 4.4A,B,C). In lacerations, the arachnoidal membranes and the underlying brain parenchyma are disrupted (e.g. due to a skull fracture), whereas in contusions the arachnoidal membranes are intact. Both conditions are accompanied by significant edema, which may result in life-threatening increase in intracranial pressure. The

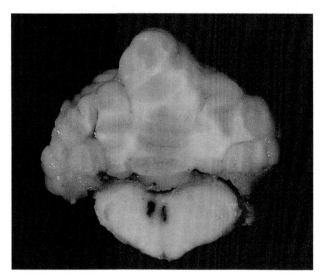

Fig. 4.5 Iatrogenic trauma. Cat. Iatrogenic laceration and hemorrhage of the brainstem resulting from two misguided attempts using a biopsy needle for CSF collection.

separation of contusion from hematoma is ambiguous since intraparenchymal hemorrhage occurs in both.

Iatrogenic trauma

A particular type of trauma is laceration and hemorrhage of the brainstem or spinal cord during CSF puncture. Such lesions may be an incidental finding during the neuropathological examination, but may also be associated with significant neurological deficits. On gross examination longitudinal hemorrhage corresponding to the needle track is observed near the midline (Fig. 4.5).

Old trauma

If an animal is well nursed during the acute post-traumatic phase it may recover depending on the site of the lesion, sometimes with only minor residual neurological deficits. In surviving animals hemorrhages and destroyed tissue are removed by macrophages. As is usually the case in massive destruction of CNS tissue, because neural tissue cannot regenerate, cystic lesions are formed with atrophy of the involved area (Fig. 4.6A,B). The edges of such cysts are often decorated with hemosiderophages (Fig. 4.6C). These are macrophages that have phagocytosed and digested the erythrocytic hemoglobin. In HE sections they contain yellow to brownish-orange granules of blood breakdown products. These *hemosiderophages* may persist throughout life in the scar tissue formed by fibrillary astrocytes. See MRI Atlas.

Diffuse traumatic axonal injury

Apart from direct mechanical disruption, axons in multiple areas of the traumatized brain may undergo degeneration called *traumatic axonal injury* (TAI), which results from shearing forces during rapid acceleration or

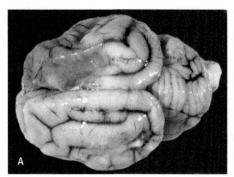
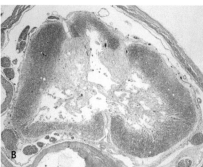
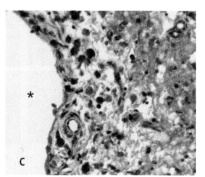

Fig. 4.6 Previous old trauma. A: Cat. A depressed area of focal, chronic encephalomalacia in the right frontal lobe with loss of tissue. Note yellowish-brown discoloration of lesion. B: Dog. Spinal cord. Chronic cystic myelomalacia following spinal cord contusion. HE. C: Dog. Cerebral cortex. A cyst (asterisk) is lined by astrogliotic tissue containing numerous hemosiderin-containing macrophages. HE.

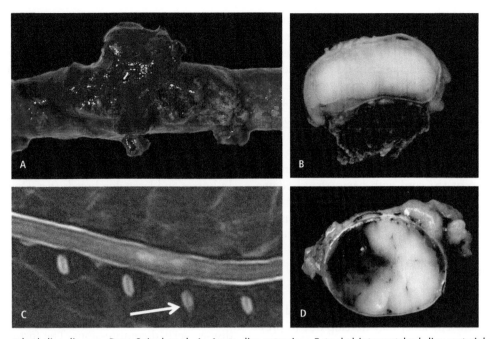

Fig. 4.7 Intervertebral disc disease. Dog. Spinal cord. A: Acute disc extrusion. Extruded intervertebral disc material and associated hematoma over the ventral surface of the cord attached to the dura. Note diffuse subdural hemorrhage. B: Chronic disc extrusion. There is ventrodorsal compression of the spinal cord due to a mass of granulation tissue, disc material and hemorrhage. C: MRI sagittal T2W sequence of the spine of a dog with an explosive disc extrusion. Focal hyperintensity of the cord and the nucleus pulposus of one disc has a comparatively diminished signal (arrow). D: Traumatically induced (explosive, high velocity) disc extrusion with severe unilateral, well demarcated focal spinal cord necrosis and hemorrhage.

deceleration. In severe cases this change may be widespread ("diffuse axonal injury"), a clinically relevant complication in cranial trauma in human beings and also known from experimental trauma in animals. The lesion starts as focal axonal swelling resulting from impaired axonal transport and progresses to axonal disconnection and Wallerian degeneration.

4.3.2 Traumatic spinal cord lesions

Intervertebral disc disease

Endogenous cord trauma associated with **intervertebral disc disease** is particularly common in dogs. Degenerative changes in the intervertebral disc occur as an aging change in non-chondrodystrophic dog breeds and very rarely in cats or other species (except humans) or prematurely at early age (2 months in Dachshunds) in chondrodystrophic breeds (Dachshund, Basset, Beagle, Pug, Pekingese, Poodles, Cocker Spaniels and others). The degenerative process in the intervertebral disc starts with degradation and loss of proteoglycans, a change from collagen type II to type I and proliferation of chondrocyte-like cells. This is associated with appearance of clefts within the intervertebral disc. In chondro-

dystrophic breeds there is loss of notochordal cells and often mineralization of the nucleus pulposus, which retains its volume. In non-chondrodystrophic breeds there is rather atrophy of the disc. Associated degeneration and weakening of the annulus fibrosus may result in rupture of the annulus fibrosus and *extrusion* of degenerated disc material in the extradural space (Hansen type I, Fig. 4.7A,B). Alternatively, the weakened annulus fibrosus containing degenerated nucleus pulposus *protrudes* in the spinal canal (Hansen type II herniation). Most of these herniations occur spontaneously without history of previous trauma between the T10 and L3 vertebrae but also in the cervical area. Whereas the relatively large extradural space around the cervical, cranial thoracic and caudal lumbar spinal cord segments may accommodate a relatively large amount of herniated disc material without causing significant compression, herniated disc material in the upper lumbar and lower thoracic spine quickly causes significant compression and neurological deficits due to the small extradural space at these sites.

On postmortem examination a disc extrusion (Hansen type I) is easily recognized. In view of the relatively small volume of the nucleus pulposus, surprisingly large amounts of extradural material are frequently found attached to the dura because of extensive hemorrhage and inflammatory reaction. In chronic extrusions, the nucleus pulposus material may get organized by granulomatous inflammation and fibrous tissue that adheres the disc material firmly to the dura (Fig. 4.7B). Disc protrusions are characterized by bulging of the intervertebral disc, which maintains a smooth surface and generally does not adhere to the dura. Along with compression, acute and large disc extrusions often also cause contusion of the cord with hemorrhage, edema and extensive necrosis of gray and white matter (Fig. 4.2). Rarely, pulposus material penetrates the dura mater and can even enter the cord tissue.

Spinal trauma

Fractures, **subluxations** and **luxations** of the spine cause contusion but are also frequently associated with cord compression. The latter may develop due to presence of bone fragments, narrowing of the canal resulting from instability, massive extradural hemorrhage or delayed stenosis of the canal as a result of callus formation. Trauma may also cause extrusion of a degenerated intervertebral disc causing similar pathology as described above (contusion and compression). In recent years extrusion of healthy nucleus pulposus tissue ("**explosive disc**", "high-velocity disc extrusions") following traumatic rupture of the annulus fibrosus has been increasingly recognized as a frequent event in spinal trauma. This type of disc herniation may also occur following intensive exercise. The extruded nucleus pulposus may even perforate the dura. The lesions can be extremely destructive, strongly lateralized and well demarcated resembling an ischemic infarct (Fig. 4.7C,D). It is not associated with compression, because the gelatinous nucleus pulposus diffuses in the epidural space and hence does not accumulate. See MRI Atlas.

Spinal malformations

In canine toy breeds, such as Miniature Poodles, Maltese and Yorkshire Terriers, **atlanto-axial subluxation** with dorsal displacement of the axis leads to cervical spinal cord compression and severe ambulatory problems. The cause of the dorsal displacement in toy breeds includes malformation (aplasia, hypoplasia) of the dens or its postnatal progressive degeneration, and absence of the transversal ligament of the atlas. In other dog breeds, atlanto-axial subluxation may occur with incomplete ossification of the atlas. Furthermore, it may result from traumatic injury causing fracture/avulsion of the dens or rupture of the transversal ligament.

Abnormal vertebrae (**hemivertebrae**, *wedge vertebrae, centrum defects, block and transitional vertebrae*) may cause stenosis of the spinal canal with spinal cord compression as well as kyphosis and scoliosis, especially in small dog breeds. Arachnoidal cysts are discussed in chapter 5.3.8.

Wobbler syndrome (cervical spondylomyelopathy, cervical stenotic myelopathy)

In horses and large dog breeds (e.g. Dobermann, Great Dane), static or dynamic stenosis of the cervical spinal canal causes spinal cord compression, neck pain, paresis and ataxia (known as **Wobbler syndrome**). The definition of **cervical spondylomyelopathy** and its pathogenesis are controversial. Genetic, dietary etiologies and congenital anomalies (such as congenital vertebral canal stenosis in Dobermanns) have been proposed.

Static stenoses have been divided into osseous- and disc-associated compressions. The former are observed predominantly in young adult animals and have their origin in vertebral malformations that are frequently associated with degenerative changes of the facet joints that narrow the spinal canal. Furthermore, synovial cysts secondary to the degenerative synovial joint changes and hypertrophy of the *ligamentum flavum* may complicate the compression. Disc-associated compressions occur in adult dogs that are born with a congenital vertebral canal stenosis. These dogs are prone to spinal cord compression due intervertebral disc protrusions because of the relatively small extradural space. Disc-associated compressions generally occur at the transition between C5–C6 and C6–C7. *Dynamic compression* of the spinal cord occurs with cervical extension and flexion over a compressive lesion within the spinal canal and significantly contributes to spinal cord damage in cervical spondylomyelopathy.

Neuropathological changes in the spinal cord depend on the duration and severity of compression. They may vary from focal axonal degeneration and edema to marked malacia, gliosis and atrophy of gray and white matter (Fig. 4.8C).

Synovial cysts

Spinal synovial cysts arising from the intervertebral joints and bulging in the spinal canal may be causative for or contribute to cervical spondylomyelopathy. They are a frequent cause of spinal cord compression in riding horses. In this species, they occur at the level of the vertebral articulations C4–C7 and result from chronic inflammation of the intervertebral joints (Fig. 4.8B). In dogs, they can be associated with cervical stenotic mye-

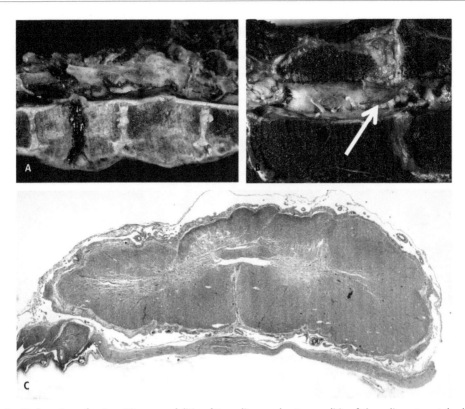

Fig. 4.8 A: Dog. Sagittal section of spine. Discospondylitis of two discs and osteomyelitis of the adjacent vertebral bodies. B: Horse. Synovial cyst of the articular facet joint (arrow) in the cervical spinal canal. C: Dobermann. Chronic canine wobbler syndrome. Marked dorsoventral flattening and atrophy particularly on the left side, cystic poliomyelomalacia with gliosis. HE.

lopathy (see above), but may occur along the entire spinal cord.

Discospondylitis

Discospondylitis is mostly a problem in dogs resulting from hematogenous embolic infection of the disc by bacteria (e.g. *Brucella canis*) or fungi (e.g. *Aspergillus tereus*), frequently at multiple sites. Typically the infection and associated inflammation lead to lysis of the disc and osteomyelitis of the adjacent endplates of the vertebral bodies (Fig. 4.8A). In the chronic stage sclerosis and spondylosis occur. There is usually only moderate stenosis of the canal.

Abscess of the spine

Bacterial infection with abscess formation in the spine is an important cause of spinal cord compression in livestock animals.

Tumors

Neoplastic disease of the spine and other tissues surrounding the cord are discussed in Chapter 7.

4.3.3 Trauma in the peripheral nervous system

General

Peripheral nerve injury is a frequent complication in trauma of the extremities such as fractures and luxations. Superficial nerves can be directly traumatized. **Neuropraxia** occurs in crush injuries in which the nerve remains intact but with interruption of conduction resulting from compression/ischemia. There is no Wallerian degeneration and function returns within hours to weeks. More severe is **axonotmesis**, where axons are destroyed but anatomical continuity of the connective tissues of the nerve remains preserved. This leads then to Wallerian degeneration and retrograde changes as explained in Chapter 1. Regeneration occurs but takes months to years depending on the distance from the nerve's target. The most severe type of injury with rupture and loss of continuity of the nerve or extensive destruction of the connective tissue structures is called **neurotmesis**. Histological changes consist of axonal swelling and fragmentation, loss of myelin sheaths,

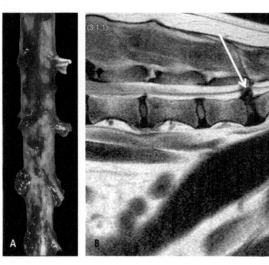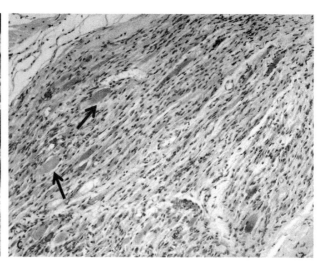

Fig. 4.9 Peripheral nervous system trauma. A: Dog. Ventral view of the cervical intumescence with brachial plexus avulsion. Four nerve roots of the right side are avulsed and replaced by hemorrhagic stumps. B: Dog. Cauda equina compression. Sagittal MRI T1W of L7–S1 disc protrusion in a dog with complete loss of signal of the cauda equina and dural sac at the level of the disc lesion. C: Dog. Chronic cervical nerve root compression. Marked loss of nerve fibers, edema and hyperplasia of Schwann cells. Many remaining axons are swollen (arrows). HE.

invasion of macrophages in the degenerating fibers and Schwann cell proliferation.

Brachial plexus avulsion

Avulsion of the brachial plexus is the most frequent cause of monoplegia in small animals. Extreme sudden abduction of a frontlimb during an accident can pull one or more spinal nerve roots of the brachial plexus completely or partially out of the spinal cord (*avulsion*, Fig. 4.9A). In cases of complete interruption the prognosis is bad because regeneration is not possible.

Avulsion of cauda equina nerves

Cauda equina nerve avulsion (most commonly pudendal and coccygeal nerves) is often associated with fractures/subluxations in the lumbosacral area or avulsion of the tail (the latter particularly in cats).

Compression of cauda equina

This lesion, commonly called **cauda equina syndrome** is a frequent neurological problem especially in large-breed dogs. The cause is stenosis of the lumbosacral canal and/or associated intervertebral foramina resulting from pathology in the intervertrebral disc (L7/S1), intervertebral joints, vertebral bone or associated ligamentous structures (Fig. 4.9B). The pathophysiology of nerve compression within the confined space of the spinal canal is similar to what has been described for spinal cord compression. Depending on severity and

duration, lesions range from disseminated degeneration of fibers to extensive loss of nerve fibers and fibrosis.

Cervical spinal root compression

Compression of cervical nerve roots with radicular pain (*"root signature"*), lameness and muscle atrophy in the affected limb is quite common in dogs. The lesions are usually associated with cervical disc disease, instability and other causes of hypertrophy of the soft tissues leading to stenosis of the intervertebral foramina. Lesions range from mild loss of fibers to complete nerve root degeneration and fibrosis (Fig. 4.9C).

Further reading

Pathophysiology of CNS trauma

Drew LB, Drew WE. The contrecoup-coup phenomenon: a new understanding of the mechanism of closed head injury. Neurocrit Care 2004;1:385–390.

Greve MW, Zink BJ. Pathophysiology of traumatic brain injury. Mt Sinai J Med 2009;76:97–104.

Nag S, Kapadia A, Stewart DJ. Review: molecular pathogenesis of blood-brain barrier breakdown in acute brain injury. Neuropathol Appl Neurobiol 2011;37:3–23.

Okada M, Kitagawa M, Ito D, Itou T, Kanayama K, Sakai T. Magnetic resonance imaging features and clinical signs associated with presumptive and confirmed progressive myelomalacia in dogs: 12 cases (1997–2008). J Am Vet Med Assoc 2010;237:1160–1165.

Sande A, West C. Traumatic brain injury: a review of pathophysiology and management. J Vet Emerg Crit Care (San Antonio) 2010;20: 177–190.

Brain trauma

Barkhoudarian G, Hovda DA, Giza CC. The molecular pathophysiology of concussive brain injury. Clin Sports Med 2011;30:33–48

Maruta J, Lee SW, Jacobs EF, Ghajar J. A unified science of concussion. Ann N Y Acad Sci 2010;1208:58–66.

Luján Feliu-Pascual A, Garosi L, Dennis R, Platt S. Iatrogenic brainstem injury during cerebellomedullary cistern puncture. Vet Radiol Ultrasound 2008;49:467–471.

Meythaler JM, Peduzzi JD, Eleftheriou E, Novack TA. Current concepts: diffuse axonal injury-associated traumatic brain injury. Arch Phys Med Rehabil 2001;82:1461–1471.

Intervertebral disc disease

Bergknut N, Rutges JP, Kranenburg HJ, Smolders LA, Hagman R, Smidt HJ, Lagerstedt AS, Voorhout G, Hazewinkel HH, Grinwis GC, Creemers LB, Meij BP, Dhert WJ. The dog as an animal model for intervertebral disc degeneration? Spine 2012;37:351–358.

Brisson BA. Intervertebral disc disease in dogs. Vet Clin North Am Small Anim Pract 2010;40:829–858.

De Risio L, Adams V, Dennis R, McConnell FJ. Association of clinical and magnetic resonance imaging findings with outcome in dogs with presumptive acute noncompressive nucleus pulposus extrusion: 42 cases (2000–2007). J Am Vet Med Assoc 2009;234:495–504.

McKee WM, Downes CJ, Pink JJ, Gemmill TJ. Presumptive exercise-associated peracute thoracolumbar disc extrusion in 48 dogs. Vet Rec 2010;166:523–528.

Spinal malformations

Warren-Smith CM, Kneissl S, Benigni L, Kenny PJ, Lamb CR. Incomplete ossification of the atlas in dogs with cervical signs. Vet Radiol Ultrasound 2009;50:635–638.

Westworth DR, Sturges BK. Congenital spinal malformations in small animals. Vet Clin North Am Small Anim Pract 2010;40:951–981.

Wobbler syndrome

da Costa RC. Cervical spondylomyelopathy (wobbler syndrome) in dogs. Vet Clin North Am Small Anim Pract 2010;40:881–913.

Sale CS, Smith KC. Magnetic resonance imaging features of cervical stenotic myelopathy in 21 dogs. Vet Radiol Ultrasound 2001;42:20–27.

Other causes of cord compression

Dickinson PJ, Sturges BK, Berry WL, Vernau KM, Koblik PD, Lecouteur RA. Extradural spinal synovial cysts in nine dogs. J Small Anim Pract 2001;42:502–509.

Forterre F, Kaiser S, Garner M, Stadie B, Matiasek K, Schmahl W, Brunnberg L. Synovial cysts associated with cauda equina syndrome in two dogs. Vet Surg 2006;35:30–33.

Tipold A, Stein VM. Inflammatory diseases of the spine in small animals. Vet Clin North Am Small Anim Pract 2010;40:871–879.

Cauda equina syndrome

Meij BP, Bergknut N. Degenerative lumbosacral stenosis in dogs. Vet Clin North Am Small Anim Pract 2010;40:983–1009.

Worth AJ, Thompson DJ, Hartman AC. Degenerative lumbosacral stenosis in working dogs: current concepts and review. N Z Vet J 2009;57:319–330.

5

Congenital malformations

Congenital malformations of the CNS are structural abnormalities of prenatal origin present at birth. In general, they seriously interfere with postnatal viability or normal physical function. Broadly across domestic animal species, such malformations may account for up to 5% of all neonatal deaths and for an undetermined incidence of abortions.

5.1 Pathophysiology

5.1.1 Ontogeny of the CNS

Some knowledge of the mechanism and sequence of normal mammalian embryological development is critical to even a basic understanding of CNS malformations. The CNS develops from primitive neuroectoderm with initial staged neurulation finally resulting in closure to form the neural tube. Neural crest cells then separate from the tube to form neurons of peripheral autonomic ganglia and sensory nerve roots. From a subependymal germinal cell layer, there is a massive proliferation in successive waves of immature neurons and then glioblasts, which migrate along radial glial processes guided to predetermined locations in gray and white matter. Functional cell maturation then follows with populations of postmitotic neurons, astrocytes and oligodendrocytes forming myelin with increasing morphological and functional complexity. During this development all these cells have different vulnerability to various teratogenic agents at different stages of maturation leading to a vast array of acquired malformations, depending as much on the time of insult as on any specific teratogen.

5.1.2 Etiology

The major classification of malformations into two groups is based on presumed differences in etiology. Primary malformations are caused by spontaneous or inherited single point gene mutations or chromosomal abnormalities. A rapidly increasing number of such mutations is being characterized, including the proteins they code for, leading to a fundamental molecular understanding of many developmental abnormalities. In contrast, secondary malformations are those acquired from exposure to known teratogens, including transplacental viral infections, ionizing radiation, hyperthermia, known toxic or some therapeutic chemicals, hypothyroidism, vitamin deficiencies, plant toxins etc., although the cause of many malformations still remains enigmatic. Thus, an etiologic classification of all animal CNS malformations is not possible with currently available information. Classifications are essentially based upon morphologic descriptions against a background of normal fetal CNS development. This allows then a broad interpretation of the pathogenesis of particular malformations. Current evidence suggests that most defects are probably the result of interactive combinations of both genetic and environmental factors.

Critical features of teratogenesis that largely determine the type of fetal CNS malformation are:

- a longer period of development and maturation and therefore greater time for susceptibility to injury compared to other organ systems;
- most severe defects occur in the first trimester during this critical period of morphogenesis;
- there is changing individual cell susceptibility to various insults at different stages of development;
- the type of malformation depends more on the critical timing of the insult in relation to ontogenesis than the nature of the insult;
- because domestic animal species are born at different stages of CNS maturation, postnatal myelination and neuronal cell trafficking can still provide targets of opportunity for teratogens.

Veterinary Neuropathology: Essentials of Theory and Practice, First Edition. Marc Vandevelde, Robert J. Higgins, and Anna Oevermann.
© 2012 John Wiley & Sons, Ltd. Published 2012 by John Wiley & Sons, Ltd.

5.2 General strategy for diagnosing anomalies of the CNS

- The typical clinical presentation is an immature animal with neurological signs occurring immediately after birth or within the first weeks or months of life. Signs are usually non-progressive with compensation in some animals that survive for longer periods of time. In some malformations signs may progress rapidly. In others (e.g. Arnold Chiari, syringomyelia) signs may occur later in life.
- The basic neuropathological pattern is deviation of normal anatomy. The detection of such anomalies is in most cases not a problem. Malformations may be apparent from the outside or be revealed by sectioning the brain and cord. Some malformations may be quite subtle and require a good knowledge of neuroanatomy.
- The next step is to place the detected lesion in one of the major malformation categories. This morphological classification is set in the context of CNS ontogeny as briefly described above: certain types of gross malformations occur as a result of interference with normal sequences at certain stages of fetal CNS development. These categories include:
  - defects of neural tube closure;
  - defects of forebrain induction;
  - neuronal migration disorders and sulcation defects;
  - disorders of proliferation or size;
  - encephaloclastic defects;
  - cerebellar and spinal malformations;
  - congenital hydrocephalus and cysts.

5.3 Common malformations

The following is only meant to be a guide to the classification system for common malformations in animals and not an exhaustive documentation of all anomalies reported.

5.3.1 Neural tube closure defects

Interference with neurulation, with failure of complete closure of the neural groove to form a neural tube (CNS dysraphism) at various sites and stages, results in various neural tube defects (NTDs) of the brain and/or spinal cord. In NTDs there can be focal defective induction of mesodermal tissue forming the cranial vault and spinal vertebrae resulting in the lesions of cranium bifidum and spina bifida respectively.

Anencephaly

Anencephaly is an uncommon malformation in puppies and calves and of unknown cause, with the complete lack of the development of the brain. There is also no induction of the calvarium. Anencephaly is probably preceded by exencephaly, with complete exposure of the dysraphic neural plate, which then degenerates resulting in anencephaly. Anencephaly must be differentiated from holoprosencephaly, in which the cerebral hemispheres fail to develop but the structures of the midbrain, brainstem and cerebellum are intact. Exposure of amniotic fluid to CSF results in elevated maternal serum levels of α-fetoprotein which is a commonly used diagnostic tool for most forms of human NTDs in conjunction with ultrasound or MRI. Numerous gene mutations have been associated with anencephaly in humans and mice.

Cranium bifidum

With **cranium bifidum** there is a focal osseous defect in the cranial vault through which there is eversion of some of the underlying brain and meninges into a large CSF-containing fluctuant subcutaneous sac called a **meningoencephalocele** (Fig 5.1A). A **cranial meningocele** results from the same process but without the concurrent eversion of any brain tissue. Both occur mainly in the frontal midline region in piglets, kittens and calves.

Spina bifida

In **spina bifida** with absence of one or more segments of the dorsal arch, usually in the lumbosacral segments, there is a number of possible malformations (schematic representation in Fig. 5.1B):

- **Spina bifida occulta** is the least clinically severe variant with skin covering a segmental loss of the dorsal arch but without dorsal herniation of the meninges or spinal cord (Fig. 5.1B,b).
- In **spina bifida aperta** the still open neural tube is visible in the spinal canal through a contiguous defective closure in the overlying skin (Fig. 5.1B,a).
- A **meningocele** results from an arachnoid- and dura mater-lined, fluid-filled subcutaneous sac protruding from the spinal canal through the segmental defect or absence of one or more dorsal arches (Fig 5.1B,d).
- A **meningomyelocele** is a more severe variant with inclusion of spinal cord in the herniated cyst (Fig 5.1B,c).

Various forms of spina bifida occur in calves, lambs, foals, and in English Bulldogs. Hydromyelia and syringomyelia are often found in the underlying spinal cord (see Hydrocephalus below). In **spinal dysraphism** in Weimaraners the spine is intact but a variety of midline anomalies can be found in the cord (fig 5.1D).

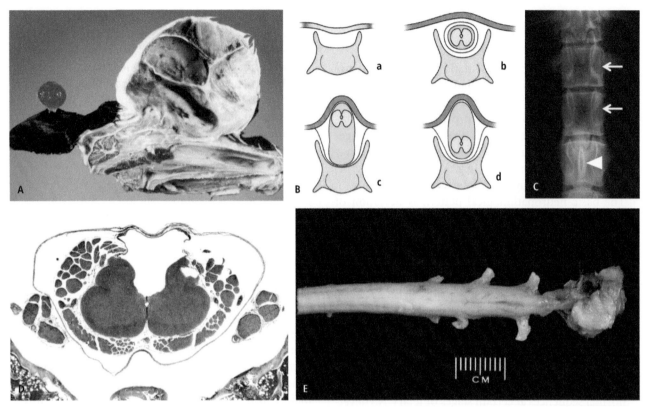

Fig. 5.1 Neural tube closure defects. A: Newborn calf. Head. Meningoencephalocoele. There is partial protrusion of the parietal lobes through a midline defect in the overlying calvarium [cranial bifida], into a large subcutaneous sac lined by meninges once dilated with CSF. B: Diagram of common types of dysraphic malformations of the spinal cord associated with spina bifida a: spina bifida aperta with a lack of closure of the neural tube b: spina bifida occulta c. meningomyelocoele d: meningocoele. C: English bulldog. Spina bifida occulta. Dorso-ventral Xray of thoracolumbar vertebrae, with loss of the dorsal arch and dorsal process over two vertebrae (arrows), compared to adjacent vertebrae with normal dorsal spinous process (arrow head). D: Weimaraner puppy. Spina bifida, absent dorsal arch with a syringomyelic cavity in dorsal columns, HE. E: Kitten with spinal bifida and myelomeningocoele in lower lumbar segments. Note the disorganized tissue mass comprised of cord and meninges.

5.3.2 Defects of forebrain induction

Holoprosencephaly

The forebrain (prosencephalon) arises from bilateral vesicular evaginations of the rostral neural tube in extremely complex patterns of development. In animals one of the more common malformations of this process is **holoprosencephaly**, in which there is variable failure in cerebral hemispheric sagittal cleavage. A small monoventricular cerebrum remains undivided into two hemispheres. The spectrum of subtypes of holoprosencephaly range from a complete absence of development, **holoprosencephaly** (Fig 5.2A), to a minimal abnormality such as agenesis of the olfactory bulbs or lobes. Usually holoprosencephaly is associated with midline facial

abnormalities, e.g. cyclopia, a proboscis and loss of many facial bones including the premaxilla (Fig. 5.2A). Mid- and hindbrain and cerebellum are usually normal (Fig. 5.2B). In man, there is a wide variety of fetal teratogens, including diabetes, infections and alcohol, as well as chromosomal abnormalities and several genetic mutations in different loci. In animals, holoprosencephaly is most commonly seen in fetal lambs, associated with cyclopia and other characteristic facial defects, following a narrow window of opportunity during early pregnancy (around 14 days) of maternal exposure to the plant *Veratrum californicum*. Experimentally the alkaloids cyclopamine and jervine inhibit cholesterol synthesis. Inhibition of the *Patched receptor* associated with low cholesterol levels may then inhibit transcrip-

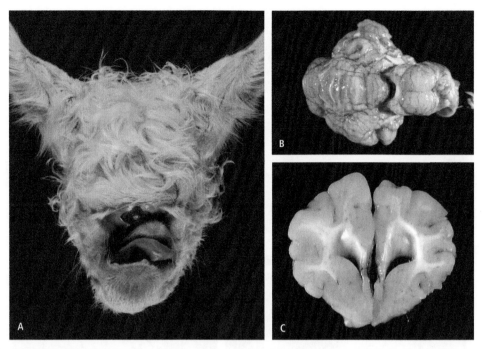

Fig. 5.2 Defects of forebrain induction. A: Neonatal alpaca. Head. Phenotype for holoprosencephaly with cyclopia, maxillary dysplasia and mandibular micrognathia (Reproduced with permission from Dr A. Mete, CAHFS UC Davis.) B: Alpaca brain. Holoprosencephaly with no development of the cerebral hemispheres and thalamus. Rostrally there is a small melanin-pigmented cyst while the mid- and hindbrain and cerebellum are intact. C: Neonatal dog. Brain. There is agenesis of the corpus callosum and hydrocephalus. There is pachygyria of the opposing midline cortex corresponding to the normal precingulate gyri. Note also the characteristic abnormal "bat wing" shape of the lateral ventricles.

tion of the *Sonic hedgehog gene Shh*, responsible for a key signaling molecule in early forebrain induction in mammals.

Agenesis of the corpus callosum

Agenesis of the corpus callosum occurs in young dogs and in most other domestic animals, usually in conjunction with a variety of other malformations including hydrocephalus, agenesis of the septum pellucidum and often abnormal gyral patterns in opposing parasagittal midline gyri (Fig. 5.2C).

5.3.3 Neuronal migration disorders and sulcation defects

This group contains primary malformations with genetic defects resulting in interference with the normal migration of postmitotic neuroblast and glioblast populations, derived from the subependymal plate zone. The neuroblasts are guided by radial glial processes by receptor-dependent signaling to form the layers of the mature cerebral cortex and subsequently the glioblasts to form the white matter of the cerebral hemipheres.

Agyria (lissencephaly) and pachygyria

Agyria, or the more common designation **lissencephaly**, is a malformation with a complete lack of the normal number and thickness of cerebral hemispheric gyri (Fig. 5.3A). On transverse sections of brain there is a thickened cortex with an underlying reduction in the white matter. In lissencephaly there is characteristically a thin heterotopic laminar layer of white matter embedded within the cortex (Fig. 5.3B). Bilateral hydrocephalus of the lateral ventricles is common. There are at least four genetic mutations associated with different human phenotypes of lissencephaly. Lissencephaly is common in Lhaso Apso dogs and manifested from birth by severe cognitive dysfunction, but the genetic defect is unknown. However, as a word of diagnostic caution, rodent and rabbit brains normally lack any gyral formation.

In **pachygyria** there are abnormally fewer but widened gyral convolutions with shallow sulci (Fig. 5.3C). On transverse sections the cortex is abnormally thickened with reduced neuronal layers and the underlying white matter is reduced in thickness; focal neuronal heterotopias are often embedded in this white matter.

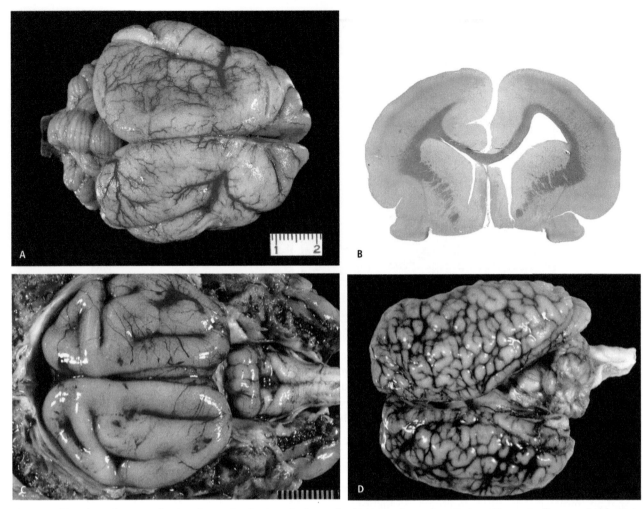

Fig. 5.3 Disorders of neuronal migration and sulcation. A: 6-month-old Lhaso Apso dog. Brain with agyria (lissencephaly). Note the lack of any hemispheric gyral formation and slight collapse of cerebral hemispheres suggestive of some degree of hydrocephalus. B: Same dog, transverse section through the cerebral hemispheres with complete lack of gyral formation. Note thickened cortex and and a bilateral midcortical laminar layer of aberrant white matter. The subependymal white matter is relatively thin and there is bilateral slightly asymmetrical hydrocephalus. HE-LFB stain. C: Newborn goat. Brain. Pachygyria. Normal cortical gyri are replaced by fewer greatly thickened gyral convolutions bilaterally in the cerebral hemispheres. There is also a severe cerebellar hyoplasia. D: Calf brain. Polymicrogyria. There are multifocal random areas of small disorganized cortex with smaller gyri in the cerebral hemispheres.

Polymicrogyria

Polymicrogyria is due to excessive cortical folding with gyral fusioning with an increase in numbers of smaller irregularly convoluted cortical gyri. The microgyrial patterns of distribution can be focal, random, bilateral and/or symmetrical (Fig. 5.3D). Clinical blindness has been associated with occipital lobe involvement in the dog. On transverse sections the cortex can be extremely convoluted but thinner and more laminated than normal. It has a multifactorial etiology in people, seen with familial genetic syndromes, metabolic diseases, infectious agents and ischemia.

5.3.4 Disorders of proliferation or size

Megalencephaly

Megalencephaly is an absolute increase in the size of the brain while **megaloencephaly** refers to an enlargement of the head irrespective of cause, e.g. congenital hydrocephalus.

Microoencephaly

Microoencephaly is a congenital defect resulting in a brain of smaller than usual size and weight, due to relative lack of both gray and white matter, mainly affecting

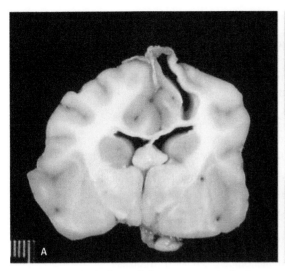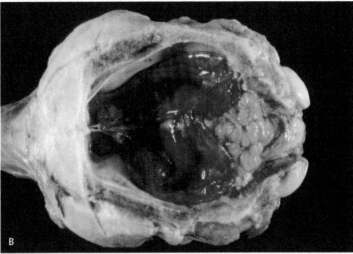

Fig. 5.4 Encephaloclastic defects. A: Dog. Brain. Porencephaly. There is a single, once fluid-filled, cyst in both white and gray matter but without connections to either the ventricle or subarachnoid space. B: Neonatal calf. Hydranencephaly. This calf was transplacentally infected with modified live bluetongue virus at 60 days' gestation. The cerebral hemispheres have been essentially destroyed and there are residual cystic meningeal sacs, which have collapsed. The cerebellum and brainstem appear normal.

the cerebrum. It can be found in conjunction with cerebellar anomalies from teratogenic virus infections in lambs, calves and piglets. Cerebral convolutions are very simplified and have abnormal anatomical gyral patterns.

5.3.5 Encephaloclastic defects

These are classified as secondary malformations which occur probably as a result of an acquired transplacental and destructive process in pre-existing brain tissue.

Porencephaly

Porencephaly is a usually single, cystic, fluid-filled cavity of varying size, in the wall of the cerebral hemispheres, usually in one frontal lobe (Fig. 5.4A). Uncommonly, there may be connections between the cyst and with both or either the ventricular and subarachnoid space. Typically it involves mainly white matter. Occasionally the cystic cavities may be bilateral and symmetrical as occurs with both fetal Border disease infection, swayback with *in utero* copper deficiency, and in fetal hyperthermia. The cystic wall is smooth surfaced and surrounded histologically by normal brain tissue and not lined by ependyma.

Hydranencephaly

Hydranencephaly is caused by a more globally destructive event within pre-existing tissue of the cerebral hemispheres in which there is massive bilateral symmetrical necrosis with almost complete loss of pre-existing tissue and replacement by huge fluid-filled sacs contained by the intact leptomeninges (Fig. 5.4B). Sometimes there

can be residual peripheral evidence of an inflammatory or ischemic process with gitter cells, mineralization and gliosis in any surviving brain parenchyma. The lateral ventricles remain intact. Many fetal transplacental virus infections, including those of wild and modified *bluetongue, Wesselbron, Akabane, Cache River Valley, bovine virus diarrhea* and *Border disease* are associated with hydranencephaly in ruminants. Hydranencephaly has been associated with *feline parvovirus* infection (see Table 5.1). Experimental induction of hydranencephaly by timed transplacental bovine fetal infection of bluetongue virus (at 50–70 days' gestation) suggests selective viral homing, targeting and subsequent endothelial cell cytolysis in the germinative subependymal zone with ischemia as the precipitating event in tissue destruction. The ependymal lining of the lateral ventricles remains intact though there maybe *ex vacuo* dilation of the lateral ventricles. In contrast, transplacental bovine fetal infection at between 75 and 100 days' gestation induces porencephaly, illustrating that teratogens can cause different malformations presumably due to a temporal change in cell susceptibility to viral infection.

5.3.6 Malformations in the caudal fossa and spinal cord

A rather large group of anomalies in the brainstem, cerebellum and spinal cord is difficult to classify according to the scheme described above, because of their complexity with simultaneous occurrence of diverging types of lesions. Such malformations are collectively discussed in this section.

Table 5.1 Some important fetal teratogenic virus infections in different species.

VIRUS	SPECIES	CNS LESIONS
Feline panleukopenia virus (*Parvovirus*)	Kitten	Cerebellar hypoplasia, dysplasia, Purkinje cell loss, hydranencephaly
Classical swine fever virus (*Pestivirus*)	Piglet	Dysmyelinogenesis, cerebellar hypoplasia
Bovine virus diarrhea virus (BVDV) (*Pestivirus*)	Calf, lamb	Hydrocephalus, cerebellar hypo- or aplasia, prosencephaly in calves; hypomyelination, porencephaly in lambs
Akabane virus, Cache Valley virus (*Orthobunya virus*)	Lamb, calf	Hydranencephaly, arthrogryposis, cerebellar hypoplasia, porencephaly
Bluetongue virus (*Orbivirus*)	Lamb, calf	Hydranencephaly
Canine parvovirus (*Parvovirus*)	Puppy	Cerebellar hypoplasia, dysplasia
Chuzan virus (*Orbivirus*)	Calf	Hydranencephaly, cerebellar hypoplasia
Aino virus (*Orthobunyavirus*)	Calf	Arthrogryposis, hydranencephaly, cerebellar hypoplasia
Border disease virus (*Pestivirus*)	Lamb	Porencephaly, hypomyelination
Wesselbron virus (*Flavivirus*)	Calf	Hydranencephaly, porencephaly

Cerebellar agenesis

In **complete cerebellar agenesis** there is complete absence of any cerebellar tissue. This malformation is well known in calves, particularly of the Simmental breed. Characteristically, these calves are unable to stand after birth or even to right themselves in a sternal position. In **cerebellar vermal agenesis** there is a selective agenesis of the vermal lobules even though the lateral lobes appear morphologically intact and of normal size (Fig. 5.5A).

Granule cell hypoplasia or aplasia

Granule cell hypoplasia can be classified as either a primary genetic or secondary malformation. Anatomically all or parts of the cerebellum can be affected. This group of cerebellar disorders is common in many pure-breed dogs but presents with a bewildering range of clinical signs, onset, progression and lesions. The underlying genetic basis identified for a similar range of human spinocerebellar ataxias transformed both the classification and pathogenesis of these diseases and such information and similar resolution can be expected in the dog eventually.

Cerebellar hypoplasia and dysplasia

Cerebellar folial hypoplasia, where only parts of the cerebellar folial cortex are affected, is one of the most common malformations in the dog and ruminants.

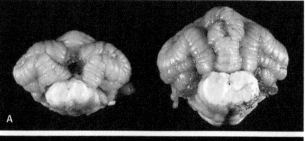
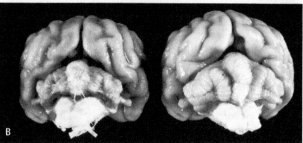

Fig. 5.5 A: Puppy with selective cerebellar vermal agenesis compared with an age-matched control normal dog on right. B: Dog. Cerebellar hypoplasia. In the brain on the left there is hypoplasia affecting both the vermis and lateral lobes without any apparent pattern compared with an age- and breed-matched control cerebellum (right).

Equine cerebellar hypoplasia and dysplasia occurs as a familial entity in Arab and Arabian crossbred foals. The folial dysplasia with massive disorganization of the Purkinje cell layer and a hypoplastic granule cell layer is most likely the result of defective signaling of the radial

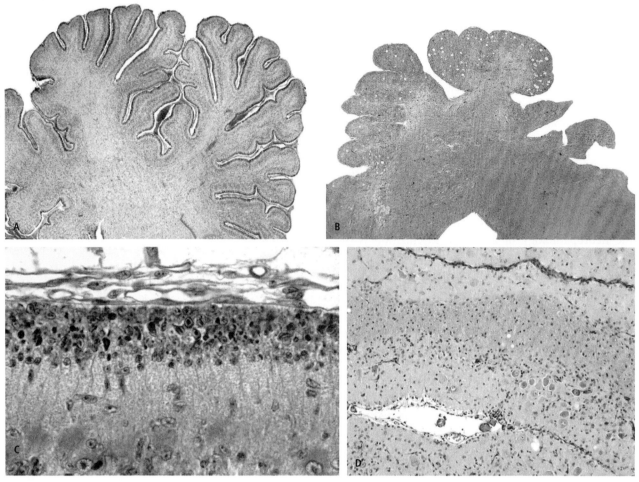

Fig. 5.6 Cat. Virus-induced cerebellar hypoplasia. A: Kitten. Normal neonatal cerebellum including the folial cortex. HE. B. Kitten with extreme cerebellar hypoplasia and dysplasia from *in utero* transplacental feline panleukopenia virus infection. HE. C: Newborn kitten. Cerebellum. Feline panleukopenia virus intranuclear viral inclusion bodies and cytolysis of the subpial neuroblast layer. HE. D: Kitten. Extreme cerebellar folial dysplasia and hypoplasia with almost non-existent granular layer and dysplastic disorganized Purkinje cells. HE.

glia, which provide a scaffold for the normal inward migration of neuroblasts from the subpial layer to populate the granule cell layer. In turn the resultant interference with subsequent and dependent Purkinje cell migration leads to their aberrant location. A similar pathogenesis has been demonstrated in the homozygous Weaver (Wv/Wv) mouse. It remains to be determined whether there may be an overlap between this disease and cerebellocortical degeneration in Arabian horses (discussed in Chapter 8).

Certain types of cerebellar hypoplasias or dysplasias are due to specific **maternal transplacental teratogenic viral infections** (Table 5.1). At defined gestational windows of opportunity, in dogs, cats, calves and piglets, a maternal viral infection is transmitted transplacentally to the fetus and selectively targets subpial neuroblast cell precursors prior to their centripetal migration to form the cerebellar folia. The viral-induced cytolysis results in massive loss of subpial neuroblasts, which were destined to populate the granular cell layer, which therefore becomes hypoplastic and dysplastic (Fig. 5.6). Migration of Purkinje cells to their destination is disrupted and disorganized due to the distortion of receptor-mediated signaling from the defective granular layer, which completes the spectrum of widespread cerebellar folial dysplasia and hypoplasia. Sometimes there is histological evidence of non-suppurative encephalitis. Such grossly obvious cerebellar hypoplasia/dysplasia can affect all or parts of the vermis and lateral lobes (Fig. 5.5B). Such lesions result from transplacental fetal virus infection with feline panleukopenia virus (parvovirus) in kittens (fig 5.6), canine parvovirus in puppies, pestivirus infection (bovine virus diarrhea virus) in calves and with classical swine fever virus (pestivirus) in piglets.

Cerebellar hypoplasia and hypomyelination occurs in piglets from sows treated with an organophosphate insecticide (Neguvon) during the second half of gestation. Piglets are born with a congenital tremor syndrome. The CNS of affected piglets shows various degrees of cerebellar hypoplasia mostly involving Purkinje cells and generalized hypomyelinogenesis. Viral -induced hypomyelinogensis is discussed in Chapter 3, the neuropathology of abnormal myelination is discussed in Chapter 8.

Dandy-Walker syndrome

Dandy-Walker syndrome is a rare midline defect of the cerebellum most commonly identified in the foal, calf and lamb and of unknown etiology. It has also been reported in dogs. The three essential lesions to confirm a diagnosis are cerebellar vermal agenesis, cystic dilation of the expanded fourth ventricle and enlargement of the caudal fossa (Fig. 5.7). Hydrocephalus and polygyria of cerebral convolutions can occur concurrently.

Arnold Chiari malformation

The **Arnold Chiari malformation** in people is classified into three different phenotypes of cerebellar deformities

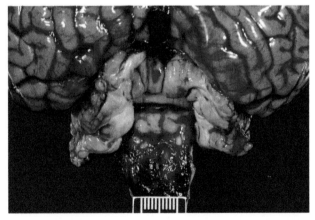

Fig. 5.7 Neonatal foal. Dandy-Walker syndrome. There is marked vermal cerebellar agenesis with cystic distension of the fourth ventricle.

commonly associated with hydrocephalus, and meningomyelocele with spina bifida. In the most comparable malformation in dogs (Arnold Chiari type II), the caudal fossa is shallow and of reduced volume with elongation of the cerebellar vermis and of the medulla with their combined displacement into the cervical spinal canal (Fig. 5.8). In the Cavalier King Charles Spaniel with Arnold Chiari-like type II malformation, using three-dimensional MRI, the caudal fossa is proportionately smaller than in other breeds while the ratio of the parenchymal tissue volume to that of the caudal fossa is critically higher. In these dogs with associated syringomyelia, the width of the syrinx directly correlates with the increased size of the fourth ventricle of the caudal fossa. See MRI Atlas.

Defects of the spinal cord

These include **myelodysplasia** usually associated with spina bifida (see above) and **diastematomyelia** which means complete duplication of the spinal cord which is sometimes seen in foals and calves. **Diplomyelia** occurs in foals and calves where there is histologically a dysplastic mixture of gray and white matter of two partially merged spinal cords (Fig. 5.9A). **Segmental aplasia**, where whole segments of the cord and vertebral column are lacking, can occur at any level, preferentially in the lumbar segments, e.g. **sacrococcygeal agenesis** in Manx cats (Fig. 5.9B) or **perosomus elumbis** in calves, in which the whole lumboscral and coccygeal spine is absent.

5.3.7 Congenital hydrocephalus and other anomalies of CSF pathways

Hydrocephalus is one of the most common congenital anomalies in all domestic animals especially in the dog. Hydrocephalus is defined as the enlargement of all or part of the ventricular system in the brain and spinal cord, due in most cases to the rate of production of cerebrospinal fluid exceeding its rate of removal. There is a wide spectrum of ventriculomegaly associated with hydrocephalus. Knowledge of the normal intraventricular anatomy and of the sites of production, flow and absorption of cerebrospinal fluid is essential to interpret the various causes and manifestations of hydrocephalus (see Chapter 1). Also critical to the evolution of most forms of hydrocephalus is a constant or episodic period of raised intraventricular pressure. Hydrocephalus can be classified by different criteria but we will start with the concept of it either being communicating with no detectable pathological lesions or non-communicating

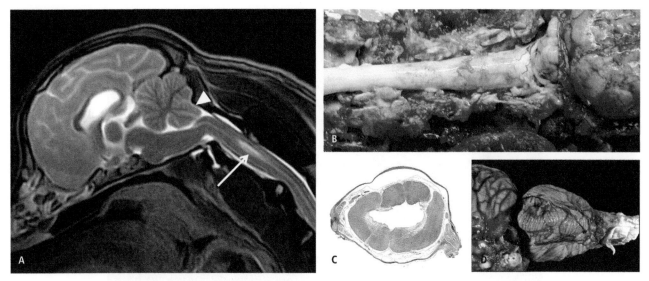

Fig. 5.8 Dog. Cavalier King Charles Spaniel. Brain and cervical spinal cord. Arnold Chiari-like type II malformation. A: MRI. Sagittal section. A T2W image illustrates the abnormal cerebellar crowding in the small-sized caudal fossa with herniation of vermis through foramen magnum (arrowhead), and a syrinx in the cervical spinal cord (small arrow). B: Same case. Brain and cervical spinal cord. There is marked enlargement of cranial cervical cord segments associated with hydro- and syringomyelia. C: Same dog. Transverse section of CSF-filled syringomyelic cavity in cervical spinal cord. D: Newborn calf. Arnold Chiari-like malformation with massive cerebellar coning through the foramen magnum on to the cervical spinal cord segments.

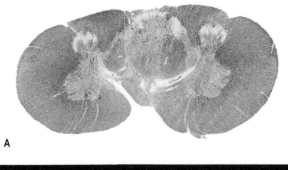

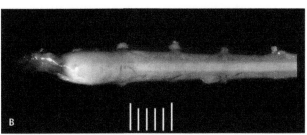

Fig. 5.9 A: Neonatal foal. Spinal cord. Diplomyelia. Transverse section through the lumbar spinal cord illustrating the severe dysplasia, partial duplication and disorganization of both white and gray matter. HE-LFB. B: Manx cat. Lumbar cord. Segmental agenesis of the lumbar spinal cord distal to L4 segment.

(either partial or completely obstructive) due to defined lesions.

Communicating hydrocephalus

Communicating hydrocephalus is not common and usually assumes the form of bilateral and symmetrical dilation of the ventricular system without any detectable macro- or microscopic lesions (Fig. 5.10). Most toy breed (Chihuahua, Yorkshire Terrier, Shi Tzu etc.) and some brachycephalic breed (e.g. Boxer) dogs from birth have much larger intraventricular volumes compared with their cohorts but this distension may be just a normal physiological finding. However, if clinical neurological signs occur then such ventriculomegaly would be classified as a primary malformation of communicating idiopathic hydrocephalus.

Non-communicating hydrocephalus

The secondary teratogen-induced type of **non-communicating hydrocephalus** is generally a result of partial or complete obstruction to normal CSF flow at any of several critical stricture points within the intraventricular pathways or in the extraventricular subarachnoid space (Fig. 5.11). Diagnostic neuroimaging

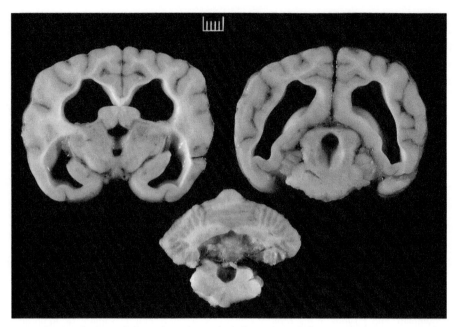

Fig. 5.10 Puppy. Communicating hydrocephalus. There is marked distension of the ventricular system and no apparent gross or microscopic lesion to account for the obstruction.

(MRI) is extremely useful for clinical detection and for identification of intra- or extraventricular sites of obstruction based on the specific pattern of ventriculomegaly (Fig. 5.10). The major intraventricular sites of potential obstruction include either of the interventricular foramina between the lateral and third ventricles, the mesencephalic aqueduct (Fig. 5.11C,D), or lateral foramina of the fourth ventricle. Fusion of the rostral colliculi is also observed associated with stenosis of the aqueduct (Fig 5.11C). The main extraventricular site for lesions is in the subarachnoid space of the brain and spinal cord where the arachnoid villi mediate CSF transfer into the dural venous sinuses. The timing, site and degree of obstruction in the fetus determines the severity of the hydrocephalus and effect, e.g. of prenatal doming of the skull due to increased intraventricular pressure inhibiting the normal closure of sutures of the cranial vault. Acquired congenital hydrocephalus is considered a secondary malformation due to the fetal lesions from a wide variety of teratogens. Transplacental viral (see Table 5.1) or protozoal (e.g. *Neospora* and *Toxoplasma* sp) infections can result in fetal aqueductal subependymal gliosis and stenosis, porencephaly, ependymitis and possibly loss of arachnoid villi in the subarachnoid space, all of which can result in some form of congenital hydrocephalus. Rarely neonatal tumors of probable fetal onset (e.g canine thalamic leiomyosarcoma) can result in obstructive hydrocephalus.

Hydrocephalus *ex vacuo*

A third form of congenital or post natal hydrocephalus is classified as **compensatory** or *ex vacuo* **hydrocephalus,** in which primary loss of brain tissue leads to a local distension of the ventricle into the lesion site of cavitation. This form of hydrocephalus is not necessarily dependent on any change in hydrostatic pressure or in obstruction/production of CSF.

Secondary lesions of hydrocephalus

The sequence of pathological effects of hydrocephalus starts with increased ventricular hydrostatic pressure proximal to the site of obstruction, flattening, loss and increased permeability of the lining ependymal cells, periventricular interstitial edema with demyelination and axonal atrophy and eventual loss in subependymal white matter and induced ventriculomegaly. The cortex is last and least affected (Fig. 5.10 and Fig. 5.11). Externally the gyri may appear flattened. The lesions are irreversible. A common secondary effect with bilateral lateral ventricular hydrocephalus is loss of the septum pellucidum (Fig. 5.10 and Fig. 5.11). Rapidly progressing hydrocephalus with high intraventricular pressure in young puppies may lead to rupture of the ependyma with formation of CSF-filled clefts and diverticula in the brain parenchyma as well as hemorrhage, especially in the area of the caudate nucleus and capsula interna

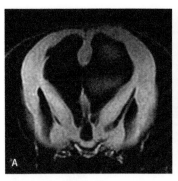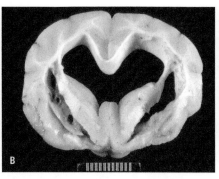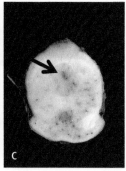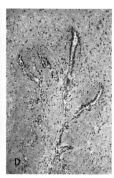

Fig. 5.11 A: Puppy. Brain. Congenitally acquired hydrocephalus. MRI with a FLAIR sequence illustrating the bilateral symmetrical hydrocephalus in lateral ventricles and secondary diverticula through the basal nuclei and internal capsule. B: Same puppy. Brain at same slice level. There is massive enlargement of the ventricles. In the area around the internal capsule there is obvious bilateral cleft formation as a result of pressure-induced rupture of the ependymal lining and ischemic necrosis of the tissue. The yellow–brown discoloration indicates old hemorrhage. C: Dog with obstructive hydrocephalus, midbrain. There is fusion of rostral colliculi and stenosis of the mesencephalic aqueduct, which inhibits normal CSF flow caudally with subsequent rostral distension of the lateral ventricles. D: Same dog as in C. Mesencephalic aqueduct. Histologically there is loss of patency of the collapsed aqueduct due to destruction of most of the ependymal lining and subependymal gliosis. HE.

(Fig. 5.11B). Because of variable degrees of associated suppurative and non-suppurative inflammation these lesions are also known as **hydrocephalus associated with periventricular encephalitis**.

Hydromyelia

Congenital **hydromyelia** is a focal or generalized dilation of the central canal most common in lumbar segments. Thinning or compression of the ependymal cell lining and loss of cilia can be the result of increased sustained intraventricular pressure within the central canal as often occurs with hydrocephalus. Alternatively, it may result from proximal strictures or occlusions of the central canal associated with concurrent malformations, for example Arnold Chiari malformations (ACM, see above).

Syringomyelia and syringobulbia

Syringomyelia is defined as a cystic fluid-filled tubular cavity within the spinal cord extending over several segments. As mentioned in Section 5.3.1 it may occur as a primary inherited malformation most commonly associated with NTDs. Acquired syringomyelia is usually preceded by hydromyelia and results from rupture of the ependymal cell lining and secondary cavitation into either gray or white matter of the cord. Chronically the cavities can be lined by reactive astrogliosis. This lesion has been most intensively studied in Cavalier King Charles Spaniels (CKCS) with ACM (Fig. 5.8C) but this syndrome has been reported in a wide variety of dog breeds. In ACM in CKCS, syrinx formation has been attributed to altered CSF dynamics due to compression of the subarachnoid space after obstruction of the foramen magnum by the herniated cerebellar tissue (Fig. 5.8). See MRI Atlas. **Syringobulbia** results from the formation of fluid-filled slit-like cavities in the medulla, which usually communicate with the lumen of the fourth ventricle.

Arachnoidal and ependymal cysts

These are CSF-filled cavities (strictly speaking not true cysts) arising from the arachnoid membrane or recesses of the ventricles, some of which maybe of congenital derivation. Ependymal cysts are extremely rare in animals (see MRI Atlas) but arachnoidal cysts are relatively common in the meninges of the spinal cord of dogs. **Spinal arachnoidal cysts** may compress the spinal cord leading to often fluctuating but generally progressive signs. The diagnosis is best based on MRI. At necropsy such cysts usually collapse following exposure and removal of the CNS. The main finding at the site of the cyst is a compressed spinal cord, the lesions of which are discussed in Chapter 4 on Trauma. A further common location of cysts in dogs is the space dorsal to the roof of the midbrain (consisting of the colliculi or lamina quadrigemina) between the occipital lobes and cerebellum. This space also contains an extension of the third ventricle (suprapineal recess) and the pineal gland. Cysts in this area are usually called **quadrigeminal cysts**. Large cysts may cause seizures or cerebellar signs. These lesions are easily detected on MRI (Fig. 5.12A). Some of

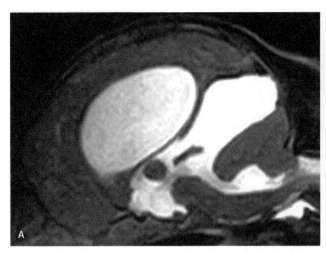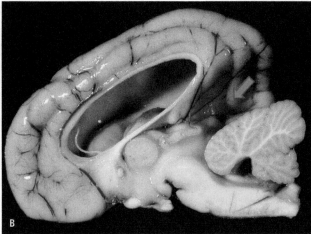

Fig. 5.12 Puppy with quadrigeminal cyst. A: Sagittal MRI with the T2W image revealing the patent connection between the lumen of the quadrigeminal cyst and the third ventricle. The cerebellar vermis is herniated through the foramen magnum. B: Gross image of the same puppy as in A. The cyst has collapsed but leaves a markedly enlarged space (arrow) with obvious induced compression of the occipital lobes and cerebellum with cerebellar coning. There is also dilatation of the lateral ventricle.

them communicate with the third or fourth ventricle (and may be partially lined by ependyma). At necropsy they collapse but leave an enlarged space resulting from compression atrophy of the occipital lobes and cerebellum (Fig. 5.12B). See MRI Atlas.

Further reading

Neural tube closure defects

M. Huisinga *et al.* Anencephaly in a German Shepherd dog. Vet Pathol 2010;47:948–951.

Kiviranta AM, Lappalainen AK, Hagner K, Jokinen T. Dermoid sinus and spina bifida in three dogs and a cat. J Small Anim Pract 2011;52:319–324.

Defects of forebrain induction

Welch KD, Panter KE, Lee ST, Gardner DR, Stegelmeier BL, Cook D. Cyclopamine-induced synophthalmia in sheep: defining a critical window and toxicokinetic evaluation. J Appl Toxicol 2009;29: 414–421.

Neuronal migration disorders and sulcation defects

Saito M *et al.* Magnetic resonance imaging features of lissencephaly in 2 Lhaso Apsos. Vet Radiol Ultrasound 2002;43:331–337.

Jurney C, Haddad J, Crawford N, Miller AD, Van Winkle TJ, Vite CH, Sponenberg P, Inzana KD, Cook CR, Britt L, O'Brien DP. Polymicrogyria in Standard Poodles. J Vet Int Med 2009;23: 871–874.

Encephaloclastic defects

Montgomery DL, Van Olphen A, Van Campen H, Hansen TR. The fetal brain in bovine viral diarrhea virus-infected calves: lesions, distribution, and cellular heterogeneity of viral antigen at 190 days gestation. Vet Pathol 2008;45:288–296.

Bielefeldt-Ohmann H, Tolnay AE, Reisenhauer CE, Hansen TR, Smirnova N, Van Campen H. Transplacental infection with non-cytopathic bovine viral diarrhoea virus types 1b and 2: viral spread and molecular neuropathology. J Comp Pathol 2008;138:72–85.

Vercauteren G, Miry C, Vandenbussche F, Ducatelle R, Van der Heyden S, Vandemeulebroucke E, De Leeuw I, Deprez P, Chiers K, De Clercq K. Bluetongue virus serotype 8-associated congenital hydranencephaly in calves. Transbound Emerg Dis 2008;55: 293–298.

Cerebellar hypoplasia

Résibois A, Coppens A, Poncelet L. Naturally occurring parvovirus-associated feline hypogranular cerebellar hypoplasia – a comparison to experimentally-induced lesions using immunohistology. Vet Pathol 2007;44:831–841.

Dandy Walker syndrome

Wong D, Winter M, Haynes J, Sponseller B, Schleining J. Dandy-Walker-like syndrome in a quarter horse colt. J Vet Int Med 2007;21:1130–1134.

Chiari malformation, Syringomyelia

Driver CJ, Rusbridge C, Cross HR, McGonnell I, Volk HA. Relationship of brain parenchyma within the caudal fossa and ventricle size to syringomyelia in cavalier King Charles spaniels. J Small Anim Prac 2010;51:382–386.

Park C, Kang BT, Yoo JH, Park HM *et al.* Syringomyelia in three small breed dogs secondary to Chiari-like malformation: clinical and diagnostic findings. J Vet Sci 2009;10:365–367.

Wolfe KC, Poma R. Syringomyelia in the Cavalier King Charles spaniel (CKCS) dog. Neurology 2010;51:95–102.

Hydrocephalus

Rekate HL A contemporary definition and classification of hydrocephalus. Semin Ped Neurol 2009;16:9–15.

Thomas WB Hydrocephalus in dogs and cats. Vet Clin Small Anim 2010;40:143–159.

Wünschmann A, Oglesbee M. Periventricular changes associated with spontaneous canine hydrocephalus. Vet Pathol 2001;38: 67–73.

Arachnoidal and ependymal cysts

Skeen TM, Olby NJ, Muñana KR, Sharp NJ. Spinal arachnoid cysts in 17 dogs. J Am Anim Hosp Assoc 2003;39:271–282.

Matiasek LA, Platt SR, Shaw S, Dennis R. Clinical and magnetic resonance imaging characteristics of quadrigeminal cysts in dogs. J Vet Intern Med 2007;21:1021–1026.

Wyss-Fluehmann G, Konar M, Jaggy A, Vandevelde M, Oevermann A. Cerebellar ependymal cyst in a dog. Vet Pathol 2008;45: 910–913.

This book is accompanied by a companion website which is maintained by the Division of Diagnostic Imaging, Dept of Clinical Veterinary Medicine, Vetsuisse Faculty, University of Bern, Switzerland.

www.wiley.com/go/vandevelde/veterinaryneuropathology

6

Metabolic–toxic diseases

In this group of diseases, the lesions are caused by either toxins or deficiencies. Intoxications are caused by exposure to organic (e.g. pesticides) and inorganic (e.g. lead) compounds, or naturally occurring plant, microbial or animal poisons. Deficiencies result from inadequate intake of certain minerals and vitamins. Endogenous intoxications or deficiencies may occur when metabolically important organs such as the liver or kidney fail to function properly.

These diseases generally cause acute neurological signs and bilateral, usually symmetrical, lesions involving specific anatomic areas of the brain and/or spinal cord. The strikingly selective vulnerability may be due to factors including regional differences in vascular perfusion patterns or the differences in distribution/concentration of receptors for toxic molecules. Lesions vary according to the etiology and stage of the disease. The precise molecular mechanisms of cellular damage to primary targets such as neurons, glial cells or blood vessels are, however, poorly understood. Intriguingly, the same toxins or deficiencies may induce different types of patterns and lesions in different species. Much can be learned in this respect from experimental toxicology.

6.1 General strategy for diagnosis of metabolic–toxic lesions

6.1.1 The major patterns

The typical clinical presentation is of an animal (of any age) with peracute/acute onset of signs and a frequently fatal outcome. The disease may affect a single animal or more likely occur as an outbreak. There are three major types of gross or microscopically detected lesions, which are (1) malacia, sometimes with hemorrhage; (2) selective necrosis or loss of neurons, axons or myelin; and (3) spongy state. Most of these diseases result in lesions that occur in an anatomically restricted bilaterally symmetrical pattern although sometimes they can be unilateral.

6.1.2 Further differential diagnosis

A classification of the differential diagnosis of candidate diseases based on each of the three major morphological patterns and lesion types is shown in Fig. 6.1.

- With malacia as the predominant lesion, the specific anatomical distribution pattern (e.g. cerebral cortex, subcortical white matter, white matter, spinal cord) provides diagnostically important etiological information (see Fig. 6.1). Malacic lesions caused by metabolic–toxic problems have to be differentiated from other conditions as shown in Fig. 6.1.
- In cases of selective lesions without marked destruction and loss of the normal tissue architecture determine whether either neurons, axons or myelin are primarily involved. Since this type of lesion is also found in degenerative diseases, see Fig. 8.1.
- When spongy state of the tissue is the most striking change, determine first whether there are any underlying cellular changes since spongy change can be a reactive event to, for example, neuronal necrosis. Spongy state also occurs in other categories of diseases. Consult Fig. 6.14 for the differential diagnosis of spongy state in the CNS.
- From the morphological classification, there is some overlap between lesions of toxic–metabolic cause and those included as degenerative diseases. This overlap is not surprising as most degenerative diseases involve

Veterinary Neuropathology: Essentials of Theory and Practice, First Edition. Marc Vandevelde, Robert J. Higgins, and Anna Oevermann.
© 2012 John Wiley & Sons, Ltd. Published 2012 by John Wiley & Sons, Ltd.

Table 6.1 Overview of metabolic-toxic diseases of the CNS according to major lesion patterns.

PATTERN	METABOLIC	TOXIC
Malacia (see Fig. 6.1)		
Gray matter	Thiamin deficiency in ruminants Thiamin deficiency in carnivores Water deprivation (pig, bovine) Hippocampal sclerosis (dog, cat) Seizures (dog, cat) Hypoglycemia (all)	Sulfur (ruminants) Carbamate (carnivores) Lead (all) Mercury (all) Selenium (pig) Cyanide (dog, cat) Hydrogen sulfide (ruminants, pigs) Metronidazole (dogs, cat) Nigropallidal encephalomalacia (horse) Annual ryegrass staggers (ruminants) *Aeschynomene indica* (pig) Feline hippocampal necrosis
White matter	Swayback (sheep)	Equine leukoencephalomalacia
Both		Enterotoxemia (ruminants, pig) CO (all)
Selective changes (see Fig. 8.1)		
Neurons	Enzootic ataxia (goat, sheep) Equine motor neuron disease	*Aspergillus clavatus* (ruminants) *Phalaris* grass staggers (ruminants, horse) *Crysocoma tenuifolia* (sheep) Dysautonomia (horse, cat, dog) Toxic lysosomal storage (ruminants)
Axons	Cobalamin deficiency (cat) Vitamin A deficiency (pig) Vitamin E deficiency (dog, horse)	Zamia staggers (ruminants) Sorghum (horse, ruminants) *Halinium braziliense* (sheep) Perennial ryegrass staggers (ruminants, horse) *Tribulus terrestris* (sheep) Organophosphates (all) Tri-nitro (pig)
Myelin	Hound ataxia Irradiated feed (cat)	
Spongy state (see Fig. 6.14)		
	Liver failure (all) Renal failure (all)	Hexachlorophene (dog, cat) Ammonia (ruminants, pig) Closantel (goat, sheep) Bromethalin (dog, cat) *Helichrysum argyrosphaerum* (ruminants) *Stypandra* sp (ruminants) Sporadic brain edema in Swiss cattle

genetically determined metabolic abnormalities of specific cell populations or cell organelles. Therefore, anamnestic and clinical data are also important for etiological clarification. Whereas degenerative diseases generally occur in young animals, possibly as familial clusters, metabolic–toxic diseases are acquired and may affect animals of any age. Furthermore, degenerative diseases commonly have an insidious onset and a slowly progressive course in contrast to metabolic–toxic diseases with their more acute onset and rapid clinical progress.

- Although some toxic–metabolic disorders can be diagnosed from specific topography and type of lesions, determining the etiology requires an analysis of combined anamnestic, clinical and pathological data.

6.2 Encephalomalacias/myelomalacias

Encephalomalacia is defined as grossly observable softening of the brain and is a descriptive term for necrosis. It can be the result of many different types of insults. Malacia may affect the gray matter (polioen-cephalomalacia, poliomyelomalacia), the white matter (leukoencephalomalacia) or both (encephalomalacia).

Common to these diseases is their acute or peracute onset and extensive tissue destruction resulting in grossly detectable malacia in a bilateral, often symmetrical distribution pattern. Note that malacia is a final common pathway of a variety of insults including toxins, deficiencies and ischemia. In peracute cases, there may be no macroscopic lesions yet and microscopic changes may be very subtle. For the differential diagnosis of malacia see Fig. 6.1.

6.2.1 Polioencephalomalacia (PE) or cerebrocortical necrosis (CCN)

General morphological features

In many toxic–metabolic disorders the cerebral cortex (including hippocampus) is primarily affected and this is commonly called either cerebrocortical necrosis or polioencephalomalacia. However, other areas such as basal and thalamic nuclei, colliculi and cerebellar cortex may also be involved. Grossly and externally, the brain may be acutely swollen with cortical gyri appearing flattened and wider than normal, while the sulci are

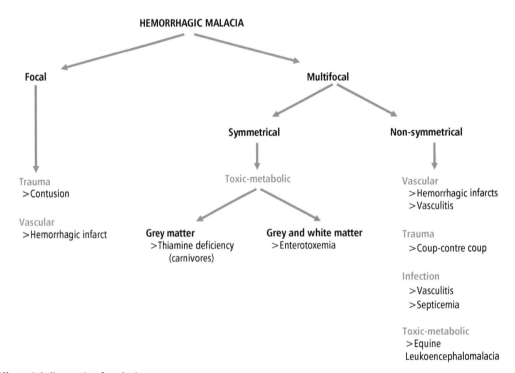

Fig. 6.1 Differential diagnosis of malacia.

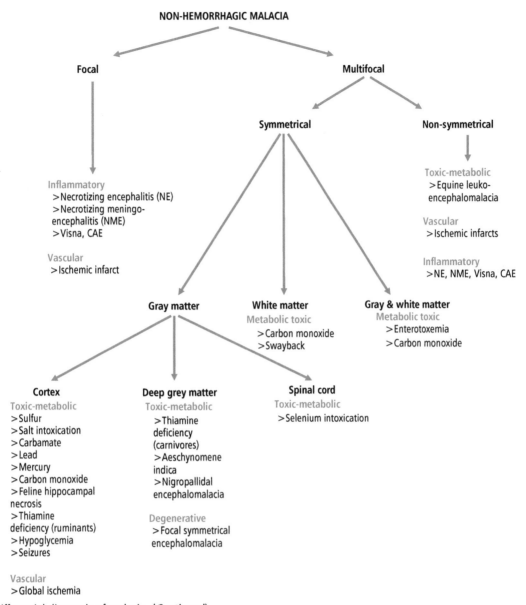

Fig. 6.1 Differential diagnosis of malacia. (*Continued*)

compressed. Additionally, a bilaterally symmetrical yellowish discoloration of the gray matter may be observed (Fig. 6.2A). In severe cases, brain edema causes subtentorial herniation of the occipital lobes and cerebellar vermal herniation through the foramen magnum. Later there is a strict line of demarcation of the malacic gray matter from the underlying intact white matter. Chronically, cystic fluid-filled cavities are observed.

Histologically, acutely there is edema and acidophilic neuronal necrosis (Fig. 6.3A,B), of varying severity. These neurons initially have a swollen granular cytoplasm and centrally placed karyorrhectic nuclei (see Chapter 1). Astrocytes become reactive and have vesicular nuclei. There is also prominent vascular endothelial hypertrophy and hyperplasia (Fig. 6.3A,B). Edema and neuronal necrosis can occur in a band-like (*pseudolaminar*) pattern parallel to the gyral surface (Fig. 6.3A) or can affect the full thickness of the cortex. After approximately 2–3 days blood-derived macrophages infiltrate the necrotic neuropil and become are actively phagocytic as gitter cells (Fig. 6.4C). In chronic cases, the fluid-filled cystic spaces are bordered and traversed by astroglial processes.

PE or CCN in large animals

CCN or PE in cattle and sheep is caused by a variety of toxins and deficiencies. Currently, **sulfur intoxication** (due to consumption of sulfate-rich diets or water) and dietary **thiamin deficiency** are incriminated as major causes in sheep and cattle; thiamin inactivation may also be involved in sulfur intoxication. Since under physiological conditions rumenal bacteria are able to produce thiamin, thiamin deficiency in ruminants is a relative deficiency due to imbalances between thiamin-producing and thiamin-destroying bacteria. It occurs mainly in cattle fed concentrated feed with high carbohydrate content and little roughage, resulting in rumenal acidosis and overgrowth of thiaminase-producing bacteria (e.g. *Clostridium sporogenes*, *Bacillus thiaminoolyticus*). Additionally, grazing of thiaminase-containing plants (e.g. bracken fern, nardoo) or exposure to the coccidiostatic amprolium, a thiamin antagonist, may result in cerebrocortical necrosis. Neuronal necrosis is observed mainly in the cortex (Fig. 6.3), but may sometimes also affect other areas, including basal and thalamic nuclei, colliculi and brainstem nuclei. In acute cases, a macroscopic diagnosis of CCN may be confirmed by bright green fluorescence of affected cortex of either fresh or formalin-fixed brain exposed to ultraviolet light (Wood's lamp) (Fig. 6.2B). Necrotic areas appear green due to autofluorescence.

In acute **lead poisoning**, initial microscopic changes include vascular congestion with endothelial hypertrophy and capillary hyperplasia. **Salt poisoning** of swine and ruminants (also **water deprivation encephalopathy**, "water intoxication") occurs rarely following excessive salt intake. More commonly the PE is the

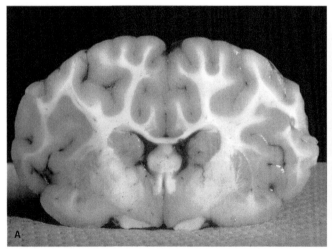
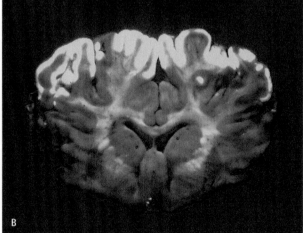

Fig. 6.2 Polioencephalomalacia. Sheep. A: Cerebrum at level of basic nuclei. Note the bilaterally symmetrical yellowish-tan discoloration of the cortical gray matter in the parietal cortex. B. Same level as in A. Transverse section of fresh brain under UV light. Strong greenish autofluorescence of the bilaterally symmetrical lesions in the cerebral cortex.

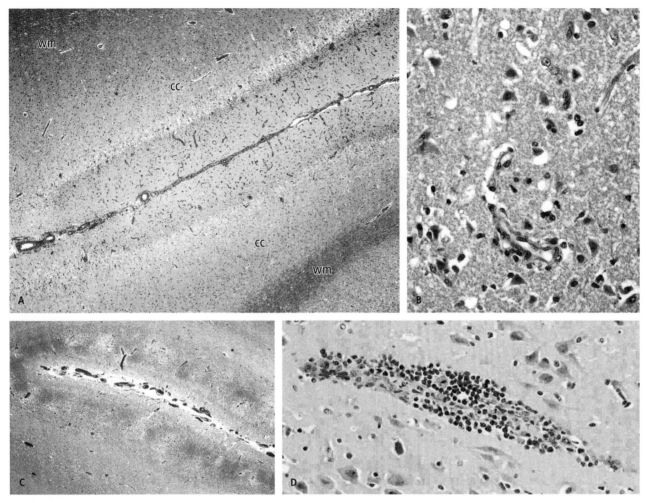

Fig. 6.3 Polioencephalomalacia. A. Bovine. Cerebrum with two cortical gyri on either side of meningeal sulcus. Marked change in staining intensity, partial spongy state and hypercellularity of both superficial cortical layers in a band-like pattern ("pseudolaminar") (cc, cerebral cortex; wm, white matter). HE. B: Sheep. Cerebral cortex. Acute cerebrocortical necrosis. Widespread acidophilic neuronal necrosis. Perineuronal edema. Capillaries are prominent due to endothelial hypertrophy and hyperplasia. HE. C: Pig. Chronic polioencephalomalcia in salt intoxication. Most of the cortex is completely malacic and basophilic due to massive infiltration with macrophages replacing the necrotic parenchyma. HE. D: Pig. Acute polioencephalomalacia in salt intoxication. Prominent perivascular cuffing containing eosinophils and some acidophilic necrotic neurons. HE.

result of sustained water deprivation (e.g. broken pipes, freezing) resulting in hyperosmolarity of the brain. If animals have subsequently excessive water intake, water follows the osmotic gradient into the brain leading to cerebral edema and necrosis. Lesions are of polioencephalomalacia (Fig. 6.3C), and in pigs there are also pathognomic eosinophilic cell infiltrates in the parenchyma and perivascular spaces (Fig. 6.3D).

Organomercurial poisoning occurs after consumption of contaminated feed. In cattle and pigs, in addition to PE, cerebellar granule and Purkinje cell necrosis, it

causes degeneration of cardiac Purkinje cells and fibrinoid necrosis in the walls of the leptomeningeal arteries. Other known but rare causes of PE include **hypoglycemia** (e.g. pregnancy toxemia of ewes, newborn piglets), **manure gas intoxication** (hydrogen sulfide), **closantel intoxication**, **cyanide poisoning** and **peracute *Phalaris* poisoning** (see below).

PE or CCN in small animals

Sporadic PE of unknown cause in dogs and cats is clinically characterized by severe seizures and also

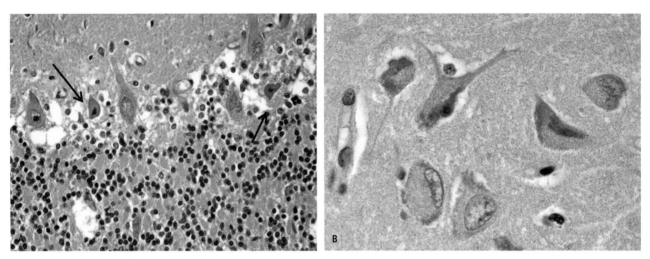

Fig. 6.4 Carbamate poisoning. Dog. A: Cerebellum. Purkinje cells showing acidophilic neuronal necrosis in the cerebellar cortex (arrows). HE. B: Cerebral cortex. Pyramidal neurons are chromatolytic with peripherally displaced nuclei. HE.

status epilepticus. It remains uncertain whether such PE is the cause or the result of seizure activity. The currently accepted mechanism of seizure-induced acidophilic neuronal necrosis is that due to excessive neurotransmitter-induced excitotoxicity. Although light-microscopic lesions are commonly absent in dogs with "idiopathic" seizures, acidophilic neuronal necrosis in the hippocampus, piriform lobe and other sites in the cerebral cortex and cerebellum – predilection areas in epileptic humans and some animal seizure models – can occur in animals with status epilepticus or severe cluster seizures.

In **hypoglycemia**, neuronal injury is due to excitotoxicity as a result of energy deprivation with aspartate acting as the main excitatory amino acid. Cerebral cortex and hippocampus (in rodents particularly the dentate gyrus) have been defined as predilection sites for hypoglycemic injury of neurons, but there are also reports of involvement of basal nuclei and cerebellum. Therefore, hypoglycemia cannot be reliably discriminated from ischemia based on light microscopy. The latter is discussed in Chapter 2 (vascular disorders). Hypoglycemia occurs with functional β-cell tumors of the pancreas or with iatrogenic insulin overdosage. Furthermore, it is commonly seen in puppies of miniature dog breeds (Chihuahua, Yorkshire Terrier, Miniature Poodle) during their first months of life. In these dogs, polioencephalomalacia is associated with microvacuolar hepatocellular degeneration.

Cyanide poisoning has been reported as a cause of PE in dogs and cats. Although *carbamates* (e.g. aldicarb) are widely used as pesticides, data on the lesions of **carbamate intoxication** are unavailable. In the dog, we have seen acute brain edema and PE beginning with widespread neuronal chromatolysis and acidophilic necrosis of Purkinje cells (Fig. 6.4A,B). The mode of action is similar to the one of organophosphates but the binding to acetyl cholinesterase is reversible. Extensive acidophilic neuronal degeneration in cerebrum, cerebellum and brainstem occurs in **organic mercury poisoning**, particularly in cats. Experimental induction of the lesions in cats led to the identification of organic mercury as the etiology of the infamous *Minamata disease* in people in Japan due to the ingestion of contaminated sea food.

Feline hippocampal necrosis

In domestic cats, **hippocampal necrosis** is a relatively frequent neurological disorder in several European countries. The cause is unknown but cluster analysis indicated a toxic environmental factor. Cats typically exhibit aggressive behavior and complex focal seizures. The lesions are mainly restricted to the hippocampus bilaterally (Fig. 6.5A), but may also extend into the parahippocampal and piriform cortex. There is neuronal chromatolysis (Fig. 6.5B) followed by acidophilic neuronal necrosis (Fig. 6.5C) and, in severe cases, complete hippocampal necrosis. In chronic cases, there is vascular proliferation and both micro- and astrogliosis. In some cases these lesions are accompanied by remarkable perivascular mononuclear cuffing that may occur in the acute phase. See MRI Atlas.

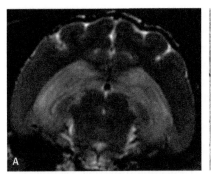 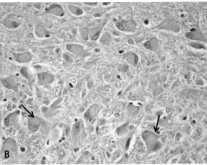 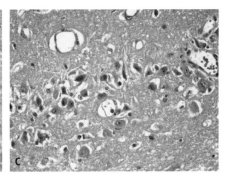

Fig. 6.5 Hippocampal necrosis. Cat. A: T2W MRI sequence. Note the bilateral diffuse hyperintensity of the hippocampi. (Reproduced with permission from Dr. Frank Steffen.) B: Initial changes of hippocampal necrosis consist of neuronal swelling and chromatolysis in the pyramidal cell layer. Neuronal nuclei are displaced to the periphery. Nuclei of astrocytes are swollen (arrows). HE. C: Acidophilic neuronal necrosis of most pyramidal neurons. Capillaries are distended and show endothelial hypertrophy. HE.

Hippocampal sclerosis

Hippocampal sclerosis is well known in humans with temporal lobe epilepsy. The lesion is characterized by necrosis and loss of neurons in the pyramidal cell layer of the hippocampus unilaterally or bilaterally. It is believed that neuronal loss is due to severe and prolonged seizures, particularly severe febrile seizures during childhood. However such a correlation is not always present: hippocampal sclerosis can occur without seizures and vice versa. Hippocampal sclerosis and atrophy (Fig. 6.6A,C) can be found in dogs and cats with a long history of generalized seizures refractory to antiepileptic treatment. Atrophy and asymmetry of the hippocampi can be seen either on MRI or macroscopically in severe cases. In contrast to PE associated with seizures as described above, there are no malacic lesions. In most cases, lesions are only detected microscopically and

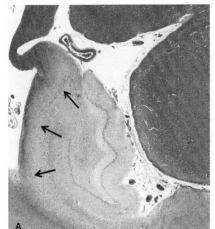 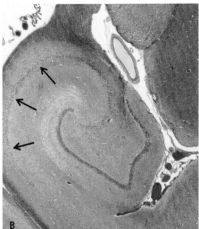 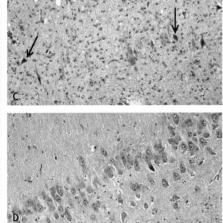

Fig. 6.6 Hippocampal sclerosis. Dog with chronic seizures. A: Pyramidal neurons are lost and replaced by a band of gliosis (arrows). HE. B: Compare with the normal canine hippocampus. Note the pyramidal neuron layer (arrows). HE. C: The density of neurons in the pyramidal cell layer is severely reduced. Reactive astrocytic gliosis is prominent. Most of the remaining neurons are shrunken and deeply basophilic (neuronal atrophy, arrows). HE. D: Normal appearance of the pyramidal neuron layer in the canine hippocampus. HE.

consist of diffuse loss of pyramidal cells in the hippocampus of varying severity with extensive gliosis (Fig. 6.6C). As this is a progressive disease, remaining neurons may exhibit acidophilic neuronal damage.

6.2.2 Polioencephalomalacia of subcortical structures and brainstem

Thiamin deficiency in carnivores

In contrast to ruminants, carnivores are dependent on an adequate dietary supply of vitamin B1. Dietary thiamin deficiency can occur with ingestion of food containing thiaminase (e.g. fish) or deficient in thiamin or if thiamin is inactivated by preservation procedures (e.g. by heating or sulfur dioxide). In wild and farmed foxes and mink, thiamin deficiency is called **Chastek's paralysis**. In domestic carnivores, **thiamin-deficiency encephalopathy** occurs relatively commonly in starved cats, but is very rare in dogs. As in ruminants, thiamin deficiency causes necrosis of the gray matter (polioencephalomalacia) but the topography and nature of lesions is different. The periventricular gray matter is bilaterally symmetrically affected and the caudal colliculi, medial vestibular nuclei and lateral geniculate bodies are consistent target regions (Fig. 6.7A,B). See MRI Atlas.

The diagnosis can frequently be made macroscopically if the characteristic, bilaterally symmetrical hemorrhages in the brainstem are present (Fig. 6.7A,B). Histologically, there is PE with edema and varying degrees of hemorrhage, capillary endothelial hypertrophy and hyperplasia with a proteinaceous exudate (Fig. 6.7C). In chronic lesions, neuronal loss, vacuolation of the neuropil and intense astrogliosis are found.

Equine nigropallidal encephalomalacia

Equine nigropallidal encephalomalacia (yellow star thistle poisoning) has been described in the USA, South America and in Australia, where horses in arid areas feed on pastures containing *Centaurea solstitialis* (yellow star thistle) or *C. repens* (Russian knapweed). After prolonged ingestion horses show abnormal tongue and mouth movements, with difficulty in prehension, swallowing and drinking. In the brain characteristic lesions evident both on MRI and grossly are of bilaterally symmetrical acute malacic or chronic cystic polioencephalomalacia in the substantia nigra and the globus pallidus (Fig. 6.8A,B). Unilateral lesions can occur. Microscopically, well demarcated necrosis is infarctive in type with widespread acute acidophilic neuronal necrosis and glial cell necrosis but some surviving blood vessels. *Repin* has been postulated as the causative neurotoxin but the pathogenesis is unknown. The malacic nature of the lesions is very different in extent and type from the selective loss of dopaminergic

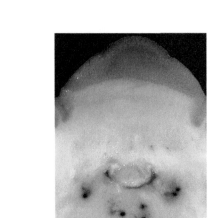
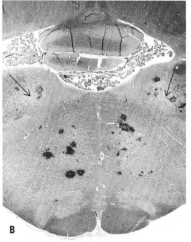
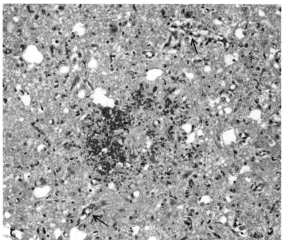

Fig. 6.7 Thiamin deficiency. Cat. Brainstem. A: Bilateral and almost symmetrical foci of hemorrhage and malacia in the brainstem. B: Section of the same brain with bilateral hemorrhages. In some nuclei foci of pallor and spongy state indicating edema and necrosis (arrows). HE. C: Hemorrhage and edema in the caudal colliculus. Neuronal loss is accompanied by marked astrocytic gliosis and microgliosis. Capillaries are prominent due to endothelial hypertrophy (arrows). HE.

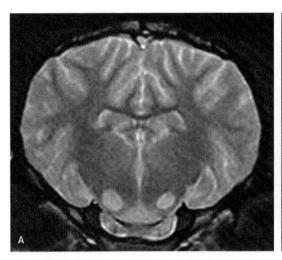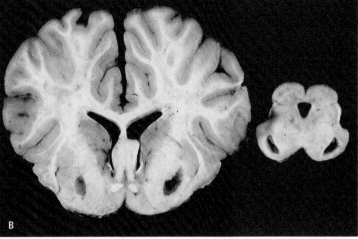

Fig. 6.8 Nigropallidal encephalomalacia. Horse. A: T2W MRI sequence showing bilateral and symmetrical hyperintensity in the substantia nigra. B: Same case as in A. Bilaterally symmetrical and well demarcated areas of polioencephalomalacia with brownish discoloration and cystic malacia in the globus pallidus (left section) and substantia nigra of the midbrain (right).

neurons in the substantia nigra in human Parkinson's disease.

PE with *Aeschynomene indica*

Aeschynomene indica is a weed, which frequently grows in rice paddies in South America, Africa, Asia and Australia. Intoxication has been reported in pigs fed rice contaminated with seeds. The pathogenesis is unknown. Neurological signs occur within hours of ingestion and are initially not associated with neuropathological changes. In more protracted cases, histologically there are bilaterally symmetrical areas of malacia in vestibular, cerebellar, oculomotor and red nuclei, substantia nigra, putamen and cortex. Acute lesions include edema, congestion and hemorrhage, which are followed by necrosis, infiltration with gitter cells and capillary prominence with endothelial hypertrophy.

Annual ryegrass staggers

A tremorgenic syndrome in ruminants, horses and pigs called **annual ryegrass staggers** is caused by corynetoxin. This toxin is produced by *Rathayibacter toxicus*, a bacterium that is carried by the nematode *Anguina agrostis*, which parasitizes annual ryegrass (*Lolium rigidum*). Ingestion of infected ryegrass causes vascular injury with secondary proteinaceous edema and ischemic damage in the cerebellum with necrosis and loss of Purkinje cells.

Metronidazole toxicity

Metronidazole is widely used in the treatment of infections with anaerobic bacteria or protozoa. **Metronidazole neurotoxicity** has been frequently reported in men, dogs and cats, but the pathogenesis is currently not known. There is little information on the neuropathology, likely because metronidazole toxicity is reversible when drug administration is discontinued and fatal cases are rare. In humans, peripheral neuropathies and reversible bilaterally symmetrical MRI changes in the brain, mainly affecting the cerebellar nuclei, are reported. In dogs and cats, metronidazole poisoning causes ataxia, nystagmus, head tilts, tremors and seizures. The few available reports describe Purkinje cell degeneration/loss and axonal degeneration in the cerebellovestibular white matter tracts of dogs. One report on metronidazole intoxication in a cat describes demarcated, rather non-symmetrical areas of necrosis in the thalamus, midbrain and medulla.

Encephalomalacias due to genetic mutations

Note that symmetrical encephalomalacia can also be caused by genetic disorders (see Chapter 8).

6.2.3 Poliomyelomalacia

Poliomyelomalacia due to iatrogenic **selenium poisoning** occurs in pigs. Characteristic lesions affect the cervical and lumbar intumescences of the spinal cord (Fig. 6.9). There is focal and bilaterally symmetrical necrosis

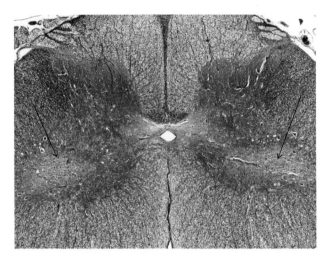

Fig. 6.9 Selenium poisoning. Pig. There is bilaterally symmetrical loss of staining in the ventral horns of the cervical intumescence due to poliomyelomalacia (arrows). HE-LFB.

with gross softening and cavitation of the ventral horns. Microscopically, initial lesions include neuropil vacuolation, necrosis of glial cells, capillary hypertrophy and neuronal degeneration. In the chronic stage, the picture is predominated by neuronal loss and extensive gliosis with capillary proliferation in the ventral horns. In addition, many brainstem nuclei and cerebellar roof nuclei may be similarly affected. Similar syndromes of bilateral poliomyelomalacia affecting the ventral horns of the spinal cord have been described in other species (e.g. sheep, goats and Ayrshire calves), but their etiologies remain unknown.

6.2.4 Leukoencephalomalacias

Equine leukoencephalomalacia

Equine leukoencephalomalacia or **moldy corn disease**, a fatal neurological disorder with sudden onset, is observed in horses and donkeys worldwide that have ingested moldy corn contaminated with the fungus *Fusarium moniliforme*. The fungus produces the mycotoxin fumonisin B1, which is believed to cause vascular damage selectively in the white matter with secondary encephalomalacia. However, the exact pathogenesis is not known.

The toxin may also cause concurrent hepatic necrosis. Macroscopically, lesions are characterized by bilateral but fairly asymmetrical areas of leukoencephalomalacia in the centrum semiovale and corona radiata (Fig. 6.10A) and sometimes in the brainstem and cerebellar white matter. Acutely malacic foci are yellowish-brown to hemorrhagic, soft and progress to form fluid-filled cavities. Histologically in acute cases, vessels are necrotic with intravascular thrombi. The white matter is necrotic and massively infiltrated with gitter cells and some neutrophils. In the periphery of the necrosis, proteinaceous edema dissects the white matter and vessels are surrounded by small hemorrhages and cuffs of eosinophils, lymphocytes and neutrophils (Fig. 6.10B).

Swayback

Congenital copper deficiency affects lambs and rarely goat kids, which are born with neurological signs called **swayback**. It develops *in utero* during which time ewes are fed a copper-deficient or molybdenum-rich diet, the latter antagonizing copper solubility and absorption in the digestive tract. Affected animals are blind and show

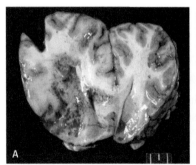
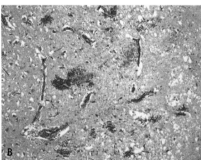
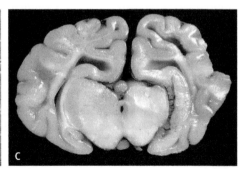

Fig. 6.10 Leukoencephalomalacia. A: Horse. Equine leukoencephalomalacia (moldy corn poisoning). Massive swelling of the left hemisphere with midline shift. There is hemorrhagic necrosis and yellowish discoloration of the white and gray matter. B: Acute lesions of equine leukoencephalomalacia are characterized by vascular damage (as indicated by the hemorrhages and fibrin exudation), acidophilic neuronal necrosis, capillary hypertrophy and hyperplasia, marked edema and necrosis. HE. C: Sheep. Swayback in a newborn lamb. Bilateral loss and cyst formation of the cerebral white matter.

severe incoordination progressing to complete immobility and death. Grossly, there is bilaterally symmetrical cavitation of the periventricular white matter in the cerebrum with associated ventricular distension (Fig. 6.10C). The histological lesion is a severe rarefaction and edema of the cerebral white matter resulting in cavitations that are traversed by axons and astrocytic processes. Neuronal necrosis can be observed in the overlying cortex. The pathogenesis is unknown.

6.2.5 Encephalomalacias involving both gray and white matter

Enterotoxemias

In enterotoxemias, the intestine is excessively colonized by toxin-producing bacteria. Enterotoxins are absorbed from the gut and distributed hematogeneously causing a systemic toxemia and resulting widespread tissue damage. In the brain, enterotoxemias present as bilaterally symmetrical encephalomalacias.

Focal symmetrical encephalomalacia (FSE) in ruminants affects mainly well nourished animals fed diets high in carbohydrate content (crops, grain), and therefore is also called overeating disease. Such diets create optimal conditions for intestinal overgrowth of

ε-toxin-producing *Clostridium perfringens* type D. The neurotoxicity is likely due to injury of microvascular endothelium and neuronal excitotoxicity of ε-toxin. In peracute cases with high toxin levels, macroscopic lesions may be absent but microscopic lesions consistent with vasogenic edema are observed. Focal symmetrical areas of malacia, sometimes hemorrhagic, affecting gray and white matter occur in subacute to chronic cases (Fig. 6.11A) in the corona radiata, basal nuclei, internal capsule, thalamus, midbrain and cerebellar peduncles. See MRI Atlas. Microscopically, these sharply demarcated areas of necrosis (Fig. 6.11B) contain vacuolated white matter, axonal spheroids and necrotic neurons and glial cells. Vascular endothelium is hypertrophic and vessels are surrounded by proteinaceous edema and hemorrhages (Fig. 6.11B). With time, numerous macrophages and neutrophils infiltrate the necrotic foci and capillaries become prominent.

Edema disease (**cerebrospinal angiopathy**) occurs in feeder pigs in the first weeks after weaning following small intestinal colonization by verotoxin-producing *Escherichia coli* (VTEC) and systemic absorption of the verotoxin (verotoxin or shiga-like toxin type 2e; Stx2e). This toxin causes widespread injury of small arteries and

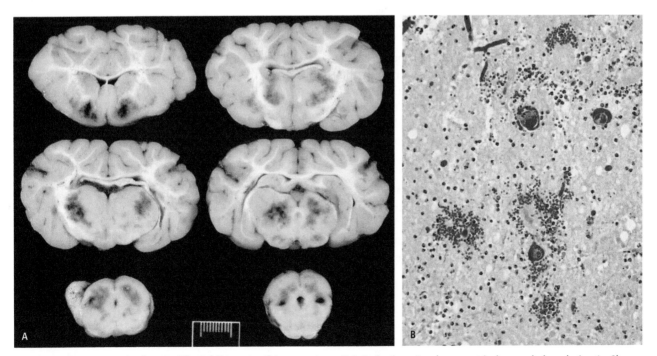

Fig. 6.11 Enterotoxemia due to *Clostridium perfringens* type D intoxication. Focal symmetrical encephalomalacia. A: Sheep. Consecutive transverse sections of the brain. Bilateral and fairly symmetrical areas of malacia and hemorrhage in basal nuclei, thalamus and midbrain. B: Same case as in A. Acute focal encephalomalacia with vascular necrosis, small hemorrhages and massive polymorphonuclear cell infiltrates. HE.

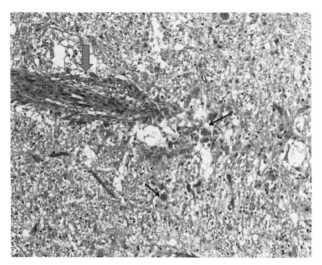

Fig. 6.12 Porcine edema disease. Pig. Chronic. A medium-sized artery has a severely thickened wall (large arrow). In the Virchow-Robin space and in the surrounding parenchyma there are many brightly eosinophilic (protein-rich) droplets (arrows). Spongy state with large and small vacuoles indicating edema and malacia. HE.

arterioles resulting in edema and ischemic damage of tissues including the brain. The pathogenesis is multi-factorial involving genetic (e.g. the expression of the F18 receptor on the intestinal epithelium), nutritional (e.g. diet changes, high-energy diets allowing proliferation of *E. coli*) and environmental (weaning) factors.

Macroscopically, bilaterally symmetrical areas of malacia with tan-grayish discoloration may be observed in the brainstem. These may extend rostrally into the basal nuclei. Microscopically, the characteristic lesion is that of a bilaterally symmetrical malacia due to necrosis of arterial smooth muscle cells. The initial lesion is a perivascular edema with protein-rich, eosinophilic droplets. Then fibrinoid vascular necrosis is accompanied by infiltration of the vascular wall and adventitia with neutrophils, lymphocytes and macrophages as well as endothelial hypertrophy. Edema and necrosis of the parenchyma are secondary to the vascular changes. In animals surviving for a prolonged time, necrotic areas are infiltrated by macrophages and arteries are thickened (Fig. 6.12).

Carbon monoxide poisoning

Fatal exposure to carbon monoxide (CO) is generated following incomplete oxidation of hydrocarbons due to lack of oxygen. It occurs for example during fires or when wood stoves are used in closed or poorly ventilated spaces. In human medicine **CO poisoning** is one of the most common intoxications. It is rarely described in

animals. The pathogenesis is not entirely understood. CO binds avidly to the binding site for oxygen in hemo-globin and myocardial hemoglobin and thus causes severe hypoxia. Neuropathological changes include bilaterally symmetrical polioencephalomalacia with acute neuronal necrosis in the cerebral cortex, caudate nucleus, globus pallidus, thalamic nuclei and cerebel-lum. Furthermore, bilaterally symmetrical demyelina-tion and sharply demarcated areas of necrosis in the deep periventricular white matter are observed in animals which survive for a longer time period.

6.3 Acquired metabolic–toxic selective lesions

Selective lesions, which to a certain extent morphologi-cally resemble the hereditary conditions described in Chapter 8, can occur as a result of intoxications or meta-bolic deficiencies. The clinical signs may be acute as in the diseases described above but also subacute to chronic and progressive. Some of these lesion patterns are also discussed in more detail in Chapter 8 on degenerative diseases.

6.3.1 Neuronal degeneration
Enzootic ataxia

In contrast to congenital copper deficiency ("swayback", see Section 6.2.4), **enzootic ataxia** results from postnatal copper deficiency. Goat kids and lambs are normal at birth, but develop progressive paraparesis and ataxia at 3–12 weeks of age. However, there may be a certain overlap between the neuropathology of swayback and that of enzootic ataxia. Histopathologically, enzootic ataxia resembles a motor neuron disease (MND) with neuronal swelling, chromatolysis and eosinophilia (Fig. 6.13A). Neuronal changes are found in the ventral horns and various brainstem and midbrain nuclei. Additionally, there is axonal degeneration with demyelination of the Wallerian type in the dorsolateral and ventromedial funiculi of the spinal cord.

Equine motor neuron disease

Equine motor neuron disease (EMND) was originally described in North America but occurs in several European countries. The condition shares clinical and neuropathological findings with all other MND (see Chapter 8.2) including chromatolysis, nuclear changes and eventually loss of spinal cord and brainstem motor neurons (Fig. 6.13B) as well as Wallerian degeneration in respective nerve roots and nerves. In EMND there is also conspicuous accumulation of lipopigment in neurons and endothelial cells. Retinal changes in EMND resemble those found in experimental vitamin E defi-

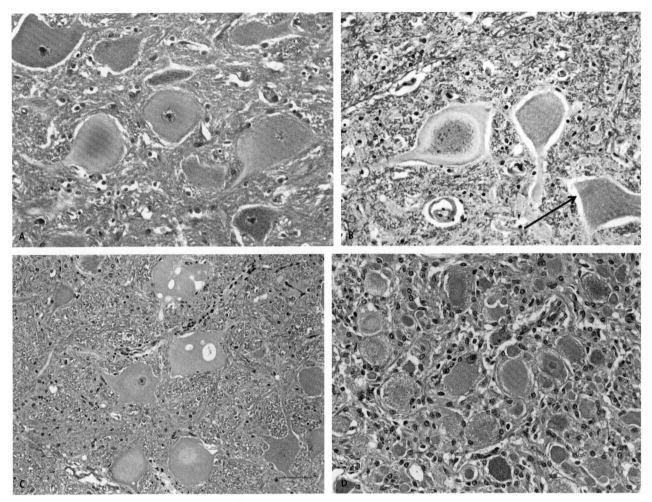

Fig. 6.13 Neuronal degeneration. A: Goat. Midbrain. Enzootic ataxia. Most motor neurons in the red nucleus exhibit various stages of chromatolysis. HE. B: Horse. Spinal cord. Equine motor neuron disease. A chromatolytic degenerating neuron in the ventral horn containing numerous eosinophilic cytoplasmic inclusions. Neurons also contain excessive lipofuschin pigment (arrow). HE. C: Bovine. Brainstem. *Aspergillus clavatus* intoxication. Large motor neurons in the brainstem are chromatolytic and swollen with pale eosinophilic cytoplasm. Some contain cytoplasmic vacuoles. HE. D: Horse. Mesenteric ganglion. Acute grass sickness. Most ganglionic neurons are chromatolytic and many contain intracytoplasmic eosinophilic spheroid inclusion bodies. Nuclei are displaced to the periphery. There are numerous axonal spheroids between the neurons. HE.

ciency in dogs, suggesting that these diseases share a common pathogenesis.

Aspergillus clavatus intoxication

A tremorgenic syndrome has been described in ruminants fed beer by-products, sprouted barley or grain contaminated with *Aspergillus clavatus*. The fungus produces various toxins including *patulin*. In *Aspergillus clavatus* intoxication, in addition to degeneration and necrosis of skeletal muscle, widespread degeneration of large motor neurons in the brainstem and spinal cord is found associated with Wallerian degeneration in the spinal cord and peripheral nervous system. Degenerated

neurons are severely swollen and chromatolytic. They show either a brightly eosinophilic, homogeneous cytoplasm or cytoplasmic pallor and contain numerous large intraneuronal vacuoles (Fig. 6.13C). Occasionally, necrotic neurons with shrunken, deeply eosinophilic cytoplasm and peripheral, karyopyknotic nuclei are observed.

Chrysocoma tenuifolia intoxication

Vacuolation and chromatolysis of spinal cord neurons, particularly motor neurons of the ventral horns, has been described in lambs in South Africa grazing *Chrysocoma tenuifolia*. Neuronal degeneration is associated with Wallerian degeneration in lateral and ventral funiculi.

Dysautonomia

Neuronal degeneration in the autonomic nervous system is the main feature of dysautonomias. Acute neuronal degeneration is seen in autonomic (sympathetic and parasympathathetic) neurons of the PNS and in the CNS. Dysautonomias have been reported in a variety of domestic animals but also in wild species. They occur sporadically and are presumably caused by hitherto undefined toxins. Clinical signs refer to autonomic dysfunction. Pathological findings in autonomic ganglionic and enteric neurons and central autonomic neurons include neuronal degeneration with swelling, chromatolysis with central eosinophilic spheroidal bodies, foamy cytoplasm and eccentric nuclei (Fig. 6.13D). All these changes lead to neuronal loss and reactive gliosis/satellite cell proliferation in chronic cases. These changes are similar in all dysautonomias.

Equine dysautonomia or **grass sickness** (**mal seco** in South America) was the first identified dysautonomia in animals. It is generally fatal and occurs mainly in grazing horses and donkeys in the UK, continental Europe and South America. Sporadic cases have been reported in the USA. Endemic areas have been identified in several countries. Depending on the severity of the lesions, there is an acute form, with animals dying within days after onset, and a milder chronic form with signs lasting for weeks and months, from which animals may recover. In addition to the neuronal degeneration in autonomic neurons, other neurons in various motor nuclei of the brainstem and spinal cord show extensive chromatolysis, although this change may not progress to neuronal degeneration. The gold-standard diagnosis is postmortem histopathology but ileal biopsies have been used successfully for antemortem diagnosis of grass sickness. Synaptophysin has been proposed as a marker for degenerated neurons in diagnosis of grass sickness. The cause of grass sickness is still unknown, although epidemiological studies of this sporadic disease have identified a number of risk factors. The most favoured, although not finally proven etiology, is a toxicoinfection with *Clostridium botulinum* type C that is acquired during grazing. Recently, high levels of heavy metals in the herbage and high representation of *Ranunculus* sp in the pasture have been associated with grass sickness.

Feline dysautonomia (**Key–Gaskell syndrome**) is a sporadic disease of cats occuring throughout the world. A large number of cases were detected during the 1980s in the United Kingdom but since then the incidence of the disease has decreased considerably. The cause of the disease remains unknown. There have been recent attempts to associate feline dysautonomia to *Clostridium botulinum* C/D toxico-infection.

Canine dysautonomia has been described worldwide, but in contrast to dysautonomias in other species more frequently occurs in the USA than in Europe. Dysautonomias have been described in other species including rabbits, hares, sheep (abomasal-emptying defect) and South American camelids.

Phalaris grass intoxication

Canary grass (*Phalaris*) poisoning has been reported worldwide and affects sheep, cattle and horses. *Phalaris* grass poisoning manifests in one of two neurological syndromes. In the peracute form, also referred to as "sudden death" or "polioencephalomalacia-like sudden death", animals die within hours. Neuropil vacuolation and swollen astrocytes with a vesicular nucleus may be observed in the deep cerebrocortical layers. Occasional necrotic neurons are present.

The second form is a tremorgenic syndrome referred to as *Phalaris* **grass staggers**. *Phalaris* contains tryptamine alkaloids structurally resembling serotonin, and it is thought that neurotoxicity is the result of agonistic interaction of the toxin with serotonergic receptors. Macroscopically, pigment accumulation representing an indolin-like molecule may be appreciated as greenish-gray discoloration of the kidney, brainstem and spinal cord. Histologically, a granular cytoplasmic pigment accumulates bilaterally symmetrically in specific neuron populations of the brainstem and spinal cord. Neuronal necrosis may be present.

Acquired lysosomal storage diseases

Acquired lysosomal storage can be induced by plant toxins in various herbivorous species. It occurs mainly in the USA, South America, Australia and Africa. Plants of the genera *Swainsona*, *Astragalus*, *Oxytropis*, *Ipomea*, *Sida* and *Turbina* contain lysosomal glycosidase inhibitors including swainsonine. These alkaloids are potent inhibitors of, for example, α-mannosidase and Golgi mannosidase II. The resulting lysosomal accumulation of mannose leads to neuronal vacuolation mimicking the lesions of inherited mannosidosis (described in Chapter 8).

Cerebellar signs in ruminants have been associated with the ingestion of *Solanum* spp. Gross lesions are absent, but histologically cytoplasmic vacuolation, degeneration and loss of Purkinje cells are observed. Ultrastructurally, these vacuoles consist of lipids, electron-dense granules and membraneous debris. Secondary axonal swelling and Wallerian degeneration occur in the cerebellar white matter.

6.3.2 Axonal degeneration

Wallerian-like long tract degeneration

Long tract degeneration of the Wallerian type throughout the spinal cord has been found in a wide variety of deficiencies and intoxications in all domestic animal species. The basic lesion is fragmentation and loss of axons, secondary demyelination and reactive phagocytosis/gliosis in a specific distribution pattern, depending on etiology and species. Very similar lesions are illustrated in Chapter 8. Plant-induced axonal degeneration in ruminants occurs following ***Tribulus terrestris* intoxication**; axonal degeneration is also seen in Zamia staggers following cycade poisoning. In horses and sheep it is associated with **sorghum poisoning**. Long tract degeneration was found in cats with **cobalamin deficiency**, in dogs with **vitamin E deficiency** and pigs with **vitamin A deficiency** or **3-nitro poisoning** (an organic arsenic compound).

Organophosphates (OPs) are widely used (anthelmintics, lubricant oils, pesticides) and are inhibitors of acetylcholinesterase. Apart from acute intoxications with abrupt onset of clinical signs, various OPs have been associated with delayed neurotoxic syndromes (organophosphate-induced delayed axonopathy). Clinical signs may develop slowly and are progressive over a few weeks. Common clinical signs are ataxia and weakness in the pelvic limbs that usually progresses to paraplegia. **Delayed organophosphate poisoning** conforms broadly to dying-back polyneuropathy in the CNS and PNS caused by inhibition of the neuropathy target esterase. Axons of long and large nerve fibers both in the central and peripheral nervous system are affected, and lesions are predominantly in the distal portions of the axons, therefore called distal axonopathy. Hence, axonal degeneration in the spinal cord is most prominent in the dorsal and superficial dorsolateral (ascending) tracts of the cervical spinal cord and in the ventral and deep lateral (descending) tracts of the lumbar spinal cord. Histologically, this axonopathy is characterized by Wallerian-type degeneration of distal axons with secondary myelin degradation. Neuronal degeneration and chromatolysis are observed in the spinal cord and brainstem.

Neuroaxonal-dystrophy-like lesions

Neuroaxonal dystrophy is defined as focal axonal swelling (spheroids) in both specific nuclei and tracts following disruption of axonal transport usually due to metabolic derangement of the neuron. The basic lesion is discussed and illustrated in Chapter 8. It may occur in the gray or white matter and is a feature of various toxic and metabolic conditions or genetically determined.

Such lesions have been associated with **Vitamin E deficiency** (likely genetically determined) in animals, particularly horses (see Chapter 8).

The ingestion of the endophytic fungus *Neotyphodium* (previously *Acremonium*) *lolii* that grows on perennial ryegrass (*Lolium perenne*) causes a tremorgenic syndrome associated with neuroaxonal-dystrophy-like lesions in domestic ruminants, horses and deer. **Perennial ryegrass staggers** occurs mainly in Australia and New Zealand, but is also described in other continents. *Neotyphodium lolii* produces neurotoxic alkaloids that are tremorgenic (lolitremes) and cause K^+-channel dysfunction. Associated neuropathologic changes include swollen axons (torpedos) within the granular cell layer of the cerebellum and vacuolar degeneration of Purkinje cells. Similar **tremorgenic syndromes** have been reported in association with feedstuffs contaminated with other fungi (e.g. *Aspergillus* spp, *Penicillium* spp., *Claviceps paspali*) able to produce tremorgenic toxins (e.g. verrucologen, penitrem A) but information on neuropathology is scarce. In dogs, such intoxications have been seen following ingestion of moldy cream cheese, moldy walnuts and garbage.

In sheep grazing *Sorghum* spp. dystrophic axons occur in the cerebellar roof nuclei, red nucleus, brainstem nuclei and spinal cord. Additionally, mild neuronal necrosis can be observed.

Halimium brasiliense

A particular type of axonal degeneration with axonal vacuolation throughout the brain and spinal cord has been reported in Brazilian sheep grazing on pastures with *Halimium brasiliense*. It is associated with white matter vacuolation and lipofuscin accumulation in neurons and astrocytes.

6.3.3 Myelin degeneration

Hound ataxia

Primary myelin degeneration has been described in **hound ataxia**, a disease of adult Harrier Hounds, Beagles and Foxhounds kept in hunting packs. The disease is characterized by gradual onset of ataxia and spastic paresis. Microscopic findings are confined to the spinal cord and are most prominent in the ventral and lateral tracts. Intact axons in vacuolated myelin sheaths and variation in myelin sheath thickness suggest a primary myelinopathy. However, some axonal degeneration is present. It has been suggested that this myelopathy is caused by methionine deficiency and altered methionine synthetase activity resulting from feeding rumen.

Irradiated feed in cats

Primary demyelination of the brain and spinal cord has been described in cats (**leukoencephalomyelopathy**) that have been experimentally given irradiated feed during pregnancy. Non-pregnant cats, male cats and their offspring did not develop neurological signs. White matter vacuolation, demyelination and remyelination with relative sparing of axons occur mainly in the lateral and ventral columns of the spinal cord, corona radiata, crus cerebri and optic nerve. Other authors describe outbreaks of leukoencephalomyelopathy in cat colonies related to irradiated feed. Non-pregnant cats were affected and, interestingly, primary axonal degeneration of Wallerian type in spinal cord and brain is described. However, the distribution is similar to that in the primary demyelination described above with lateral and ventral columns being mainly involved. The syndrome could be reproduced by giving cats irradiated feed with elevated peroxide and reduced vitamin A levels. Therefore, it is suspected that free-radical formation causes axonal degeneration of the Wallerian type. A similar leukoencephalomyelopathy has been reported in various large felid species and vitamin A deficiency has been implicated.

6.4 Spongy degeneration

Spongy state is one of the most common neuropathological changes. A wide array of mechanisms/causes can produce vacuolation of the white or gray matter. An overview of the differential diagnosis of spongy state in the CNS is presented in Fig. 6.14. In this section we cover spongy changes, also called "spongy degeneration", which occur as a primary morphological change, not associated with destructive lesions of neurons or myelin. This lesion is characterized by bilaterally symmetrical vacuolation more often in white than gray matter. The vacuoles are sharply defined and vary in size. In severe cases vacuoles may coalesce. In the acute stage there are no reactive changes: there is no axonal swelling, invasion with macrophages or gliosis. The latter may occur later in longstanding severe lesions. The basic lesion is probably cytotoxic edema (see Chapter 1 on general neuropathology) in the white matter with myelin splitting and vacuolation. The lesions can be widespread in the CNS but may target specific areas. Macroscopically, brain swelling may be observed. Myelin vacuoles are also present in the PNS.

Intoxications

Spongy degeneration of the white matter can result from **ammonia poisoning**, **hexachlorophene intoxication**, **closantel intoxication and poisoning with bromethalin-derived rodenticides**. Some plants have also been implicated: **Helichrysum argyrosphaerum intoxication** and **Stypandra sp intoxication** induce spongy degeneration in ruminants. **Sporadic brain edema** in ruminants is a sporadic condition of unknown etiology usually in adult animals, which occurs in Switzerland. The condition is characterized by status spongiosus of variable degree in the cerebral white matter and the brainstem (Fig. 6.15A). In the cerebrum, the status spongiosus follows the border between cerebral cortex and subcortical white matter. In mild cases, this status spongiosus or edema is restricted to the substantia nigra in the lateral midbrain. It occurs occasionally combined with neuronal degeneration in brainstem nuclei. The cause of this quite common brain condition of Swiss ruminants is unknown. Although it is neuropathologically similar to the vacuolation occurring in metabolic encephalopathy, liver lesions have not been demonstrated in these animals. In birds, epidemics of **avian vacuolar myelinopathy** in the USA have been associated with cyanobacteria growing on invasive exotic aquatic plants (*Hydrilla*).

Metabolic encephalopathy

Metabolic encephalopathy results from hepatic (hepatic encephalopathy) or renal (renal encephalopathy) failure. **Hepatic encephalopathy** is recognized in all domestic animal species. It may be caused either by a portosystemic shunt (congenital or acquired) or result from infectious/metabolic/toxic/degenerative liver diseases. The pathogenesis has not been entirely unraveled but it is accepted that in liver failure, bypassing or injury of hepatocytes hampers the detoxification of ammonium, which is neurotoxic at elevated concentrations. Excess ammonium enters the brain and is metabolized by astrocytic glutamine synthetase to noxious glutamine. Glutamine acts as an osmolyte causing astrocytic swelling. It is transported into mitochondria and there again split into glutamate and ammonium ("Trojan horse hypothesis"), which induces generation of free radicals that damage mitochondrial membranes, finally resulting in astrocytic dysfunction and brain edema. Additionally, inflammatory mediators contribute to astrocytic swelling and edema.

In **renal failure**, the resulting encephalopathy is thought to result from accumulation of neurotoxic metabolites, but as yet no specific neurotoxin has been identified.

Gross lesions are lacking in metabolic encephalopathy. Depending on the animal species there are varying degrees of white matter vacuolation. The spongy state with numerous clearly defined vacuoles of varying size is reminiscent of cytotoxic edema and particularly affects

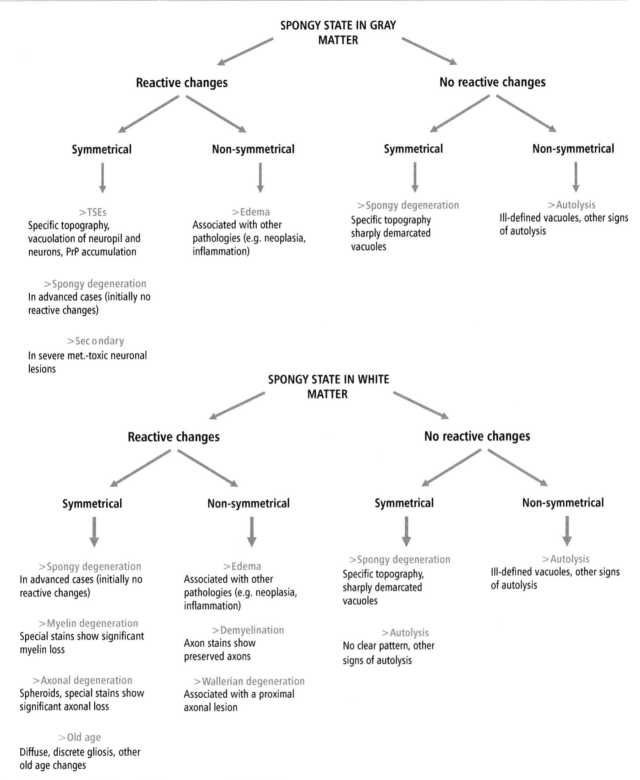

Fig. 6.14 Differential diagnosis of spongy state in the CNS.

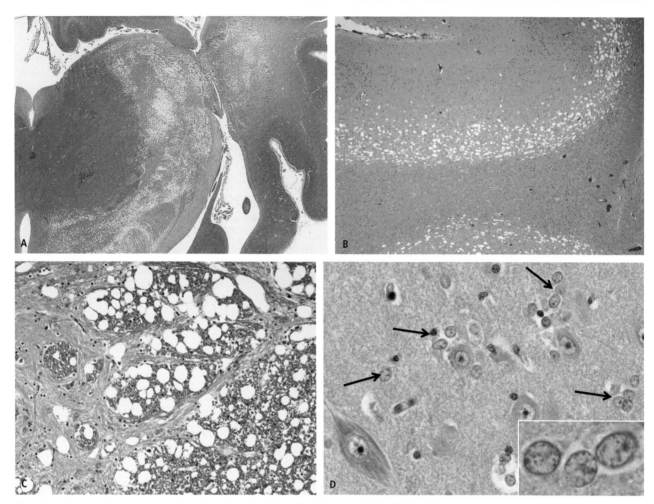

Fig. 6.15 Spongy degeneration. A: Bovine. Cross-section of forebrain. Sporadic brain edema. Massive spongy state in large areas of the white matter. HE. B: Calf. Hepatic portosystemic shunt. Cerebral cortex. Prominent vacuolation in the deep layers of the cerebral cortex. HE. C: Same case as B. Spongy state with clear, empty vacuoles in the white matter in the internal casule. HE. D: Horse. Globus pallidus. Hepatic encephalopathy. Many Alzheimer type II cells single or in small groups (arrows). HE. Inset: Their nuclei are swollen and open-faced with marginalized chromatin. HE.

boundary areas between gray and white matter in a bilaterally symmetrical pattern (Fig. 6.15B,C). In small animals this is often most prominent in the cerebellar nuclei and brainstem nuclei. In large animals there may be widespread spongy degeneration of the white matter. This is conspicuous in the subcortical white matter (Fig. 6.15B), internal capsule, thalamus, cerebellar medulla and brainstem (Fig. 6.15C). In the spinal cord, lesions are prominent in the fasciculus proprius. Additionally, in rare cases, occasional necrotic neurons, with shrunken, bright eosinophilic cytoplasma and pyknotic nuclei, may be found.

Histological changes in metabolic encephalopathy include the presence of astrocytes with swollen nuclei referred to as Alzheimer type II cells (Fig. 6.15D). Their

nuclei typically have marginalized chromatin and a clear center. Alzheimer type II cells occur as single cells, in short chains or small groups of two to six cells throughout the gray matter, particularly in the cerebral cortex and basal nuclei. The Alzheimer type II cells are also seen when spongy degeneration is only minimal or even absent, and may thus be the only change indicative of metabolic encephalopathy (particularly in horses).

6.5 Metabolic–toxic lesions of the peripheral nervous system (PNS) and skeletal muscle

Several toxins and deficiencies selectively or primarily affect the PNS. Any diagnostic assessment of the PNS requires electrodiagnostic testing, systematic sampling of proximal and distal portions of the nerves, semithin sectioning and teased fiber preparations. For the latter two methods the reader is referred to more specific literature. Here, the histopathological changes of the most common toxic–metabolic disorders affecting the PNS and skeletal muscle are briefly described.

6.5.1 Metabolic–toxic neuropathies
Salinomycin poisoning

Monovalent ionophores such as *salinomycin* are widely used as coccidiostatic drugs in poultry and as growth promoters in ruminants. These compounds are toxic in other species such as cats, horses and dogs. Salinomycin chelates monovalent cations, thereby facilitating cation transport across cell membranes. This affects the electrical potential and energy metabolism, eventually leading to structural damage to muscle (skeletal and cardiac) and axons. Animals with **salinomycin poisoning** show paraparesis to tetraplegia resulting from widespread primary axonal degeneration in the PNS involving both sensory and motor nerves. Additionally, Wallerian-type axonal degeneration is present in the dorsal tracts of the spinal cord. Outbreaks in cats have occurred as a result of errors in industrial feed production.

Axonal degeneration of peripheral nerves has been described in **vincristine poisoning** of cats. Here, focal axonal swelling and demyelination occur in motor and sensory nerves. In the more distal portions of the nerves, Wallerian degeneration is observed.

Organophosphate poisoning

Axonal degeneration in the distal portions of peripheral nerves is also a feature of **organophosphate poisoning** in several animal species. In advanced stages, peripheral nerves show Schwann cell proliferation with Büngner's bands and nerve fiber regeneration. In the PNS, this distal axonopathy produces a clinical picture of polyneuropathy in man and animals, in which sensory and motor disturbances develop in the distal limbs (feet and hands) then progress with time to involve the proximal limbs (legs and arms).

Presumptive toxic polyneuropathies of horses

A **polyneuropathy** in Norwegian horses has been described in animals on a diet of big bale hay (probably bad hay) with symmetrical weakness of the digital extensor muscles. In the sciatic nerve large swollen axons and distended myelin sheaths with myelinophages were noted. In chronic cases loss of nerve fibers and fibrosis were present. Swollen axons were also found in the lumbar spinal cord.

Similar lesions in the distal nerves of the hind limbs have been described in horses worldwide with **Australian stringhalt**, a disease with sudden onset occurring as herd outbreaks in late summer. The CNS remains unaffected. It has been associated with grazing on pastures contaminated with *Hypochaeris radicata*, *Taraxacum officinale* and *Malva parviflora*.

Metabolic neuropathies in small animals

In **canine hypothyroidism** various neurological complications have been reported including myxedema, coma, brain infarcts subsequent to atherosclerosis of the cerebral vasculature and vestibular disease. Clinical studies describe polyneuropathy – mainly apparent in the cranial nerves – and myopathy in dogs, which otherwise show no clinical signs of hypothyroidism. However, the little pathological information existing on both canine and human pathology is inconsistent, ranging from absent neuropathological changes to demyelination and axonal degeneration.

Diabetic polyneuropathy occurs in diabetes mellitus in people but also, rarely, in dogs and particularly cats. In the latter species, it is clinically characterized by paraparesis with a characteristic plantigrade posture of the hind limbs. Neuropathological changes in peripheral nerves may vary from case to case and include axon degeneration/regeneration and myelin degeneration/regeneration. These are associated with an endoneurial microangiopathy.

Paraneoplastic neuropathy is a rare complication in animals with tumors outside of the nervous system (insulinoma, carcinoma, melanoma, lymphoma). The pathogenesis is not clear; presumably there is an immune reaction against tumor antigens, which cross-reacts with normal peripheral nerve antigens. Morphologically, in paraneoplastic neuropathies there is usually a combination of axonal loss and demyelination together with reactive changes in the form of Schwann cell and endoneurial cell proliferation. In hyperinsulinemia associated with islet cell tumors, a widespread necrotizing neuropathy may occur.

6.5.2 Metabolic–toxic myopathies

The range of histopathologic changes in metabolic–toxic myopathies is limited and there is no pattern specific for a toxin or deficiency. The identification of the underlying etiology based solely on the pathologic examination is impossible and, hence, anamnestic data are crucial. In very acute cases, no gross lesions may be seen. A few days after the insult pale, dry streaks are identifiable in the swollen skeletal muscle. Interfascial edema may be present. In some cases, mineralization is seen as chalky deposits. In protracted cases, fibrosis and muscle atrophy occur.

Microscopically, myofiber degeneration is characterized by paleness, swelling and vacuolation of the cytoplasm. In frank necrosis the typical cross-striations disappear and the cytoplasm acquires a hypereosinophilic, hyaline and fragmented/flocculated aspect. Nuclei are pyknotic and undergo rhexis. Strong variation in myofiber size may be apparent with both swollen and shrunken fibers. Mineralization of myofibers may accompany these changes and can be prominent in certain intoxications. Signs of regenerative attempts may be observed including central position and proliferation of nuclei and increased basophilia of the cytoplasm. In the later phase of toxic insult, infiltration of phagocytes and reparative processes (fibrosis) become more apparent.

Monophasic lesions (all necrotic myofibers are in the same phase of degeneration/necrosis) indicate acute intoxication or exertional rhabdomyolysis. Toxins include **ionophores** (e.g. monensin, salinomycin, lasalocid, nystatin), *Cassia* spp (e.g. *Cassia occidentalis*, annual plants occurring in the United States) and **lichen** (*Xanthoparmelia chlorochroa*). **Exertional rhabdomyolysis** is frequent in horses and **capture myopathy** is seen in birds, and involves stress-related shock, metabolic acidosis and hyperthermia.

Polyphasic muscle necrosis is mainly observed in **vitamin E/selenium deficiency** (**white muscle disease**) in horses, ruminants, pigs and birds. Inadequate intake of vitamin E/selenium results in decreased sequestration and neutralization of free radicals resulting in membrane damage and subsequent myofiber necrosis. In white muscle disease, mineralization of necrotic fibers may be prominent.

Further reading

General

Bolon B, Butt MT. Fundamental Neuropathology for Pathologists and Toxicologists. Hoboken, NJ: Wiley, 2011.

Polioencephalomalacia large animals

Bourke CA, Colegate SM, Rendell D, Bunker EC, Kuhn RP. Peracute ammonia toxicity: a consideration in the pathogenesis of *Phalaris aquatica* "Polioencephalomalacia-like sudden death" poisoning of sheep and cattle. Aust Vet J 2005;83:168–171.

McKenzie RA, Carmichael AM, Schibrowski ML, Duigan SA, Gibson JA, Taylor JD. Sulfur-associated polioencephalomalacia in cattle grazing plants in the Family *Brassicaceae*. Aust Vet J 2009;87:27–32.

Sakhaee E, Derakhshanfar A. Polioencephalomalacia associated with closantel overdosage in a goat. J S Afr Vet Assoc 2010;81:116–117.

Polioencephalomalacia in small animals

Auer RN. Hypoglycemic brain damage. Metab Brain Dis 2004;19:169–175.

Frazier K, Hullinger G, Hines M 2nd, Liggett A, Sangster L. 162 cases of aldicarb intoxication in Georgia domestic animals from 1988–1998. Vet Hum Toxicol 1999;41:233–235.

Shimada A, Morita T, Ikeda N, Torii S, Haruna A. Hypoglycaemic brain lesions in a dog with insulinoma. J Comp Pathol 2000;122:67–71.

Hippocampal necrosis and sclerosis

Fatzer R, Gandini G, Jaggy A, Doherr M, Vandevelde M. Necrosis of hippocampus and piriform lobe in 38 domestic cats with seizures: a retrospective study on clinical and pathologic findings. J Vet Intern Med 2000;14:100–104.

Kuwabara T, Hasegawa D, Kobayashi M, Fujita M, Orima H. Clinical magnetic resonance volumetry of the hippocampus in 58 epileptic dogs. Vet Radiol Ultrasound 2010;51:485–490.

Pakozdy A, Gruber A, Kneissl S, Leschnik M, Halasz P, Thalhammer JG. Complex partial cluster seizures in cats with orofacial involvement. J Feline Med Surg 2011;13:687–693.

Subcortical and brainstem encephalomalacias

Chang HT, Rumbeiha WK, Patterson JS, Puschner B, Knight AP. Toxic equine parkinsonism: an immunohistochemical study of 10 horses with nigropallidal encephalomalacia. Vet Pathol 2012;49:398–402.

Finnie JW. Review of corynetoxins poisoning of livestock, a neurological disorder produced by a nematode–bacterium complex. Aust Vet J 2006;84:271–277.

Malik R, Sibraa D. Thiamine deficiency due to sulphur dioxide preservative in "pet meat" – a case of déjà vu. Aust Vet J 2005;83:408–411.

Olson EJ, Morales SC, McVey AS, Hayden DW. Putative metronidazole neurotoxicosis in a cat. Vet Pathol 2005;42:665–669.

Riet-Correa F, Timm CD, Barros SS, Summers BA. Symmetric focal degeneration in the cerebellar and vestibular nuclei in swine caused by ingestion of *Aeschynomene indica* Seeds. Vet Pathol 2003;40:311–316.

Woodruff BK, Wijdicks EF, Marshall WF. Reversible metronidazole-induced lesions of the cerebellar dentate nuclei. N Engl J Med 2002;346:68–69.

Selenium poisoning

Casteignau A, Fontán A, Morillo A, Oliveros JA, Segalés J. Clinical, pathological and toxicological findings of a iatrogenic selenium toxicosis case in feeder pigs. J Vet Med A Physiol Pathol Clin Med 2006;53:323–326.

Equine leukomalacia

Caloni F, Cortinovis C. Effects of fusariotoxins in the equine species. Vet J 2010;186:157–161.

Enterotoxemia

Dorca-Arévalo J, Soler-Jover A, Gibert M, Popoff MR, Martín-Satué M, Blasi J. Binding of epsilon-toxin from *Clostridium perfringens* in the nervous system. Vet Microbiol 2008;131:14–25.

Lonchamp E, Dupont JL, Wioland L, Courjaret R, Mbebi-Liegeois C, Jover E, Doussau F, Popoff MR, Bossu JL, de Barry J, Poulain B. *Clostridium perfringens* epsilon toxin targets granule cells in the mouse cerebellum and stimulates glutamate release. PLoS One 2010;5.pii:e13046.

Moxley RA. Edema disease. Vet Clin North Am Food Anim Pract 2000;16:175–185.

CO poisoning

Weiss AT, Graf C, Gruber AD, Kohn B. Leukoencephalomalacia and laminar neuronal necrosis following smoke inhalation in a dog. Vet Pathol 2011;48:1016–1019.

Metabolic toxic neuronal degenerations

Binder EM, Blodgett DJ, Currin JF, Caudell D, Cherney JH, LeRoith T. *Phalaris arundinacea* (reed canarygrass) grass staggers in beef cattle. J Vet Diagn Invest 2010;22(5):802–805.

Bourke CA, Colegate SM, Rendell D, Bunker EC, Kuhn RP. Peracute ammonia toxicity: a consideration in the pathogenesis of *Phalaris aquatica* "Polioencephalomalacia-like sudden death" poisoning of sheep and cattle. Aust Vet J 2005;83(3):168–171.

Divers TJ, Cummings JE, de Lahunta A, Hintz HF, Mohammed HO. Evaluation of the risk of motor neuron disease in horses fed a diet low in vitamin E and high in copper and iron. Am J Vet Res 2006;67: 120–126.

Loretti AP, Colodel EM, Driemeier D, Correa AM, Bangel JJ, Ferreiro L. Neurological disorder in dairy cattle associated with consumption of beer residues contaminated with *Aspergillus clavatus*. J Vet Diagn Invest 2003;15:123–132.

Sabater-Vilar M, Maas RF, De Bosschere H, Ducatelle R, Fink-Gremmels J. Patulin produced by an *Aspergillus clavatus* isolated from feed containing malting residues associated with a lethal neurotoxicosis in cattle. Mycopathologia 2004;158:419–426.

Grass sickness

Edwards SE, Martz KE, Rogge A, Heinrich M. Edaphic and phytochemical factors as predictors of Equine Grass Sickness cases in the UK. Frontiers in Predictive Toxicology 2010; 10.3389/fphar.2010.00122.

Hahn CN, Mayhew IG, de Lahunta A. Central neuropathology of equine grass sickness. Acta Neuropathol 2001;102:153–159.

Milne EM, Pirie RS, McGorum BC, Shaw DJ. Evaluation of formalin-fixed ileum as the optimum method to diagnose equine dysautonomia (grass sickness) in simulated intestinal biopsies. J Vet Diagn Invest 2010;22:248–252.

Waggett BE, McGorum BC, Shaw DJ, Pirie RS, MacIntyre N, Wernery U, Milne EM. Evaluation of synaptophysin as an immunohistochemical marker for equine grass sickness. J Comp Pathol 2010;142: 284–290.

Acquired lysosomal storage diseases

Armién AG, Tokarnia CH, Peixoto PV, Frese K. Spontaneous and experimental glycoprotein storage disease of goats induced by *Ipomoea carnea* subsp *fistulosa* (Convolvulaceae). Vet Pathol 2007; 44:170–184.

Dantas AF, Riet-Correa F, Gardner DR, Medeiros RM, Barros SS, Anjos BL, Lucena RB. Swainsonine-induced lysosomal storage disease in goats caused by the ingestion of *Turbina cordata* in Northeastern Brazil. Toxicon 2007;49:111–116.

Van der Lugt JJ, Bastianello SS, van Ederen AM, van Wilpe E. Cerebellar cortical degeneration in cattle caused by *Solanum kwebense*. Vet J 2010;185:225–227.

Metabolic–toxic axonal degenerations

Imlach WL, Finch SC, Dunlop J, Meredith AL, Aldrich RW, Dalziel JE. The molecular mechanism of "ryegrass staggers," a neurological disorder of K+ channels. J Pharmacol Exp Ther 2008;327: 657–664.

Jortner BS. Mechanisms of toxic injury in the peripheral nervous system: neuropathologic considerations. Toxicol Pathol 2000;28: 54–69.

Riet-Correa F, Barros SS, Méndez MC, Gevehr-Fernandes C, Pereira Neto OA, Soares MP, McGavin MD. Axonal degeneration in sheep caused by the ingestion of *Halimium brasiliense*. J Vet Diagn Invest 2009;21:478–486.

Salvadori C, Cantile C, De Ambrogi G, Arispici M. Degenerative myelopathy associated with cobalamin deficiency in a cat. J Vet Med A Physiol Pathol Clin Med 2003;50:292–296.

Irradiated feed-induced myelinopathy in cats

Cassidy JP, Caulfield C, Jones BR, Worrall S, Conlon L, Palmer AC, Kelly J. Leukoencephalomyelopathy in specific pathogen-free cats. Vet Pathol 2007;44:912–916.

Caulfield CD, Kelly JP, Jones BR, Worrall S, Conlon L, Palmer AC, Cassidy JP. The experimental induction of leukoencephalomyelopathy in cats. Vet Pathol 2009;46:1258–1269.

Duncan ID, Brower A, Kondo Y, Curlee JF, Schultz RD. Extensive remyelination of the CNS leads to functional recovery. Proc Natl Acad Sci U S A 2009;106:6832–6836.

Toxic spongy degenerations

Ecco R, de Barros CS, Graça DL, Gava A. Closantel toxicosis in kid goats. Vet Rec 2006;159:564–566.

Wiley FE, Twiner MJ, Leighfield TA, Wilde SB, Van Dolah FM, Fischer JR, Bowerman WW. An extract of *Hydrilla verticillata* and associated epiphytes induces avian vacuolar myelinopathy in laboratory mallards. Environ Toxicol 2009;24:362–368.

Hepatic encephalopathy

Albrecht J, Zielińska M, Norenberg MD. Glutamine as a mediator of ammonia neurotoxicity: a critical appraisal. Biochem Pharmacol 2010;80:1303–1308.

Prakash R, Mullen KD. Mechanisms, diagnosis and management of hepatic encephalopathy. Nat Rev Gastroenterol Hepatol 2010;7: 515–525.

Toxic peripheral neuropathies

Domange C, Casteignau A, Collignon G, Pumarola M, Priymenko N. Longitudinal study of Australian stringhalt cases in France. J Anim Physiol Anim Nutr (Berl) 2010;94:712–720.

Hanche-Olsen S, Teige J, Skaar I, Ihler CF. Polyneuropathy associated with forage sources in Norwegian horses. J Vet Intern Med 2008;22: 178–184.

Jortner BS. Mechanisms of toxic injury in the peripheral nervous system: neuropathologic considerations. Toxicol Pathol 2000;28: 54–69.

Pakozdy A, Challande-Kathman I, Doherr M, Cizinauskas S, Wheeler SJ, Oevermann A, Jaggy A. Retrospective study of salinomycin toxicosis in 66 cats. Vet Med Int 2010;2010:147142.

Van der Linde-Sipman JS, van den Ingh TS, van nes JJ, Verhagen H, Kersten JG,Beynen AC, Plekkringa R. Salinomycin-induced polyneuropathy in cats: morphologic and epidemiologic data. Vet Pathol 1999;36:152–156.

Metabolic peripheral neuropathies

Estrella JS, Nelson RN, Sturges BK, Vernau KM, Williams DC, LeCouteur RA, Shelton GD, Mizisin AP. Endoneurial microvascular pathology in feline diabetic neuropathy. Microvasc Res 2008;75: 403–410.

Mizisin AP, Nelson RW, Sturges BK, Vernau KM, Lecouteur RA, Williams DC, Burgers ML, Shelton GD. Comparable myelinated nerve pathology in feline and human diabetes mellitus. Acta Neuropathol 2007;113:431–442.

Matabolic–toxic myopathies

Barth AT, Kommers GD, Salles MS, Wouters F, de Barros CS. Coffee Senna (*Senna occidentalis*) poisoning in cattle in Brazil. Vet Hum Toxicol 1994;36:541–545.

Dailey RN, Montgomery DL, Ingram JT, Siemion R, Vasquez M, Raisbeck MF. Toxicity of the lichen secondary metabolite (+)-usnic acid in domestic sheep. Vet Pathol 2008;45:19–25.

 This book is accompanied by a companion website which is maintained by the Division of Diagnostic Imaging, Dept of Clinical Veterinary Medicine, Vetsuisse Faculty, University of Bern, Switzerland.

www.wiley.com/go/vandevelde/veterinaryneuropathology

7

Neoplasia

Nervous system tumors are classified either as primary, when derived from cells of neuroectodermal origin, or secondary, when originating from non-neural tumor cells, and which subsequently gain access to the nervous system by different routes. Up to one half of all nervous system tumors are of primary type. Although primary tumors do not spontaneously metastazise outside of the CNS, some tumors have a tendency for metastasis and dissemination within the CSF pathways (e.g. oligodendrogliomas, choroid plexus carcinomas).

All tumors behave as space-occupying mass lesions, usually with secondary manifestations of mechanical compression including hemorrhages, edema, disturbances of CSF circulation (e.g. hydrocephalus), cerebral midline shifts and herniations. Most tumors also compress or infiltrate with eventual destruction of nervous tissue.

Both primary and secondary tumors of the nervous system occur in all domestic animal species, although they are most common and best characterized and studied in the dog. Reported incidences of primary brain tumors in dogs vary up to 1.9% of all tumors. These tumors generally affect adult to old animals, but there are a few exceptions that tend to occur preferentially in young animals (e.g. medulloblastoma, other primitive neuroectodermal tumors, and ectopic nephroblastoma). There is an increase in frequency of most tumors with age (particularly after 5 years) and a notably higher predisposition for glial tumor types (up to 25 times) in some brachycephalic breeds (Boxer, English Bulldog, Boston Terrier, etc.) compared with other breeds.

In dogs, primary tumors have histological types and biological behaviour strikingly similar to those in people, although their frequencies differ in some types. Because of these shared similarities we have applied the latest human 2007 World Health Organization (WHO) classification and grading system criteria to these tumors (Table 7.1), realizing nevertheless that prospective canine studies are urgently needed to validate such extrapolation.

7.1 General strategy for diagnosis of neoplastic lesions

7.1.1 Clinic and diagnostic imaging

In the dog and cat, mass lesions are easily detected by MRI, but neuroimaging profiles alone can at best provide only a differential diagnosis of possible tumor types. However, because most primary tumors have distinguishing features such as breed, age and sites of anatomical localization, integration of such information on each tumor together with the imaging profile can provide a reasonably accurate differential clinical diagnosis. Clinically, CSF cytological analysis can also be useful in diagnosis of some tumors. However, a specific diagnosis depends finally on histological classification of both tissues and smears obtained from surgical biopsy or from CT- or MRI-guided stereotactic biopsy techniques.

7.1.2 Interpretation of gross findings

At necropsy, one is generally confronted with mass lesions, which are easy to detect when gross examination of the CNS/PNS is performed systematically and then correlated with MR images as described in Chapter 1. Diffusely growing tumors may not be recognized initially but careful evaluation will detect one or more of the features induced by the mass effect. Several gross features may help to direct the diagnosis. An overview of such features and their interpretation is shown in Fig. 7.1.

- A single mass generally suggests a primary CNS tumor, whereas multiple masses favor a provisional

Veterinary Neuropathology: Essentials of Theory and Practice, First Edition. Marc Vandevelde, Robert J. Higgins, and Anna Oevermann.
© 2012 John Wiley & Sons, Ltd. Published 2012 by John Wiley & Sons, Ltd.

Table 7.1 Outline of the human 2007 WHO classification of human nervous system tumors adapted for the histological classification and grading of canine primary nervous system tumors.

Tumors of neuroepithelial tissue

Astrocytomas
- Pilocytic astrocytoma
- Gemistocytic astrocytoma
- Subependymal giant cell astrocytoma
- Diffuse astrocytoma
- Anaplastic astrocytoma
- Glioblastoma
- Gliomatosis cerebri

Oligodendroglial tumors
- Oligodendroglioma
- Anaplastic oligodendroglioma

Mixed gliomas

Ependymal tumors
- Ependymoma
  - Cellular
  - Papillary
  - Clear cell

Choroid plexus tumors
- Papilloma
- Carcinoma

Neuronal and mixed neuronal–glial tumors
- Ganglioglioma
- Gangliocytoma
- Neurocytoma
- Paraganglioma

Embryonal tumors
- Medulloblastoma
- PNET [Neuroblastoma]

Tumors of cranial and paraspinal nerves
- Schwannoma
- Neurofibroma
- Perineurioma
- Malignant PNST

Tumors of the meninges

Meningiomas
- Transitional
- Fibrous
- Angiomatous
- Psammomatous
- Meningothelial
- Microcystic
- Chordoid
- Atypical
- Papillary
- Malignant

Granular cell tumor

Mesenchymal tumors
- Leiomyosarcoma
- Hemangiosarcoma

Lymphomas and hemopoietic tumors
- B and T cell lymphoma
- Histiocytic sarcoma

Germ cell tumors
- Germinoma
- Teratoma

Miscellaneous tumors
- Ectopic neuroblastoma

Metastatic tumors

diagnosis of a metastatic tumor. The intra- or extra-axial site of the tumor provides the first algorithm to be applied. Extra-axial tumors originate from sites on the outer surface of the CNS (e.g. lepto- or pachymeninges, nerve roots) whereas an intra-axial location indicates that the tumor has originated from within the CNS parenchyma.

- The specific anatomical location of primary tumors may suggest a certain tumor type reflecting their preferred occurrence in specific predilection sites. Such examples would be intraventricular neoplasms arising from the choroid plexus or ependyma (choroid plexus tumors or ependymomas) or meningiomas from the olfactory bulb.

- The type of demarcation from adjacent normal tissue can provide further clues. Primary CNS tumors grow in most cases as compact mass lesions (e.g. choroid

plexus tumor, meningioma), but some tumors (e.g. diffuse astrocytoma) diffusely infiltrate and obliterate the CNS architecture and thus may only be detected by the asymmetry of the cerebral hemispheres found on transverse sections.

- Tumor consistency and color are other features that may indicate specific tumor types, e.g. a gelatinous and grayish translucent appearance is common in oligodendroglioma, while choroid plexus tumors are red with a granular roughened texture; whitish yellow areas of necrosis and variegated hemorrhage are expected features of, e.g., high-grade gliomas.

7.1.3 Diagnosis

After excluding a metastatic tumor based on multiple sites and histological diagnosis, the histological classification of primary brain tumors is more challenging.

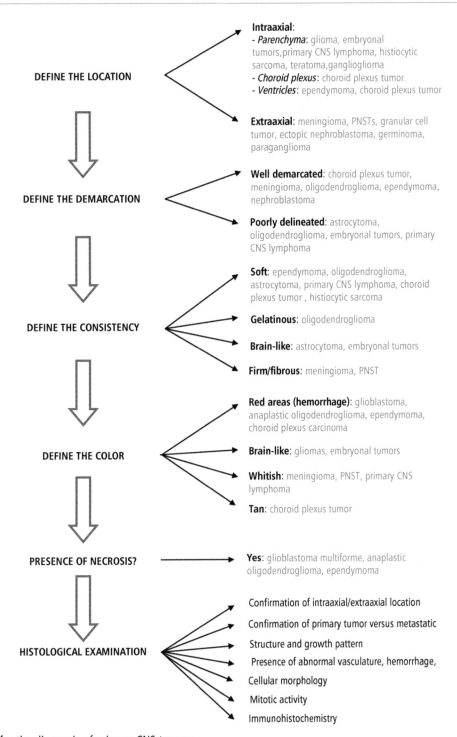

DEFINE THE LOCATION

Intraaxial:
- *Parenchyma*: glioma, embryonal tumors, primary CNS lymphoma, histiocytic sarcoma, teratoma, ganglioglioma
- *Choroid plexus*: choroid plexus tumor.
- *Ventricles*: ependymoma, choroid plexus tumor

Extraaxial: meningioma, PNSTs, granular cell tumor, ectopic nephroblastoma, germinoma, paraganglioma

DEFINE THE DEMARCATION

Well demarcated: choroid plexus tumor, meningioma, oligodendroglioma, ependymoma, nephroblastoma

Poorly delineated: astrocytoma, oligodendroglioma, embryonal tumors, primary CNS lymphoma

DEFINE THE CONSISTENCY

Soft: ependymoma, oligodendroglioma, astrocytoma, primary CNS lymphoma, choroid plexus tumor , histiocytic sarcoma

Gelatinous: oligodendroglioma

Brain-like: astrocytoma, embryonal tumors

Firm/fibrous: meningioma, PNST

DEFINE THE COLOR

Red areas (hemorrhage): glioblastoma, anaplastic oligodendroglioma, ependymoma, choroid plexus carcinoma

Brain-like: gliomas, embryonal tumors

Whitish: meningioma, PNST, primary CNS lymphoma

Tan: choroid plexus tumor

PRESENCE OF NECROSIS?

Yes: glioblastoma multiforme, anaplastic oligodendroglioma, ependymoma

HISTOLOGICAL EXAMINATION

Confirmation of intraaxial/extraaxial location

Confirmation of primary tumor versus metastatic

Structure and growth pattern

Presence of abnormal vasculature, hemorrhage,

Cellular morphology

Mitotic activity

Immunohistochemistry

Fig. 7.1 Strategy for the diagnosis of primary CNS tumors.

Essentially this still relies on the recognition of the histological similarity of neoplastic cells to either normal glial or neuronal cell phenotypes. In many tumors (especially the more malignant grades), this similarity may not be obvious. Further criteria used include the patterns of growth and infiltration, the formation of secondary structures of Scherer, cytological characteristics, and abnormal blood vessels or necrosis.

Confirmation of the histological classification can be made either by immunohistochemical visualization of cell-specific antigenic markers (Table 7.2) or less commonly by tumor-specific ultrastructural features by TEM. Recent advanced molecular genetic and biology studies in human tumors suggest that such techniques provide a more accurate classification and prognosis than that from conventional histology. However, such molecular techniques are not yet available in veterinary oncology, so here we rely on conventional histological interpretation supported mainly by immunohistochemical techniques.

Table 7.2 Some routine cell-specific antibodies for diagnostic immunohistochemical confirmation of formalin-fixed paraffin-embedded primary nervous system tumors.

TUMOR TYPE	ANTIBODY TO
Gliomas	
Astrocytomas	GFAP, Vimentin
Oligodendrogliomas	Olig2, GFAP
Ependymomas	GFAP, Vimentin, CK
Choroid Plexus tumors	CK, GFAP
Neuronal tumors	
Ganglioglioma	SYN, NeuN, NFP, GFAP
Gangliocytoma	SYN, NeuN, NFP
Neurocytoma	SYN, Olig2, NeuN
Paraganglioma	CG, SYN, NFP
Embryonal tumors	
Medulloblastoma	SYN, NeuN, GFAP, NFP, NSE
PNET	SYN, NeuN, GFAP
Tumors of peripheral nerves	
Schwannoma	S-100, GFAP, Laminin, Collagen IV
Neurofibroma	S-100, Laminin, Collagen IV
Perineurioma	Laminin, TNF, Vimentin, S-100
PNST	Vimentin, Collagen IV, Laminin
Meningiomas	CK, Vimentin
Granular cell tumor	S-100, Ubiquitin, α-1-AT
Mesenchymal tumors	
Leiomyosarcoma	Vimentin, SMA
Hemangiosarcoma	Factor VIII, CD31
Primary lymphomas	
B and T cell lymphomas	CD79a, CD3, CD18, CD20
Histiocytic sarcoma	CD1c, CD11b, CD11c, CD18
Germ cell tumors	
Germinoma	AFP, PLAP, c-kit
Teratoma	CK, Vimentin, neuronal panel
Embryonal tumors	
Nephroblastoma	WT-1, Vimentin, CK

CK: cytokeratin low and high MW(Lu 5 or AE1/AE3); SYN: synaptophysin; TNF: triple neurofilament protein; CG: chromogranin A; NSE: neuron specific enolase; α-1-AT: α-1-antitrypsin; SMA: smooth muscle actin; AFP: alpha fetal protein; PLAP: placental alkaline phosphatase; WT-1: Wilms tumor 1 antigen.

7.1.4 Grading

Most human classification and grading systems provide very reliable and accurate predictive and prognostic information resulting in the application of appropriate therapeutic protocols. These systems grade tumors according to prognostically tested significant histological features, e.g. cytological differentiation, necrosis, mitotic index, cell patterns, neovascularization etc., although the relevance of each of these criteria varies according to the tumor type. Although grading systems are being increasingly used, there is still no scientifically validated system applicable to animal nervous system tumors. Many veterinary neuropathologists now classify and grade canine nervous system tumors according to the latest human 2007 WHO classification and grading system. However, the remarkable prognostic accuracy of this proven human system awaits comparable prospective studies. Since veterinary neuro-oncologists now have neuroimaging (MRI, CT) techniques and stereotactic brain biopsy devices for *in vivo* diagnosis of tumors becoming available, it is hoped that with further education an accurate standardized grading system for such tumors will be developed.

7.2 Tumors of neuroepithelial origin

7.2.1 Astrocytomas

General features and subtypes

In dogs, astrocytomas have an overall incidence of about 15% of all primary nervous system tumors. They occur increasingly with age, and some brachycephalic breeds (Boxer, Boston Terrier, Bulldog etc.) have a much higher risk of occurrence (up to 25 times greater) than other breeds. MRI features are not exclusively diagnostic. Some astrocytoma subtypes have also been described in cats, cattle, horses and pigs. Macroscopically they can be large, unilateral, and most subtypes have usually a preferential anatomical localization and a distinctive histological appearance.

Astrocytomas are a diverse subgroup of gliomas (the other subgroup being oligodendrogliomas) with subtypes that are either well circumscribed (pilocytic, gemistocytic or subependymal giant cell) or more commonly a continuum of diffusely infiltrating astrocytomas (diffuse, anaplastic astrocytoma, glioblastoma and gliomatosis cerebri). As a general group astrocytomas share some common features – their incidence increases with age, and they generally arise supratentorially within the white matter of cerebral hemispheres and less common caudally in the thalamus, midbrain, brainstem and spinal cord. On cut surface, astrocytomas are firmer than normal brain tissue and white, but it can be difficult to pinpoint precise margins since they eventually obliterate underlying gray and white matter landmarks. Characteristically, they do not invade ventricles. There are three major astrocytoma subtypes: diffuse, anaplastic and glioblastoma (so-called glioblastoma multiforme (GBM)) in order of increasing malignancy, grades II–IV. Increased cell density, nuclear atypia, and increased numbers of normal and abnormal mitotic figures each correlate directly with more aggressive behavior (in people) and are some of the histological features used for grading. The higher-grade tumors exhibit a highly infiltrative mode of growth and expansion. Secondary structures of Scherer comprising tumor cell neuronal satellitosis, perivascular infiltration and subpial migration and accumulation are also features of higher tumor grades. Glial cell pseudopalisading around areas of necrosis and/or microvascular proliferation are exclusively characteristic of the grade IV glioblastoma. Gross features of glioblastoma can include hemorrhages, cysts and focal yellow–white areas of necrosis. The proliferative index (PI), as defined by MIB-1 immunoreactivity, ranges from between 5 and 35% for grades II–IV respectively. Most astrocytomas exhibit GFAP immunoreactivity.

Well circumscribed astrocytomas

Pilocytic astrocytoma (WHO grade I)
Pilocytic astrocytomas are extremely rare in dogs and are well circumscribed tumors, which on MRI have T2W hyperintensity and strong contrast enhancement usually with characteristic multiple small cysts. They occur mainly in the thalamus. Grossly, tumors are discrete, gray to white, often with macrocysts (Fig. 7.2A). Microscopically, they have low cellularity with a bipolar, fibrillary, predominant GFAP-immunoreactive cell but with areas of varying cell density and sometimes Rosenthal-like fibers (Fig. 7.2B). However, vascular proliferation and necrosis (both described in human pilocytic astrocytomas) have not yet been noted in the canine tumor. There can be admixed cells with a hyperchromatic and enlarged nuclei. Cysts appear empty but microscopically are lined or filled by small basophilic round cells with fibrillary processes. Mitoses are rare and PI is up to 1%.

Subependymal giant cell astrocytoma (SEGA) (WHO grade I)
These are rare, well defined, solitary, circumscribed grade I astrocytomas in the cat and dog restricted to subependymal locations medially around the lateral ventricles sometimes with distortion of the third ventricle. In the dog, SEGA also occur subependymally

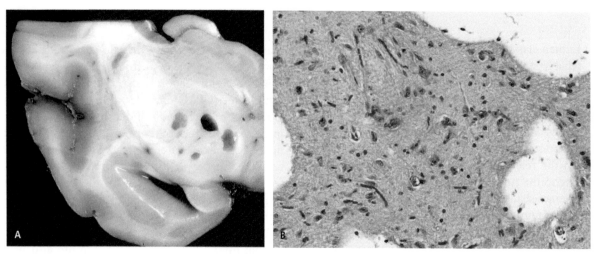

Fig. 7.2 Dog. Thalamus. Pilocytic astrocytoma. A: There is a well circumscribed whitish solid mass with multiple empty cysts of varying size. B: Elongate astrocytoma cells with marked nuclear pleomorphism and fibrillary processes with smaller cells in cyst-like spaces. HE.

with expansile growth into the fourth ventricle. This secondary intraventricular growth often results in an associated obstructive hydrocephalus. Histologically, the discrete mass is composed of gemistocytic, spindle and ganglioid-like astrocytoma cells in irregular nests separated by fibrous tissue. Many cells are large and irregular with abundant cytoplasm and prominent nuclei with some weak patchy GFAP immunoreactivity. Mitoses are absent and PI is low (<2%).

Gemistocytic astrocytoma (WHO grade II)
These uncommon astrocytomas are classified as grade II and in the dog usually occur in the cerebellum and less

often in the cervical spinal cord. MRI findings typically are of non-contrast-enhancing masses, isointense on T1W images but mildly hyperintense T2W images, suggesting intra- and slight peritumoral edema. Canine gemistocytic astrocytomas have a well defined border, are white to tan and with a roughened cut surface (Fig. 7.3A). They are composed of a distinctive population of cells most closely resembling gemistocytic astrocytes with a variable amount of angular-shaped, swollen, homogeneous and glassy eosinophilic and consistently strongly GFAP-immunoreactive cytoplasm, with multiple short processes (Fig. 7.3B). Cells have one or multiple eccentrically located nuclei with a large

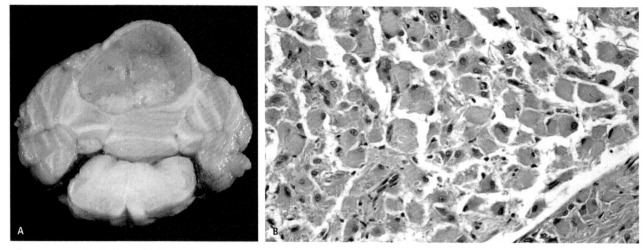

Fig. 7.3 Dog. Cerebellum. Gemistocytic astrocytoma. A: In the cerebellar cortex there is a sharply demarcated, tan-colored mass with focal yellowish areas of necrosis and small cystic spaces. B: Most of the neoplastic cells phenotypically resemble gemistocytes with an eccentric nucleus and large amount of homogeneous eosinophilic-staining cytoplasm. No mitotic figures. HE.

prominent nucleolus. Mitotic activity is minimal and the PI is <2%.

Diffusely infiltrating astrocytomas

Diffuse astrocytoma (WHO grade II)
This diffusely infiltrating glioma arises most commonly supratentorially in the frontal and temporal lobes but can occur in the brainstem and spinal cord. On MRI, diffuse astrocytomas are generally mildly hypointense on T1W and moderately hyperintense on T2W images with no or minimal contrast enhancement (Fig. 7.4A). Grossly on transverse sectioning, there is blurring of anatomical boundaries due to the infiltrating pattern of growth with initial enlargement and eventual obliteration of normal anatomical gray and white matter boundaries. Macroscopically, the tumors are firm and whitish with indistinct borders (Fig. 7.4B). Microscopically, they are composed of a uniform population of infiltrating neoplastic fibrillary astrocytes giving the impression of an increased diffuse cellularity in an otherwise normal brain (Fig. 7.5A). Smears from stereotactic biopsy characteristically have a dispersed, elongate, uniform cell population with many refractile processes (Fig. 7.5E). Cells have elongate, enlarged hyperchromatic nuclei with scant cytoplasm but whose fibrillary processes are best visualized by their uniform and relatively strong GFAP (Fig. 7.5C) and vimentin immunoreactivity. These tumor cells tend to stream in parallel alignment along white matter tracts (Fig. 7.5A). Mitotic figures are very rare or absent with minimal nuclear atypia. Their PI is about 2–4% (Fig. 7.5D). In genomic DNA extracted from nine canine grade II astrocytomas, no TP53 mutations involving exons 3–9 were found. This strongly contrasts with analogous human astrocytomas, where there is a frequency of about 60%, suggesting that alternative mechanisms of p53 inactivation are present if p53 function contributes significantly to oncogenesis of canine astrocytomas.

Anaplastic astrocytoma (grade III)
MRI is similar to grade II tumors except that they can exhibit mild to markedly non-uniform contrast enhancement or have a ring of peripheral contrast enhancement on T2W images. See MRI Atlas. These tumors arise preferentially in the same locations as grade II astrocytomas and appear grossly similar, but are characterized histologically by markedly increased cellularity and cell density; cells have minimal cytoplasm on HE but show nuclear atypia, mitotic figures and a higher proliferative activity (PI of 5–10%) (Fig. 7.5B). Nuclei vary in size and shape, are more hyperchromatic

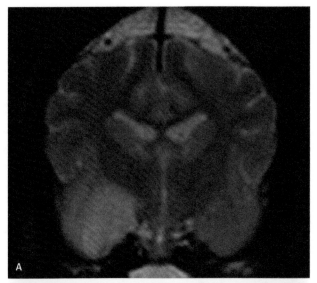

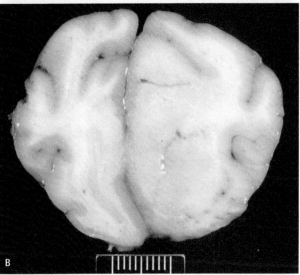

Fig. 7.4 Dog. Diffuse astrocytoma grade II. A: MRI. In the left temporal lobe on the T2W image there is mild uniform hyperintensity characteristic of a grade II astrocytoma. B: Transverse section through the frontal lobe. There is a whitish, poorly defined space-occupying mass on the right side with obliteration of normal gray and white matter boundaries and a marked left-sided midline shift.

and with prominent nucleoli, while their fibrillary cytoplasm is best defined by GFAP or vimentin immunoreactivity.

Glioblastoma (astrocytoma grade IV)
Glioblastoma, also known infamously in people as **GBM**, is common in the dog and like the human counterpart is the most malignant astrocytoma. The major predilection sites in the frontal and temporal lobes of the cerebrum parallel those of lower-grade astrocytomas. On

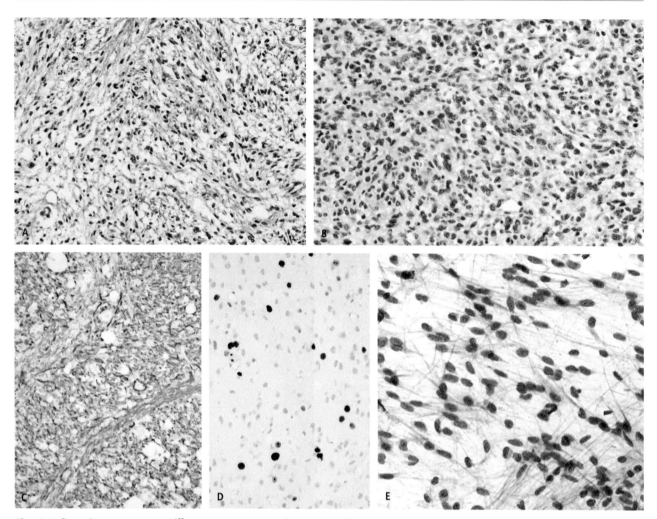

Fig. 7.5 Dog. Astrocytoma. A: Diffuse astrocytoma, grade II, with diffuse infiltration with cells with an elongate nucleus and little detectable cytoplasm often aligned within white matter tracts. HE. B: Increased cell density, prominent nuclear atypia and some mitotic figures compatible with an anaplastic astrocytoma, grade III. C: Diffuse astrocytoma with strong uniform reactivity of astrocytoma cell processes to GFAP. IHC visualized with AEC. D: Diffuse astrocytoma, grade II, with a PI of about 2% based on MIB-1 nuclear immunoreactivity. IHC. E: Smear from CT-guided stereobiopsy with elongate cells and prominent refractile processes from a diffuse astrocytoma, grade II. HE.

MRI with T1W images, there are central areas of hypodense necrosis but usually with striking partial or complete contrast ring enhancement; T2W images are heterogeneous and hyperintense, with sharp margins (Fig. 7.6A); and FLAIR images demonstrate considerable peritumoral edema. Macroscopically, there are areas of hemorrhage and necrosis within well defined boundaries (Fig. 7.6B). Microscopically, there is hypercellularity, prominent nuclear atypia, abundant normal and abnormal mitotic figures, and essential features for glioblastoma of either microvascular proliferation and/or glial cell pseudopalisading around extensive areas of coagulative necrosis (Fig. 7.7A,B). There can be widespread regional heterogeneity of neoplastic cell types with considerable nuclear and cytoplasmic pleomorphism including round, fusiform and polymorphic cells. Foci of oligodendroglial-like differentiation can occur with interstitial accumulation of myxoid material. Intravascular fibrin thrombi may be associated with areas of confluent, often serpentine, hypoxic necrosis and with acute focal hemorrhage (Fig. 7.7A). The microvascular proliferation is composed of glomeruloid-like clusters and lines of endothelial and smooth muscle cells from paracrine secretion by the tumor of growth factors VEGF and PDGF respectively. Human histological variants rarely seen in dogs include small cell GBM, astrob-

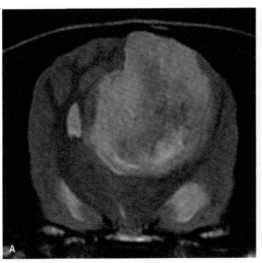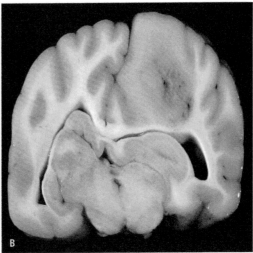

Fig. 7.6 Dog. Glioblastoma (astrocytoma, grade IV). A: MRI, T2W image. B: Transverse section of the same sharply demarcated mass with yellowish areas of necrosis, focal hemorrhage and small empty cysts. There is a massive midline shift including distortion of the hippocampus, fimbria, midbrain and lateral ventricles.

lastoma, gliosarcoma and giant cell glioblastoma. Canine glioblastomas are strongly immunoreactive to GFAP, IGFBP2 and EGFR but more variable with PDGFR-α antibodies. Extensive peritumoral tumor cell migration can lead to the formation of the so-called secondary structures of Scherer in grossly normal tissue (see Fig. 7.10C). The PI can be up to 40% with abundant normal and abnormal mitotic figures (Fig. 7.7C). Olig2 nuclear immunoreactivity can be up to 40% in each of these astrocytoma subtypes.

Gliomatosis cerebri

In people, this neoplasm is defined as a glioma characterized by a remarkably widespread, diffuse, uniform, confluent, bilateral growth in at least three cerebral hemispheric lobes of the brain, but frequently also involving the cerebellum, brainstem and spinal cord (Fig. 7.8A). Gliomatosis cerebri presents most commonly with an astrocytic phenotype, although in the original description in the dog these cells were mistakenly identified as microglial cells and the disease called microgliomatosis.

MRI findings are considered to be characteristic of an astrocytoma but with much more widely disseminated involvement. See MRI Atlas. The tumor cells have elongate, enlarged, often twisted mildly hyperchromatic nuclei without detectable cytoplasm on HE staining and with variable cell density (Fig. 7.8B,C). Formation of secondary structures of Scherer are common. Tumor cells can be immunoreactive for GFAP, and molecular genetic studies in human tumors confirm their astrocytic derivation. Gliomatosis cerebri is graded into

low-grade and high-grade tumors according to the astrocytoma grading system. An oligodendroglioma in a dog has been described with a similar diffuse infiltrating pattern to that of gliomatosis cerebri. Also a cluster of this tumor has occurred in young sibling Bearded Collie dogs in Switzerland, suggesting a familial inheritance. It is possible that these tumors are another variant of widely disseminated astrocytomas.

7.2.2 Oligodendroglioma

Oligodendroglioma is the other glioma subtype, whose incidence increases with age, and is the second most common primary tumor (20%) in the dog. It also occurs infrequently in cattle, cats and horses. Certain brachycephalic dog breeds (Boxers, Bulldogs, Boston Terriers etc.) have a remarkably higher susceptibility than other breeds. Predilection sites of oligodendrogliomas are in the frontal, parietal and temporal lobes and regionally in both white and gray matter around the lateral ventricles. Their overall frequency decreases caudally throughout the brain and spinal cord. Secondary dissemination within the ventricular system, including the central canal, and also local invasion into or widespread metastases to the meninges is common in canine and feline grade III tumors. On MRI, oligodendrogliomas are moderately hypointense on T1W, and markedly intense on T2W images. Contrast enhancement is variable with intense central non-uniform and peripheral ring enhancement expected in grade III tumors (Fig. 7.9A). See MRI Atlas. Focal or regional

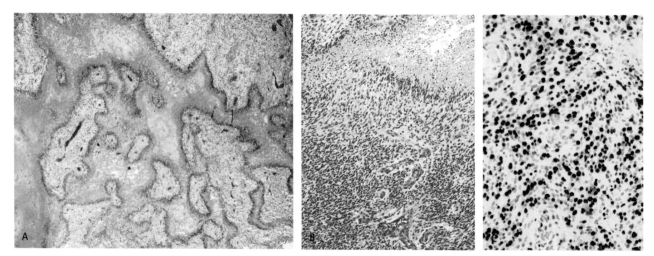

Fig. 7.7 Dog. Glioblastoma (astrocytoma, grade IV). A: Areas of serpentine necrosis bordered by glial cell pseudopalisading. B: Higher magnification illustrating the glial pseudopalisading bordering an area of necrosis and also some underlying microvascular proliferation. Both these features are characteristic of glioblastomas. HE. C: The PI is up to 30% in this glioblastoma compared with the much lower activity in a grade II tumor (see Fig. 7.5D).

contrast enhancement is distributed within the tumor often in a serpentine pattern. Intratumoral hemorrhage is common. Macroscopically, oligodendogliomas are well circumscribed, sharply demarcated, usually gelatinous or translucent, soft gray to white and have a preference for intraventricular growth from their primary site as well expansion to the cortical surface (Fig. 7.9B). Generally, there are intratumoral cystic myxoid areas, multifocal hemorrhages and whitish-yellow areas of necrosis in the grade III tumors (Fig. 7.9B).

Microscopically, oligodendrogliomas have monomorphic densely packed cells with a uniformly round

basophilic nucleus, vacuolated or eosinophilic cytoplasm and a well defined cytoplasmic border (Fig. 7.10A). If formalin fixation is delayed more than a few hours, artifactual cellular changes include a nucleus that is condensed, round, densely basophilic and surrounded by empty clear cytoplasm but with prominent cytoplasmic membranes producing a halo or "honeycomb" effect. There can be different patterns of cells arranged in rows, clusters or parallel columns. Smears from surgical or stereobiopsy are very characteristic with widely dispersed round cells with an eccentric eosionophilic cytoplasm (Fig. 7.10F). Extracellularly,

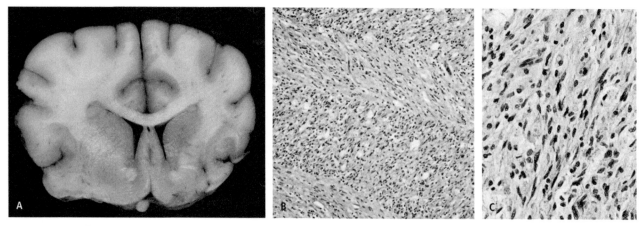

Fig. 7.8 Dog. Gliomatosis cerebri. A: Transverse section illustrating the extensive tumor cell infiltration of both hemispheres blurring the gray and white matter boundary. B: There is diffuse infiltration of the white matter tracts by elongate neoplastic cells. HE. C: Higher magnification of the very elongate pleomorphic cells some with a twisted nucleus without obvious cytoplasm. HE.

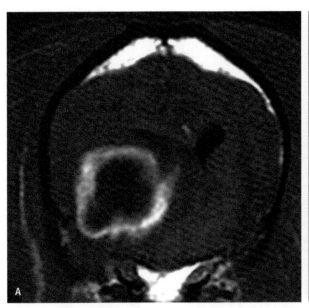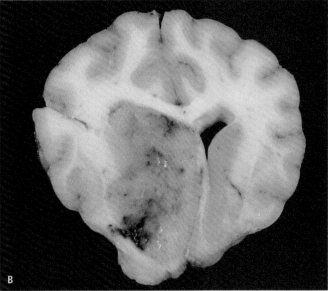

Fig. 7.9 Dog. Oligodendroglioma. A: MRI findings of T1W post-contrast enhancement with characteristic hypointense center and a bright homogeneous uniform ring-enhancing lesion. B: Transverse section through an oligodendroglioma with well demarcated borders, a grayish translucent mass with focal yellowish areas of necrosis, mucinous small cysts and multifocal hemorrhage typical of grade III tumors.

there is a bluish-staining myxoid matrix, which can form cyst-like lakes throughout the tumor (Fig. 7.10D). All tumors have thin-walled branching capillaries ("chicken-wire" vessels) (Fig. 7.10A). In contrast to the grade II oligodendrogliomas, classification of grade III tumors depends on a prominent microvascular proliferation (Fig. 7.10B) often in long curving lines, foci of dissecting or serpentine coagulation necrosis with frequent intravascular thrombosis and multifocal hemorrhage, and conspicuous abnormal and normal mitotic figures. Nuclear atypia and multiple large-walled vessels are also features; also secondary structures of Scherer are often seen peritumorally in the grade III tumors (Fig. 7.10C). From the primary site local expansion with spread into the adjacent subarachnoid space in the meninges and into the ventricular system can occur. Metastatic dissemination within the CSF pathways is also common in grade III tumors, particularly on the ependymal floor of the fourth ventricle and within the central canal of the spinal cord. In direct contrast to their low incidence in people, over 90% of canine tumors are classified as grade III tumors. GFAP immunoreactivity can identify reactive astrocytes massing at the tumor periphery as well as trapped in isolation within the tumor. There can also be a small population of minigemistocytes, which are round tumor cells lacking cellular processes but with a GFAP-positive cytoplasm. Oligodendrogliomas are generally diagnosed confidently on HE-stained sections. About 75–100% of tumor cells are also Olig2 immunoreactive, although this antibody can also immunoreact

with astrocytomas (see above) (Fig. 7.10E). Most oligodendrogliomas are also consistently and strongly immunoreactive to PDGFR-α. PI indices (MIB-1) range from 5% to beyond 15% in grade II and grade III tumors respectively. The differential diagnosis needs to exclude the very rare canine neurocytoma which can be confidently done with the latter tumor having positive immunoreactivity to synaptophysin and negative immunoreactivity to Olig2.

7.2.3 Mixed gliomas (oligoastrocytomas)

Mixed gliomas are a type of diffusely infiltrating glioma composed of a mixture of two distinct tumor populations consisting usually of both a well differentiated astrocytoma and oligodendroglioma. In the dog they represent about 5% of all the gliomas. These mixed gliomas basically have all of the features of their component tumors including MRI profile, adult onset, predilection sites and gross appearance. They can only be diagnosed histologically based on their concurrently occurring astrocytoma and oligodendroglial phenotypes, which occur in either a diffuse or biphasic (collision) growth pattern. Less commonly, there can be an ependymal component. There are currently opinions only on what tumor population fractions are required for this diagnosis but at least 30% of either type makes this diagnosis appear unequivocal. Thus, mixed gliomas can present a clinical diagnostic challenge when only needle biopsy sampled tissue is evaluated. In the most

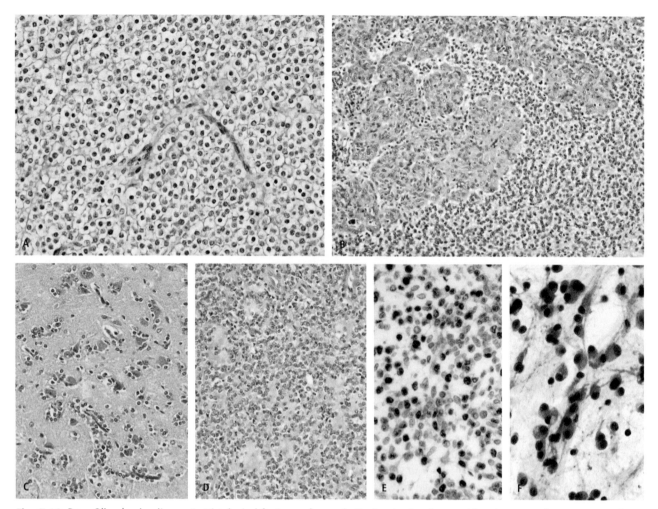

Fig. 7.10 Dog. Oligodendroglioma. A: Histological features of a grade II oligodendroglioma with uninterrupted monotonous sheets of tumor cells with a round uniform nucleus, variable amount of faintly staining or vacuolated cytoplasm, sharp cytoplasmic border, thin-walled capillaries ("chicken-wire" vessels) and interstitial accumulation of blue myxoid-staining exudate. B: Grade III oligodendroglioma with prominent microvascular proliferation, densely packed cells with nuclear atypia. C: Structures of Scherer in an oligodendroglioma with neoplastic cell infiltrates around neurons (tumor satellitosis) and perivascular invasion. These are characteristic features of high-grade infiltrating gliomas. D: Mucinous interstitial material which accumulates into cystic lakes in oligodendrogliomas but also can occur in astrocytomas. E: Olig2 nuclear immunoreactivity in an oligodendroglioma of about 60% in this tumor. IHC. F: Smear from CT-guided stereobiopsy of an oligodendroglioma with dispersed round cells with a basophilic nucleus and eccentric homogeneous eosinophilic-staining cytoplasm. HE.

common diffuse form, the astrocytoma is usually a fibrillary or less often a gemistocytic subtype and both are strongly immunoreactive to GFAP antibody. Mitotic figures are rare, there is minimal cell pleomorphism and PI is less than 2%, which together attracts a grade II classification. However, with anaplastic mixed gliomas, in which there is nuclear atypia, cellular pleomorphism, increased cellularity, mitotic figures and often microvascular proliferation, the differential diagnosis must include a glioblastoma. Differences in molecular genetics, such as 1p19q deletion in oligodendrogliomas, may be a more reliable guide in the future than any histologi-

cal distinction between glioblastoma and anaplastic mixed gliomas.

7.2.4 Ependymoma

Ependymomas arise from the ependymal lining cells of the ventricular system and are comprised of neoplastic ependymal cells usually as a supra- or subtentorial expansile mass within the lateral, third or fourth ventricle in the dog. Ependymomas are reported also in the cat, horse and cattle. Depending on their size and location, obstructive hydrocephalus and ventricular displacement may result. They have a very low frequency

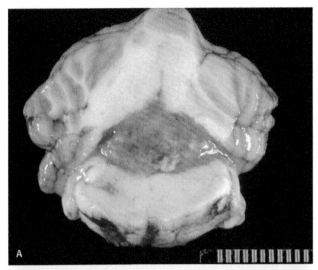

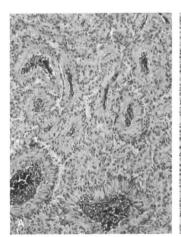

Fig. 7.11 Dog. Ependymoma. A: Cellular ependymoma occupying most of the fourth ventricle. B: Papillary ependymoma protruding into the third ventricle and with a granular papilliform appearance on cut surface.

of about 2% of all primary canine tumors. Their MRI profile is mildly hypointense on T1W, while T2W images are moderate to markedly hyperintense with intense heterogeneous contrast enhancement. Macroscopically, they are large, well demarcated, soft, tan, intraventricular masses (Fig. 7.11A) sometimes with a granular texture to the cut surface in the papillary subtype (Fig. 7.11B). There can also be focal hemorrhage, white to yellow areas of necrosis, and fluid-filled cysts. Invasion of and extension within CSF pathways or meninges may occur. Histologically, the monomorphic cells have round to oval nuclei with fine granular chromatin and a prominent nucleolus. A key feature is the formation of perivascular pseudorosettes around blood vessels with a characteristic nuclear-free perivascular zone, which is GFAP immunoreactive. Occasionally, there can be ependymal rosettes with a single layer of ependymoma cells lining a central lumen. In the dog there are three main histological subtype patterns:

- The papillary subtype is formed of finger-like or papilliform processes lined on their outer surface by ependymal cells anchored to the central blood vessel by strongly GFAP-immunoreactive fibrillary processes (Fig. 7.12A).
- The most frequent cellular subtype has round to elongate cells with dense monomorphic cellularity and nuclei-free perivascular spaces (Fig. 7.12B). Areas of necrosis without peudopalisading can occur.
- The clear cell ependymoma subtype occurs in the lateral ventricle, where it forms oligodendroglial-like cells with round nuclei, clear empty perinuclear halos and well defined cytoplasmic borders, but with

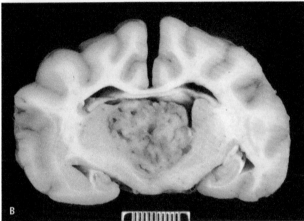
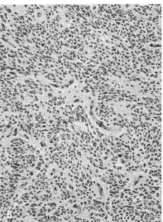
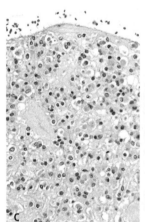
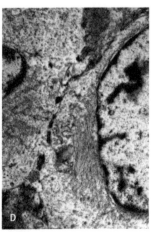

Fig. 7.12 Dog. Ependymoma. A: Papillary ependymoma subtype with characteristic papilliform pattern with tumor cells supported by a gliofibrillary stroma around a central vascular core. HE. B: Cellular ependymoma with cells interspersed between blood vessels, which sometimes have cell-free clear zones. HE. C: Clear cell ependymoma with periventricular neoplastic cells, which have round nuclei. D: Ultrastructurally adjacent neoplastic cells are connected by desmosomal junctions and have aggregations of GFAP immunoreactive intermediate filaments. Electronmicrograph (courtesy of Dr. A Traslavina).

GFAP-immunoreactive eosinophilic material eccentrically placed in the cytoplasm (Fig. 7.12C). This tumor subtype is best differentiated from an oligodendroglioma by the GFAP cytoplasmic positivity and on TEM by the intercellular zona occludens bridging between cells (Fig. 7.12D), aggregates of intermediate GFAP-immunoreactive filaments and microvilli anchored by blepharoblasts.

7.2.5 Choroid plexus tumors (papillomas and carcinomas)

Choroid plexus tumors (CPT) are intraventricular neoplasms arising from the epithelium of the choroid plexus in the lateral, third and fourth ventricles. In the dog, they comprise about 7% of all primary tumors and have been documented sporadically in the horse and cow. Most CPT occur in middle-aged dogs (median 6 years) with a breed predilection in the Golden Retriever. There is a higher frequency of carcinomas (CPC) than papillomas (CPP). Most tumors occur in the fourth ventricle with a decreasing incidence rostrally in the third and lateral ventricles. Extrusive unilateral growth through the lateral aperture of the fourth ventricle is common. On MRI, CPT may be hypo-, iso- or hyperintense on T1W images and generally hyperintense on T2W images. They are generally intensely and uniformly strongly contrast-enhancing as are the intraventricular and subarachnoid metastases characteristic of carcinomas (Fig. 7.13A,B,C,D). Development of secondary obstructive hydrocephalus and hydromyelia depends largely on the site and size of the tumor irrespective of the histological grade. For a provisional clinical diagnosis, analysis of CSF for total protein and cytology suggests that CPP grade I have a maximum protein concentration of less than 80 mg/dl compared with a minimum of 108 mg/dl for grade III CPC. Likewise critical CSF cytological evaluation has shown that at least 47% of carcinomas have exfoliated tumor cells not present with papillomas (Fig. 7.14D). A provisional clinical tumor classification and grade can be then confirmed by histological examination of highly characteristic smears and tissue from a surgical or stereotactically derived biopsy (Fig. 7.14B).

Macroscopically, CPP are granular, rough textured, circumscribed gray to reddish masses, well delineated from the ventricular wall, while CPC additionally can have areas of necrosis and focal hemorrhage and can be infiltrative and adhered to the adjacent brain (Fig. 7.13B). Primary CPC in the brain also have a predilection for metastases down the length of the spinal cord meninges or over the cerebral convexities (Fig. 7.13C,D).

Microscopically, CPP grade I recapitulate normal choroid plexus with papilliform fronds, with a dense connective tissue core around a central vessel, and covered by a single layer of cuboidal to columnar neoplastic epithelium (Fig. 7.14A). Mitotic figures are rare and the PI is less than 1%. No canine CPT with the characteristic features for the atypical human WHO grade II classification have been identified to date. CPC

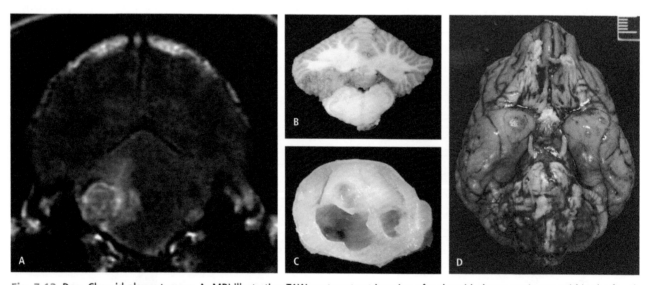

Fig. 7.13 Dog. Choroid plexus tumors. A: MRI illustrating T1W post-contrast imaging of a choroid plexus carcinoma within the fourth ventricle with contrast enhancement and with a basilar ventral metastasis. B: Transverse section of same tumor with apparent invasion of the parenchyma around the lateral aperture of the fourth ventricle. C: Spinal cord. Extensive subarachnoid metastases with local cord invasion from this carcinoma and some cyst-like structures. D: Ventral view of the brain from this tumor with extraventricular growth and numerous subarachnoid metastases on the basilar area and scattered randomly on the temporal lobes.

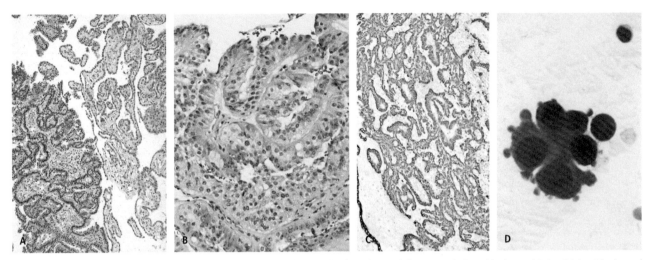

Fig. 7.14 Dog. Choroid plexus tumors. A: Comparison of the similar histology of the normal choroid plexus (right side) with that of a papilloma on the left. HE. B: Surgical biopsy of a choroid plexus carcinoma in the fourth ventricle. There is piling up of epithelial cells, mitotic figures >2 per 400X HPF and some cell sheeting. HE. C: Low and high MW (Lu5) cytokeratin immunoreactivity in a choroid plexus papilloma. IHC. D: Neoplastic epithelial cells from a cytospin preparation of CSF from a choroid plexus carcinoma. Wright's stain.

grade III are distinguished by frequent mitoses (>5 per 10 high-power fields (HPF)), nuclear atypia, increased cell density, focal loss of papillary formation with cell sheeting, necrosis and increased layering of epithelium (Fig. 7.14B). Aggressive local brain invasion is dramatic but is not included in the 2007 WHO criteria for either a grade II or III classification. CPT can be further defined by the immunoreactivity of their epithelium to CK (Lu-5) (Fig. 7.14C), E-cadherin and variably and focally to GFAP, while their connective tissue core is vimentin positive.

7.2.6 Neuronal and mixed neuronal–glial tumors

Ganglioglioma and gangliocytoma

These are both well differentiated, slow growing, extremely rare tumors in dogs and cats, comprised of mature ganglionic-like multipolar neurons (**gangliocytoma**) or also mixed with a neoplastic glial cells (**ganglioglioma**). Less well differentiated cellular blast forms are described in younger animals. Their histogenesis remains unresolved. Most have occurred in the thalamus with extension rostrally. Macroscopically, they are poorly defined often with intratumoral cyst formation.

Histologically, they are composed of increased numbers of scattered pleomorphic neurons with bizarre or binucleate forms, marginated or irregularly dispersed Nissl substance, and clusters in abnormal locations. Gangliogliomas have an increased cell density from a pilocytic-like or fibrillary-like astrocytoma cell component admixed with the neoplastic ganglion-like cells and usually with multiple cyst formation. Neurons are immunoreactive for common neuronal markers synaptophysin, NeuN and neurofilament proteins, while the glial component is GFAP immunoreactive. Mitotic figures are rare and the PI is up to 2%.

Neurocytoma

This is a rare tumor in people, and only one case has been reported in the dog. Central **neurocytomas** occur mainly in the lateral or third ventricle with an intraparenchymal component, occur in young adults and are comprised of round isomorphous cells with expressed neuronal antigenic differentiation. As a result of fixation artifact, their cytological characteristics can appear like oligodendrogliomas or clear cell ependymomas from which they can be differentiated by their strong diffuse immunoreactivity to synaptophysin and NeuN while being consistently immunonegative for Olig2 and GFAP respectively.

Paraganglioma

Paraganglioma of the CNS in the dog generally occur as well defined intradural tumors within the spinal cord presumed to arise from neural crest cell derivatives associated with regional autonomic nerves and blood vessels. In the PNS, these tumors occur in autonomic ganglia as well as in sites such as the carotid body (chemodectoma)

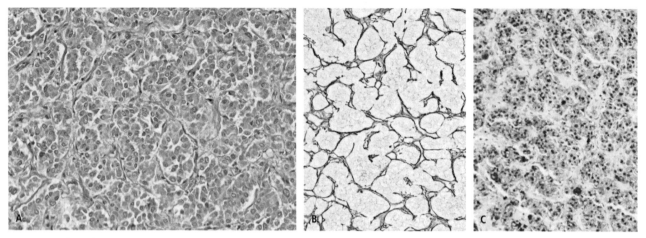

Fig. 7.15 Cheetah. Paraganglioma. A: The characteristic packeting of nests of neuroendocrine-like cells formed by a thin fibrovascular stroma. HE. B: The supporting fibrovascular stroma contains the cells within islands or nests. Reticulin silver stain. C: Strong cytoplasmic immunoreactivity to chromogranin (illustrated) and to synaptophysin is expected in most cells. IHC.

and adrenal medulla (pheochromocytoma). Microscopically, the neoplastic chief cells form typical neuroendocrine cell nests or lobules separated by a delicate fibrovascular stroma and surrounded by an outer layer of sustentacular cells (Fig. 7.15A,B). The predominant chief cells are round to polygonal with round nuclei in a finely granular wispy cytoplasm. They are strongly immunoreactive for chromogranin A and B, synaptophysin and TNF (Fig. 7.15C). There is a variable positive immunoreactivity of the peripheral sustentacular cells to S-100. A reticulin stain distinctively outlines the stromal component around each of the cell nests (Fig. 7.15B). Mitotic activity is very low and the PI less than 1%.

7.2.7 Embryonal tumors

Medulloblastoma

Medulloblastomas are rare malignant embryonal tumors of the cerebellum with a predilection for young animals and with predominant neuronal differentiation. They have been reported in the dog, cat, cow and pig. Twin calves at birth have each been reported with medulloblastomas. Macroscopically, the tumors are large, fleshy, soft, gray, well circumscribed, often located midline in the vermis and can secondarily invade the fourth ventricle and lateral cerebellar hemispheric lobes (Fig. 7.16A). See MRI Atlas. Microscopically, medulloblastomas are densely cellular, often

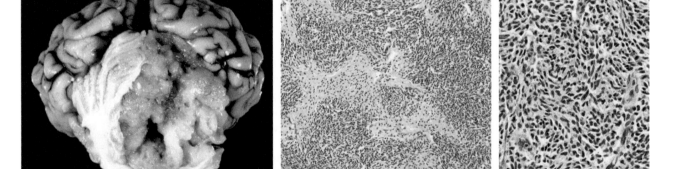

Fig. 7.16 Neonatal calf. Cerebellum. Medulloblastoma. A: The midline vermal location and subsequent growth with destruction of much of the cerebellum and intraventricular spread of a medulloblastoma. B and C: These tumors are characterized by intense basophilic staining of the nuclei of the small elongate or round cells hence their name as "small blue tumors". HE.

in sheets with ovoid, elongate to round deeply basophilic hyperchromatic nuclei and with minimal cytoplasm (so-called "small blue tumors") (Fig. 7.16B,C). Homer–Wright (neuroblastic) rosettes are sometimes found. Mitotic figures are common. Expansion into adjacent folia is common with strikingly cell dense subpial, leptomeningeal and subependymal infiltration. Other histological subtypes in animals include anaplastic medulloblastoma, nodular patterns with astrocytic islands (Fig. 7.16B) or with myogenic differentiation. Immunoreactivity for NSE, synaptophysin, chromogranin A and B, and/or TNF is confirmation of their predominant neuronal differentiation. In the nodular form GFAP immunoreactivity can be demonstrated around neuronal tumor nodules.

Primitive neuroectodermal tumors (PNET)

Primitive neuroectodermal tumors (neuroblastomas) are found in mostly young animals, are extremely rare and comprised of poorly differentiated neuroepithelial cells often with multiple divergence along neuronal, astrocytic and ependymal cell lines. Some may be so undifferentiated that they are immunonegative to all conventional antigenic markers. They are considered the supratentorial equivalent of medulloblastomas though less well differentiated. They occur in the dog, cattle and horse. They can be large, fleshy, soft, well demarcated, whitish, supratentorial masses with variable necrosis and hemorrhage. The cells have small uniform elongate to ovoid hyperchromatic, basophilic dark blue nuclei with little definable cytoplasm and poorly defined or absent cytoplasmic borders (Fig. 7.16C). True neuroblastic Homer–Wright (HW) rosettes are specifically diagnostic but are rare. Mitotic figures are common, and the PI can be up to 30%. Immunoreactivity for many neuronal and glial cell antigenic markers is highly variable and depends on the degree of differentiation. In animals because of the relatively few cases, neuroblastomas are currently classified depending on their location and/or histologic appearance as:

- olfactory neuroblastoma – arise in the olfactory neuroepithelium of nasal cavity and HW rosettes and perivascular pseudorosettes are common;
- cerebral neuroblastoma – found mainly in the frontoparietal lobes of the cerebral hemispheres.

7.3 Tumors of cranial and spinal nerves

In the peripheral nerves, tumors arise within the nerve sheaths (peripheral nerve sheath tumors, PNST) from one or more populations of endogenous cells, including Schwann cells, perineurial cells or fibroblasts. Hence, benign PNSTs are more accurately further divided according to their cell of origin by immunochemistry or ultrastructural evaluation.

7.3.1 Benign PNST

Schwannoma

These are benign slow-growing, encapsulated tumors within peripheral nerves that arise from Schwann cells. In the dog, most occur in the spinal nerve roots of the brachial plexus with much lower frequency within the cranial nerve roots V and VIII and the sciatic nerve plexus (Fig. 7.17A,B,C). Their occurrence increases with age with an overall incidence of about 5%. **Schwannomas** commonly expand by infiltration centripetally within the nerve roots, non-invasively displacing and compressing the spinal cord (Fig. 7.17A,B). They can also spread centrifugally away from their primary site microscopically. Schwannomas are firm with a rubbery texture, circumscribed, well encapsulated, smooth-surfaced, hard, whitish-gray nodular masses and usually found associated with a peripheral nerve (Fig. 7.17A,B,C). They can be molded into a characteristic dumbbell shape as the affected nerve is compressed while traversing the intervertebral foramina (Fig. 7.17A). Schwannomas can occur in subcutaneous sites. On MRI, tumors are isointense on T1W and hyperintense on T2W images and many lesions have heterogeneous contrast enhancement. See MRI Atlas.

Two histological types of biphasic cell patterns can be found within schwannomas:

- Antoni type A: the most common with compact, long, bipolar spindle cells with tapering ends forming whorls or bundles intersecting at various angles, an elongate ovoid nucleus, poorly defined cytoplasm, and with variable amount of extracellular collagen (Fig. 7.18A). Rarely in dogs there is a palisading effect with parallel arrangement of nuclei to form either a herring-bone pattern or in bundles to form Verocay bodies;
- Antoni type B: this is much less common with marked cell pleomorphism with plump or stellate cells embedded in low density in a fine eosinophilic lacy matrix.

Other histological features include acute necrosis, acute or chronic hemorrhage, foci of cartilage or osteoid, collagenous or mucoid-staining matrix, often with multifocal perivascular lymphoplasmacytic cell infiltrates. Most cellular schwannomas are comprised of just the Antoni type A pattern with marked hypercellularity and nuclear

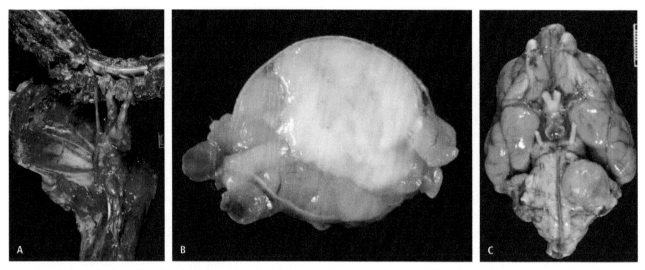

Fig. 7.17 Dog. Schwannoma of the brachial plexus. A: There are multiple spinal nerves (C7–T1), which are thickened by and contain nodular masses, which extend both centripetally into the intervertebral foramen and centrifugally into the lower spinal nerve branches. B: Spinal cord segment C7 with neoplastic infiltration of the left ventral nerve roots by this schwannoma and then subdural growth compressing the spinal cord. C: Dog. There is a large bulging but contained schwannoma of the trigeminal nerve root.

atypia. A melanocytic variant can occur in the skin not to be confused with a melanoma. A diagnosis of schwannoma can be confirmed by immunoreactivity to laminin or collagen IV both of which strongly and uniformly delineate the basal lamina outside of the cytoplasmic membrane of each neoplastic Schwann cell (Fig. 7.18C). Up to 30% of tumors can have GFAP and sometimes S-100 immunoreactivity, though the latter is much less consistent than in human schwannomas. Ultrastructurally, a continuous or segmented basal lamina can be demonstrated outside the cytoplasmic membrane.

Without immunocytochemical or ultrastructural confirmation of a basal lamina around each of the neoplastic Schwann cells, the diagnosis of either a benign or malignant PNST implies a probable origin from an endoneurial or epineurial fibroblast. Mitotic figures are minimal in schwannomas.

Neurofibroma

Neurofibromas are much less common in the dog and are intraneural encapsulated tumors or skin nodules consisting of different mixtures of cell types, which may

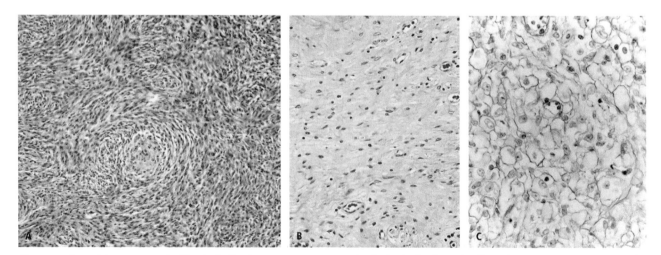

Fig. 7.18 Dog. Schwannoma. A: Histologically, these tumors are comprised of spindle-shaped cells with elongate nuclei and bipolar cytoplasmic processes, which form patterns of intersecting bundles, streams or whorls. B: Dog. Neurofibroma. These tumors have very low cell density forming spindle-shaped elongate cells (of Schwann or fibroblast cell origin) with abundant collagen arranged isomorphically. C: Immunoreactivity to laminin in the pattern of each cell bordered by a thin lamina is confirmation of a schwannoma. IHC.

include neoplastic Schwann cells, perineurial cells and/or least commonly fibroblasts. They can be found in the same locations as schwannomas but more commonly as a circumscribed mass in other individual cranial or spinal nerves.

Histologically, they are composed of cells with thin elongate wavy nuclei and fibrillary processes. They are arranged loosely and haphazardly in a stellate pattern within a mucoid or eosinophilic matrix and produce variable amounts of stromal collagen (Fig. 7.18B). Immunoreactivity to S-100 and laminin is patchy or absent depending on their Schwann cell content.

In mature cattle, similar tumors can occur in multiple sites (brachial plexus, intercostal nerves, tongue, cardiac muscle and other spinal nerve roots) and are classified simplistically as benign neurofibromatosis or multiple PNST.

Perineurioma

The canine **perineurioma** is an exceedingly rare tumor, which probably has previously been misdiagnosed as canine local hypertrophic neuropathy. An intraneural perineurioma caused focal cylindrical unilateral thickening in an L5–6 spinal nerve root in a middle-aged dog with progressive unilateral paresis. MRI revealed profound ipsilateral muscle atrophy and thickening of the nerve roots. Histologically there were distended fascicles due to widely separated axons surrounded by concentric lamellations of processes formed by neoplastic perineurioma cells in a myxoid stroma (Fig. 7.19). These cells, being modified Schwann cells, were strongly immunoreactive for laminin (Fig. 7.19). Ultrastructurally, the

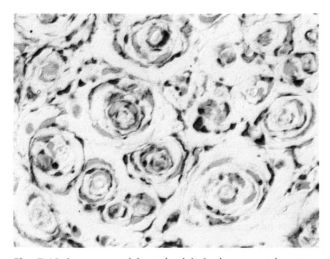

Fig. 7.19 Immunoreactivity to laminin in the concentric pattern formed by neoplastic perineurioma cells of Schwann cell derivation confirms a diagnosis of perineurioma. IHC.

processes were connected by junctional complexes and surrounded by a continuous basal lamina.

7.3.2 Malignant peripheral nerve sheath tumors (MPNST)

A **malignant PNST** is usually defined as a tumor with nerve sheath differentiation and neoplastic cell invasion beyond the confines of the epineurium. Grossly, these tumors lack an epineural tumor capsule and may aggressively invade the surrounding structures. Foci of hemorrhage and necrosis are common. Intradural tumors may show brain or spinal cord invasion. Histologically, MPNSTs vary widely in appearance. They originate within nerve fascicles but generally invade the surrounding structures. Mitotic figures are common in malignant PNST with a PI of up to 6%.

7.4 Tumors of the meninges

7.4.1 Meningioma

Meningiomas are probably derived from cells of either the leptomeninges or from various cell types forming arachnoid granulations. They are the most common intracranial and intraspinal primary CNS tumor in both dogs (40% of all primary tumors) and cats, and are reported sporadically in horses, cattle and sheep. In dogs and cats, there is an increasing frequency with age. Golden Retriever and Boxer breed dogs tend to be most susceptible. As in people there is a strikingly decreasing incidence in their localization from the olfactory bulbs caudally, which correlates directly with the decreasing density of arachnoid villi. Canine menigiomas are most common over the cerebral convexity, less so parasagitally and intraventricularly and intraorbitally, but can also form plaque-like lesions from the basilar meninges and dura mater. Cats can have multiple well demarcated tumors of varying size usually restricted to the cerebral convexity. MRI characteristics include T1W iso- to hyperintense profiles, while contrast enhancement on T1W images is always strong and in either hetero- or homogeneous patterns, and most tumors have sharply defined borders (Fig. 7.20A). On FLAIR sequences, either peritumoral or more diffuse interstitial edema is characteristic in surrounding white matter. On MRI, the intradural extramedullary masses were strongly contrast enhancing many with so-called dural tails (Fig. 7.20A). See MRI Atlas.

Macroscopically, canine meningiomas are well defined, lobulated, firm, often granular, white to tan-colored masses with a broad-based attachment to the meninges (Fig. 7.20B). Supratentorial meningiomas are more common over the meningeal-covered

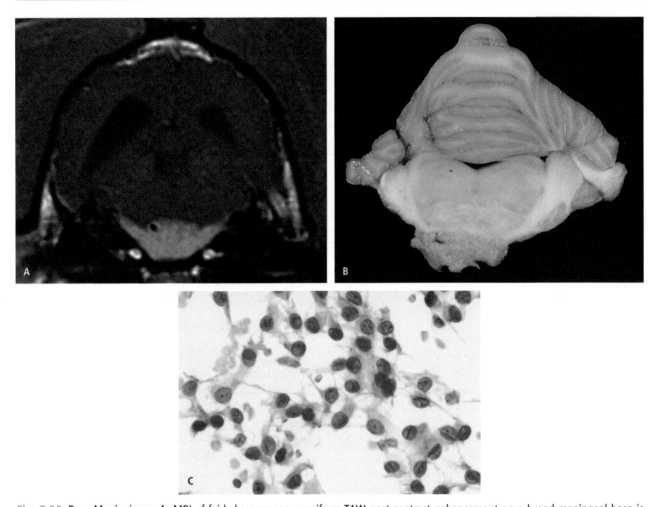

Fig. 7.20 Dog. Meningioma. A: MRI of fairly homogeneous uniform T1W post-contrast enhancement on a broad meningeal base is highly suggestive of a meningioma. B: Transverse slice from the tumor in A with a meningioma adhered to the ventral left side of the brainstem. C: Smear from CT-guided stereobiopsy of a canine meningioma. Round to elongate cells with some with intranuclear cytoplasmic evaginations and longitudinal nuclear folds. HE.

convexities than those in basilar or parasagittal sites. Most expand intra-axially with or without brain invasion. In the basilar meninges, predilection sites are the suprasellar meninges, while subtentorially plaque-like or globular masses can expand dorsally into the brain stem. Intra-axial meningiomas induce extensive peritumoral vasogenic edema. In the cat, meningiomas are usually supratentorial, globular, well defined, hard, solid, yellow–gray, intra-axial masses, which expand by compression and which can occur in varying sizes simultaneously in multiple sites. Uncommonly meningiomas, arising from the telea choroidea of the choroid plexus, develop in the lateral or fourth ventricles. Cytological evaluation of smear preparations from biopsy techniques also has proved to be diagnostically very accurate for meningiomas irrespective of histological classification (Fig. 7.20C).

Histologically, because of their striking gross and microscopical similarities to human tumors, canine meningiomas are currently classified and graded by criteria of the 2007 human WHO system. Grade I tumors exhibit a diverse array of subtypes histologically, although this does not reflect their common clinical behavior, while grade II atypical and grade III malignant tumors have fewer histologically classified categories.

Meningiomas are the most common primary CNS tumor in the spinal canal of dogs. Most occur from C1–4 cord segments and decrease in frequency caudally. These tumors are much less amenable to the well recognized histological classification of intracranial meningiomas because of their histological diversity. Most tumors in the cervical cord are grade I while those more caudally are grade II. For a detailed histological classification of

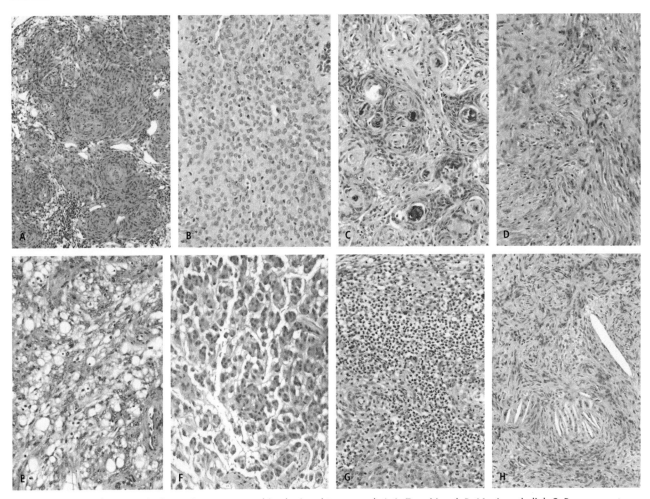

Fig. 7.21 Dog and cat. Meningioma. Some common histologic subtypes grade I. A: Transitional. B: Meningothelial. C: Psammomatous. D: Fibrous. E: Microcystic. F: Chordoid grade II. G: Transitional meningioma with focal polymorphonuclear cell accumulations. H: Feline meningioma with whorls, cholesterol clefts, mineralization and fibrous spindle cell population.

these tumors the reader is referred to the human 2007 WHO system.

Grade I meningiomas

With meningiomas there is a very diverse array of histological subtypes which is often complicated by different patterns occurring within one tumor. Tumors are therefore classified by their predominant histological pattern.

The most common histologic subtypes in dogs are:

- transitional – common with islands or nests in whorls or crescents (Fig. 7.21A) and not infrequently with focal accumulations of polymorphonuclear leukocytes (Fig. 7.21G);
- meningothelial – common with sheets of cells with no underlying pattern (Fig. 7.21B);

- psammomatous – large numbers of psammoma bodies (Fig. 7.21C);
- fibrous – streams of elongate cells with prominent extracellular collagen fibers (Fig. 7.21D);
- angiomatous – dominant vascular component;
- microcystic – widespread intracellular and interstitial vacuolation (Fig. 7.21E).

Grade II meningiomas

Histological canine subtypes identified include:

- chordoid – cords or columns of eosinophilic vacuolated cells in a mucoid basophilic matrix (Fig. 7.21F);
- atypical – with nuclear atypia, areas of necrosis, sheet-like patterns of cells, more than 4 mitotic figures per 10 HPF (400X) and increased cellular density with smaller cells.

Grade III meningiomas

These tumors are classified as:

- malignant – characterized by mitotic figures >20 per 10 HPF (400X) and with extreme anaplastic cytological features compared with the atypical subtype;
- papillary subtype – distinctive but rare in the dog.

Diagnosis

In human meningiomas, immunoreactivity to epithelial membrane antigen (EMA) is found in the vast majority of meningiomas and considered a reliable antigenic diagnostic marker but unfortunately this antigen is not expressed in dogs. Canine meningiomas are strongly and uniformly immunoreactive for vimentin and some express focal reactivity to CK (Lu-5). However, the most reliable confirmation of a diagnosis of a canine meningioma still relies on TEM with the highly distinctive and consistent features of interdigitating cytoplasmic membranes with normal and abnormal gap and desmosomal junctions. Early loss of tumor suppressor genes NF2, 4.1B and TSLC1 is a frequent occurrence in canine meningiomas. Exonic mutational frequency of the TP53 gene is only 3.0%.

Histologically, in striking contrast to the dog, all cat meningiomas have a remarkably consistent and uniform histological pattern, with prominent whorling of elongate cells in a collagen-rich matrix rather similar to a fibrous meningioma, elongate linear patterns of focal mineralization, often prominent necrosis, some clusters of cholesterol cleft-like crystals but few psammoma bodies (Fig. 7.21H). Their lack of nuclear atypia and mitotic figures, relative uniform cell type and density and benign behavior are most consistent with a grade I tumor.

7.4.2 Granular cell tumor

Granular cell tumors (GCT) in the dog are of uncertain histogenesis; in the CNS they occur in the neurohypophysis of the pituitary gland, combined with meningiomas, or as primary monomorphic tumors mainly superficially over the cerebral hemispheres. In humans, GCT are described concurrently within astrocytomas and oligodendrogliomas. Grossly, most canine tumors occur in meningeal sites diffusely over the cerebral convexities, intra-axially within the frontal lobe and infrequently within the pituitary gland as focal mass lesions. Exclusive involvement of lumbar spinal nerves has been reported. The GCT profile on MRI is distinctive and diagnostically exclusive with robust hyperintensity on both T1W and T2W images and with T1W strong uniform contrast enhancement (Fig. 7.22A). There is usually a broad-based meningeal attachment. Grossly, GCT are either firm, well demarcated, non-encapsulated lesions or involve thickened meninges. Microscopically, solid sheets of the large polygonal granule cells have an eccentrically placed nucleus with a very granular, eosinophilic, abundant cytoplasm containing distinctive periodic acid-Schiff (PAS) positivity resistant to diastase digestion (Fig.

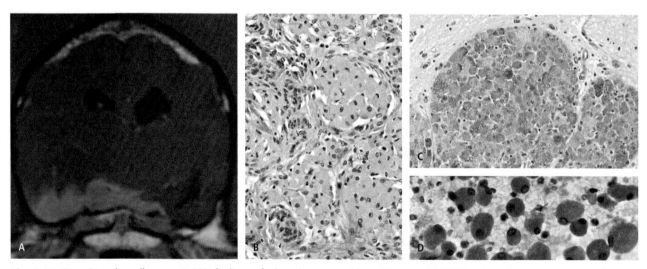

Fig. 7.22 Dog. Granular cell tumor. A: MRI findings of a broad meningeal-based tumor with T1W post-contrast enhancement. B: Some of these tumors have a concurrent meningioma component. C: Granular cell tumors have diastase-resistant PAS staining. D: This tumor can be diagnosed by the characteristic granular cells in CSF cytological analysis or from biopsy smears as large round cells with an eccentric nucleus and intensely eosinophilic and granular cytoplasmic content.

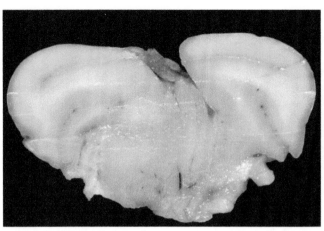
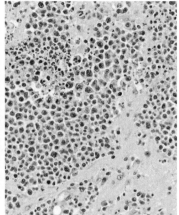
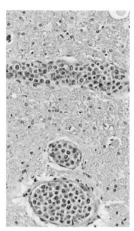

Fig. 7.23 Dog. Lymphoma. A: Primary CNS lymphoma as a single mass lesion without any extraneural involvement. B: Histologically, the cells are either lymphoblastic or more cytologically mature lymphocytes and characterized by extensive individual necrosis, high mitotic rate and spread by perivascular infiltration. C: Endotheliotrophic (angiocentric) lymphoma with intravascular accumulation and thrombosis resulting in secondary infarction.

7.22B,C). The characteristic cells are readily identified in smears from stereotactic-guided biopsy tissue and from CSF cytological preparations (Fig. 7.22D). The cells are S-100, ubiquitin and α-1-antitrypsin immunoreactive but are immunonegative for GFAP and routine canine-specific leukocyte and macrophage markers. Ultrastructurally, the granules appear to be derived from autophagic lysosomes irrespective of their varied tissue location.

7.4.3 Mesenchymal tumors

Primary mesenchymal tumors of the CNS are rare in animals. In the dog, primary leiomyoma, leiomyosarcoma and hemangioblastoma have been described.

7.5 Lymphomas and hematopoietic tumors

Lymphomas may occur in the CNS as either primary or metastatic tumors.

7.5.1 Primary T and B cell lymphomas

Primary lymphomas are single mass lesions within the CNS in the absence of any extraneural involvement as defined by a rigorous necropsy examination. They are rare tumors (3% of all primary tumors) in the dog and cat, and occur less often in cattle and the pig. Primary lymphomas mainly target supratentorial deep-seated sites close to the ventricular system as in human tumors, but they can occur also in the midbrain and

spinal cord. Pituitary gland involvement is not uncommon. On MRI, most primary lesions are either iso- or hypointense on unenhanced T1W images, mildly hyperintense on T2W images and typically have some peritumoral edema. See MRI Atlas. Macroscopically, they are grayish, soft and poorly defined and can have areas of whitish yellow necrosis (Fig. 7.23A). Microscopically, lymphomas form dense sheets of cells, which at their periphery-characteristically expand from neoplastic perivascular infiltration (Fig 7.23B). Concentric bands of reticulin within angiocentric infiltrates are highly suggestive of lymphoma. Intratumoral necrosis is common. The nuclei are large, round to angular, densely basophilic often with a prominent nucleolus and heterochromatin, minimal cytoplasm and characteristically have a high mitotic rate and with a striking degree of individual cell necrosis (Fig. 7.23B). The PI can be up to 75%. Most primary lymphomas can be identified clinically from characteristic CSF cytology. Immunoreactivity for antibodies to CD79a and CD3 can suggest either B or T cell canine lymphomas respectively but ideally this provisional diagnosis must be confirmed by demonstration of clonal B or T cell receptor rearrangements. Most canine lymphomas are of B cell origin while T and B cell phenotypes are common in the cat. No underlying immunosupression has been detected in dogs.

7.5.2 Intravascular lymphoma

This is usually a B cell lymphoma, which has a predilection for the lumens of small vessels (synonyms

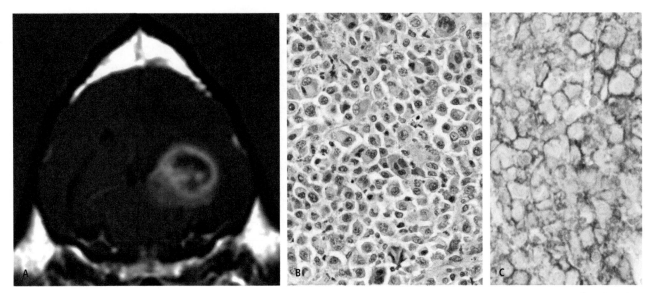

Fig. 7.24 Dog. Primary CNS histiocytic sarcoma. A: MRI with T1W post-contrast ring enhancement which can be confused with a high-grade glioma. B: Histology with cells with eccentrically placed, oval to reniform pleomorphic nuclei, multinucleate cells and numerous mitotic figures. HE. C: CD18 immunoreactive neoplastic histiocytes. CD18 IHC.

are angiocentric, endotheliotropic, intravascular lymphoma) in various organs but sometimes exclusively within the nervous system (Fig. 7.23C). In the dog, cat and sheep, primary CNS vascular involvement leads to secondary induced thrombosis with occlusion of vessels and widespread infarction particularly of the cerebral cortex. T cell lymphomas have been seen in both dogs and cats, and non-T, non-B cell lymphomas have been seen in the dog.

7.5.3 Metastatic lymphoma

In contrast to primary CNS lymphomas, CNS metastates of systemic lymphomas are restricted to the dura and leptomeninges, but may show some secondary parenchymal invasion. Histopathologically, metastatic lymphomas are identical to primary lymphomas.

7.5.4 Primary CNS histiocytic sarcoma

Primary histiocytic sarcoma of the CNS, without demonstrable extraneural lesions, occurs in intracranial and intraspinal sites in older dogs with a predilection for certain breeds including Bernese Mountain Dog, Rottweiler, Dobermann, Pembroke Welsh Corgi and some Retrievers (Golden, Flat-coated and Labrador). The lesions form single, large, broad-based masses, mainly intracranial and less commonly within the spinal cord, originating either subdurally or within the leptomeninges and usually with secondary deep focal infiltration into the underlying brain or spinal cord.

MRI is not exclusively diagnostic, with T1W isointensity and T2W hyperintensity and sometimes with marked homogeneous contrast ring enhancement (Fig. 7.24A). However, the broad-based meningeal involvement and signs of a dural tail requires consideration of of a meningioma as a differential radiological diagnosis. A diagnosis can be made from examination of either CSF cytospin smears or stereotactically derived biopsy tissue based on the characteristic cellular features of histiocytic sarcomas.

Histologically, neoplastic histiocytic cells have eccentrically placed oval to reniform, pleomorphic nuclei with eosinophilic cytoplasm and sharp cytoplasmic borders (Fig. 7.24C). Phagocytosis of nuclear debris and cells is evident in their cytoplasm. Bi- or multinucleate giant cells are frequent. Both normal and abnormal mitotic figures are numerous (Fig. 7.23C). The PI is between about 10 and 40%. CD1c, CD11b and CD11c are considered to be definitive canine diagnostic markers on frozen fresh tissue while CD18 immunoreactivity on FFPE tissue is circumstantial evidence for this diagnosis (Fig. 7.24B).

7.6 Germ cell tumors

7.6.1 Germinoma

Canine **germinomas** occur in lateral suprasellar sites or the thalamus and are derived from extraneuraxial gonadal germ cells. On MRI, they appear as a solid isodense mass with uniform T1W post-contrast

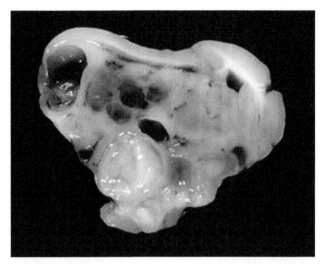

Fig. 7.25 Rabbit. Intracranial teratoma in frontal lobe. Transverse section with multiple variegated masses with characteristic fluid-filled cysts.

enhancement. Macroscopically, they have an irregular rough border, are infiltrative, closely attached to the meninges and gray colored. In both their location and MRI profile they must be differentiated from meningiomas. Histologically, they consist of large cells in sheets or lobules separated by a thin fibrovascular stroma with large nuclei and copious homogeneous faint-staining cytoplasm. Infiltrating T lymphocytes can accumulate in large numbers within the fibrovascular stroma in a biphasic tissue pattern. Some clusters of germinoma cells are immunoreactive with antibody to c-kit and also exhibit nuclear reactivity to OCT4.

7.6.2 Teratoma

Intracranial mature **teratomas** are comprised of disorganized mixtures of fully differentiated mature tissues from cell lines including ectodermal, mesodermal and endodermal derivation; grossly, they usually include cyst formation (Fig. 7.25). They occur in a wide variety of animals and in birds. Brain, choroid plexus, glandular tissue, cartilage, osteoid tissue, fat, hair follicles, skeletal and smooth muscle, bone with hemopoietic tissue etc. can be found in varying proportions within these mass lesions often in the cerebral hemispheres. Immature teratomas contain less well differentiated areas.

7.7 Embryonal tumors of non-neuroepithelial origin

7.7.1 Thoracolumbar spinal cord tumor (ectopic nephroblastoma)

This putative **ectopic nephroblastoma**, located between T9 and L3 spinal cord segments, occurs mainly in large-breed dogs (e.g. German Shepherd Dog, Golden Retriever, Boxer) between 5 and 48 months of age (median 14 months). Intraspinal metastases or a second primary site have occurred at L4–6. The incidence is less than 1% of all primary tumors. It remains uncertain whether the tumor originates within either an intradural extramedullary or intramedullary site. MRI and contrast myelography have indicated both possibilities (Fig. 7.26A). Grossly, there is a pinkish-gray discolored bulging mass, which can be restricted to either site, up

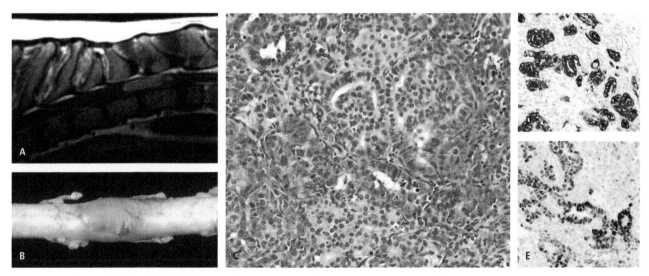

Fig. 7.26 Dog. Ectopic nephroblastoma spinal cord. A: MRI of T2W image with a subdural single well demarcated hyperintense mass at L2 segment. B: Dorsoventral aspect of the cord with a large well defined brownish subdural mass. C: Histologically, there is widespread tubular and acinar formation somewhat resembling renal glomeruli embedded in a more compacted cell population. HE. D: CK-immunoreactive epithelial cells forming acini. IHC Lu5. E: Strong immunoreactivity of the acinar cells to WT1 suggestive of a renal tissue origin for this tumor. IHC WT-1.

to 2 cm long, as well as possible extradural growth (Fig. 7.26B). Microscopically, there is a mixture of both a glandular epithelial and a more solid mesenchymal stromal pattern. The glandular pattern consists of tubules and acinar structures sometimes containing a glomeruloid-like component resembling fetal glomeruli (Fig. 7.26C). Mitotic figures are numerous particularly in the epithelial cell component which also has a high PI of about 30%. These epithelial cells are also immunoreactive to antibodies to CK (Lu-5) (Fig. 7.26D) and to WT-1, the Wilm's nephroblastoma tumor gene product (Fig. 7.26D). The second pattern is composed of sheets or interlacing fascicles of spindloid cells with ovoid nuclei and minimal cytoplasm, which are immunoreactive only for vimentin. A canine renal Wilm's tumor with a spinal cord metastases has been described once. The pathogenesis remains an enigma. These tumors have not been reported in people.

7.8 Secondary or metastatic tumors

In a recent institutional large case series, the overall incidence in dogs of secondary tumors was about equal to that of primary tumors of the CNS. Most secondary tumors are considered to arise from hematogenously disseminated metastases from primary extraneural tumors in descending order of frequency of **hemangiosarcomas** (29%, Fig. 7.27A), **carcinomas** (12%, Fig. 7.27B) (mammary, lung and kidney), **metastatic lymphomas** (12%), **nasal tumors, disseminated histiocytic sarcomas, malignant melanomas** as well as many individual miscellaneous tumors. See MRI Atlas.

Local extension

Secondary tumors can also arise by local extension particularly in the spinal cord from, for example, **osteosarcomas, chondrosacromas** and **histiocytic sarcomas**, while secondary extension from the nasal cavity through the cribiform plate is seen with **chondro- and fibrosarcomas, nasal carcinomas** and **neuroendocrine carcinomas**. Intracranial **multilobular bone tumors** can arise from the cranial vault. Embryonal **rhabdomyosarcomas** can arise from the deep intraorbital sites before secondary extension into the brain. Most canine **pituitary tumors** arise from the adenohypophysis (25%) with secondary midline dorsal extension into the hypothalamic region.

Hematogenous spread

Hemangiosarcoma is consistently the most common type of metastatic CNS tumor in dogs (29%) with a breed predilection for both Boxers and Golden Retrievers.

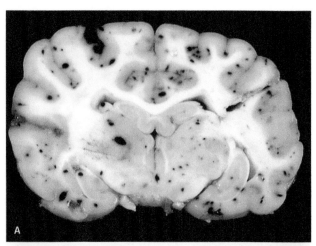

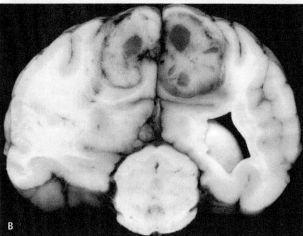

Fig. 7.27 Dog. Metastatic CNS lesions. A: Metastatic hemangiosarcoma with preferential distribution of lesions in the gray matter. B: Multiple foci of a metastatic mammary adenocarcinoma.

Most secondary tumors have multiple sites of varying size and in accordance with hematogenous access tend to involve gray rather than white matter (Fig. 7.27A). Metastatic lymphomas characteristically have widespread meningeal dissemination, while vascular occlusion from endotheliotropic lymphomas leads to multifocal infarction. Although an unknown percentage of secondary tumors are solitary lesions, multiple sites are usually indicative of metastatic spread. On MRI, hemangiosarcomas have mixed signal intensity on both T1W and T2W images with marked, non-uniform or peripheral contrast enhancement, depending on the degree of hemorrhage. Other tumor types do not have characteristic diagnostic profiles. However, most metastases retain their primary histological characteristics, although, for example, pulmonary carcinomas may mimic choroid plexus tumors. Focal hemorrhage and necrosis are common. Immunohistochemistry is often useful to distinguish primary from secondary tumors in the CNS or to confirm the site of origin of a suspected metastasis.

Further reading

General

Louis DN, H. Ohgkaki, OD Wiestler, WK Cavenee. (eds) The WHO Classification of Tumours of the Central Nervous System, 4th ed. Lyon, France: IARC, 2007.

Vernau KM, Higgins RJ, Bollen AW, Jimenez DF, Anderson JV, Koblik PD, LeCouteur RA. Primary canine and feline nervous system tumors: intraoperative diagnosis using the smear technique. Vet Pathol 2001;38:47–57.

Wisner ER, Dickinson PJ, Higgins RJ. Magnetic resonance imaging features of canine intracranial neoplasia. Vet Radiol Ultrasound 2011;52,Suppl.1:52–61.

Glial tumors

Higgins RJ, Dickinson PJ, LeCouteur RA, Bollen AW, Wang H, Wang H, Corely LJ, Moore LM, Zang W, Fuller GN. Spontaneous canine gliomas overexpression of EGFR, PDGF alpha and IGFBP2 demonstrated by tissue microarray immunophenotyping. J NeuroOncol 2010;98:49–55.

Lipsitz D, Higgins RJ, Kortz GD, Dickinson PJ, Bollen AW, Naydan DK, LeCouteur RA. Glioblastoma multiforme: clinical findings, magnetic resonance imaging and pathology in five dogs. Vet Pathol 2003;40:659–669.

Porter B, de Lahunta A, Summers B. Gliomatosis cerebri in six dogs. Vet Pathol 2003;40:97–102.

Snyder JM, Lipitz L, Skorupski KA, Shofer FS, Van Winkle TJ. Canine intracranial primary neoplasia: 173 cases. J Vet Int Med 2006;20: 669–675.

Stoica G, Levine J, Wolff J, Murphy K. Canine astrocytic tumors: a comparative review. Vet Pathol 2011;48:266–275.

Wong M, Glass E, DeLahunta A, Jackson B. Intracranial anaplastic astrocytoma in a 19 week old boxer dog. J Small Anim Pract 2011;52:325–328.

York D, Higgins RJ, LeCouteur RA, Wolfe AN, Grahn R, Olby N, Campbell M, Dickinson PJ. TP53 mutations in canine brain tumors. Vet Pathol 2012;24:14–22.

Choroid plexus tumors

Ide T, Uchida K, Kikuta F, Suzuki K, Nakayama H. Immunohistochemical characterization of canine neuroepithelial tumors. Vet Pathol 2010;47:741–750.

Nentwig A, Higgins RJ, Francey T, Doherr M, Zurbriggen A, Oevermann A. Aberrant E-cadherin, β-catenin and GFAP expression in canine choroid plexus tumors. JVDI 2012; in press.

Westworth DR, Dickinson PJ, Vernau W, Johnson EG, Bollen AW, Kass PH, Sturges BK, Vernau KM, Lecouteur RA, Higgins RJ. Choroid plexus tumors in 56 dogs (1985–2007). J Vet Int Med 2008;22: 1157–1165.

Neuronal tumors

Kuwamura M, Kotera T, Yamate J, Kotani T, Aoki M, Hori A. Cerebral ganglioneuroblastoma in a golden retriever dog. Vet Pathol 2004;41: 282–284.

Kuwamura M, Kotera T, Yamate J, Kotani T, Aoki M, Hori A. Extraventricular neurocytoma of the spinal cord in a dog. Vet Pathol 2008;45:63–66.

Uchida K, Nakayama H, Endo Y, Kai C, Tatewaki S, Yamaguchi R, Doi K, Tateyama S. Ganglioglioma in the thalamus of a puppy. J Vet Med Sci 2003;65:113–115.

Embryonal tumors

Headley SA, Koljonen M, Gomes LA, Sukura A. Central primitive neuroectodermal tumor with ependymal differentiation in a dog. J Comp Pathol 2009;140:80–83.

Kitagawa M, Koie H, Kanayamat K, Sakai T. Medulloblastoma in a cat: clinical and MRI findings. J Small Anim Pract 2003;44: 139–142.

Steinberg H, Galbreath EJ. Cerebellar medulloblastoma with multiple differentiation in a dog. Vet Pathol 1998;35:543–546.

PNS tumors

Gaitero L, Añor S, Fondevila D, Pumarola M. Canine cutaneous spindle cell tumors with features of peripheral nerve sheath tumors: a histopathological and immunohistochemical study. J Comp Pathol 2008;139:16–23.

Higgins RJ, Dickinson PJ, Jimenez DF, Bollen AW, Lecouteur RA. Canine intraneural perineurioma. Vet Pathol 2006;43:50–54.

Schoniger S, Summers BA. Localized, plexiform diffuse and other variants of neurofibroma in 12 dogs, 2 horses and a chicken. Vet Pathol 2009;46:904–915.

Meningiomas

Dickinson PJ, Surace EI, Cambell M, Higgins RJ, Leutenegger CM, Bollen AW, LeCouteur RA, Gutmann DH. Expression of the tumor suppressor genes NF2, 4.1B, and TSLC1 in canine meningiomas. Vet Pathol 2009;46:884–892.

Ide T, Uchida K, Suzuki K, Kagawa Y, Nakayama H. Expression of cell adhesion molecules and doublecortin in canine anaplastic meningiomas. Vet Pathol 2011;48:292–301.

Petersen SA, Sturges BK, Dickinson PJ, Pollard RE, Kass PH, Kent M, Vernau KM, Lecouteur RA, Higgins RJ. Canine intraspinal meningiomas: imaging features, histopathologic classification and long-term outcome in 34 dogs. J Vet Intern Med 2008;22: 946–953.

Sturges BK, Dickinson PJ, Bollen AW, Koblik PD, Kass PH, Kortz GD, Vernau KM, Knipe MF, Lecouteur RA, Higgins RJ. Magnetic resonance imaging and histological classification of intracranial meningiomas in 112 dogs. J Vet Intern Med 2008;22:586–595.

Granular cell tumor

Higgins RJ, LeCouteur RA, Vernau KM, Sturges BK, Obradovich JE, Bollen AW. Granular cell tumor of the canine CNS: two cases. Vet Pathol 2001;38:620–627.

Rao D, Rylander H, Drees R, Schwarz T, Steinberg H. Granular cell tumor in a lumbar spinal nerve of a dog. J Vet Diagn Invest 2010; 22:638–642.

Mesenchymal tumors

Cantile C, Baroni M, Tartarelli CL, Campani D, Salvadori C, Arispici M. Intramedullary hemangioblastoma in a dog. Vet Pathol 2003;40: 91–94.

Zabka TS, Lavely JA, Higgins RJ. Primary intra-axial leiomyosarcoma with obstructive hydrocephalus in a young dog. J Comp Pathol 2004;131:334–337.

Lymphomas and hemapoetic tumors

Lapointe JM, Higgins RJ, Kortz GD, Bailey CS, Moore PF. Intravascular malignant T-cell lymphoma (malignant angioendotheliomatosis). Vet Pathol 1997;34:247–250.

McDonough SP, Van Winkle TJ, Valentine BA, vanGessel YA, Summers BA. Clinicopathological and immunophenotypical features of canine intravascular lymphoma (malignant endotheliomatosis). J Comp Pathol 2002;126:277–288.

Tzipory L, Vernau KM, Sturges BK, Zabka TS, Highland MA, Petersen SA, Wisner ER, Moore PF, Vernau W. Antemortem diagnosis of localized central nervous system histiocytic sarcoma in 2 dogs. J Vet Int Med 2009;23:369–374.

Van Wettere AJ, Linder KE, Suter SE, Olby NJ. Solitary intracerebral plasmacytoma in a dog: microscopic, immunohistochemical and molecular features. Vet Pathol 2009;46:949–951.

Germ cell tumors

Chenier S, Quesnel A, Girard C. Intracranial teratoma and dermoid cyst in a kitten. J Vet Diagn Invest 1998;10:381–384.

Valentine BA, Summers BA, deLahunta A, White CL, Kuhajda FP. Suprasellar germ cell tumors in the dog: a report of five cases and a review of the literature. Acta Neuropathol 1988;76:94–100.

Nephroblastoma

Brewer DM, Cerda-Gonzalez S, Dewey CW, Diep AN, Van Horne K, McDonough SP. Spinal cord nephroblastoma in dogs:11 cases (1985–2007). JAVMA 2011;238:618–624.

Metastatic tumors

Snyder JM, Lipitz L, Skorupski KA, Shofer FS, Van Winkle TJ. Secondary intracranial neoplasia in the dog; 177 cases (1986–2003). J Vet Int Med 2008;22:172–177.

This book is accompanied by a companion website which is maintained by the Division of Diagnostic Imaging, Dept of Clinical Veterinary Medicine, Vetsuisse Faculty, University of Bern, Switzerland.

www.wiley.com/go/vandevelde/veterinaryneuropathology

8

Degenerative diseases

This chapter covers a complex group of diseases, which are broadly characterized by selective degeneration and loss of cells or cell components (e.g. axons, myelin sheaths) in a bilaterally symmetrical fashion. These diseases have usually a slowly progressive course and, with some exceptions, commonly start at a young age. Most are either suspected to be or are of confirmed genetic origin. In some, a breed or familial susceptibility for presumably environmental factors modifying degeneration appears to exist.

The pathophysiology of most degenerative diseases is only partly understood. However, in recent years considerable progress has been made. In a rapidly growing number of degenerative diseases in humans and in domestic animals, the genetic defect has been localized and characterized. In several the corresponding protein defect is known and in some the biochemical disease mechanism has been unraveled with the promise of specific therapies in the foreseeable future. Since this is a widely diverging group of diseases, pathogenetic aspects will be referred to in the respective sections of this chapter where appropriate.

Hundreds of different degenerative diseases have been recognized in domestic animals. Rapid progress in the molecular genetic characterization of these diseases will affect their diagnosis and future classification. At present there is no standardized terminology to name these diseases, which makes this field somewhat confusing. In this chapter, we classify these diseases according to their main cellular target and/or lesion patterns. In the CNS, we distinguish the following major groups: neuronal degenerations, axonal degenerations, myelin disorders, storage diseases, spongiform encephalopathies, spongy degenerations and selective symmetrical encephalomalacias. At the end of the chapter we very briefly discuss some degenerative diseases in peripheral nerves and muscles.

8.1 General strategy for differential diagnosis of degenerative lesions

8.1.1 Recognizing the major patterns

- The typical presentation is an animal, generally at a young age, with slowly progressive symmetrical neurological signs.
- The lesions are often subtle and not visible on macroscopic examination (or MRI). To search for degenerative lesions, systematic sampling as explained in Chapter 1 is essential. It is very important to include spinal cord sections because several diseases, e.g. axonopathies, are much easier to detect in cross-sections of the cord. HE sections must be systematically scanned for neuronal, glial, axonal or myelin changes.
- The lesions are almost always bilateral and symmetrical: they are often found in selected areas or with a specific pattern of distribution and require systematic careful histological examination.
- The major specific patterns are: loss of neurons/ axons/myelin, pallor of white matter, spongy state, intracellular storage and malacia. Since these are slowly progressive diseases, signs of active degeneration may be minimal since the rate of removal of dead cells by macrophages keeps pace with the degenerative process. For the same reason, macrophages seldom accumulate in large numbers. However, degeneration is often indicated by an associated astrogliosis. Thus, hypercellularity is an important marker of these diseases.

8.1.2 Further analysis

- When abnormalities are found, proceed diagnostically according to Table 8.1, which lists the prevailing

Veterinary Neuropathology: Essentials of Theory and Practice, First Edition. Marc Vandevelde, Robert J. Higgins, and Anna Oevermann.
© 2012 John Wiley & Sons, Ltd. Published 2012 by John Wiley & Sons, Ltd.

Table 8.1 Major degenerative lesion patterns.

DEGENERATIVE PATTERNS IN GRAY MATTER

Pattern	Interpretation	Disease examples
Neuronal changes/ Neuronal loss	Neuronal degenerations	
	Motor neurons	Hereditary canine spinal muscular atrophy
	Purkinje cells	Cerebellocortical atrophy in Arabian foals
	Granule cells	Cerebellar granule cell degeneration in Collie dogs
	Other neurons	Multisystem neuronal degeneration in Cocker Spaniels
Accumulation of axonal spheroids	Neuroaxonal dystrophy	NAD in Rottweiler dogs
Spongy state	Spongiform encephalopathy	Scrapie in sheep
	Spongy degeneration	1-2-Hydroxyglutaric aciduria in Staffordshire Terriers
Accumulation of material in neurons	Storage disease	GM1 gangliosidosis in Siamese cats
Malacia	Selective symmetrical encephalomalacia	Alaskan Husky encephalopathy

DEGENERATIVE PATTERNS IN WHITE MATTER

Pattern	Interpretation	Disease examples
Pale staining white matter, spongy state	Axonopathy	Hereditary ataxia in Jack Russell Terriers
	Myelin disease	Leukoencephalomyelopathy in Leonberger dogs
Accumulation of axonal spheroids	Axonopathy	Progressive axonopathy in Boxer dogs
Spongy state	Spongy degeneration	Citrullinemia in Friesian Holstein cattle
Malacia	Leukodystrophy	Afghan dog myelopathy
Pallor of white matter	Dysmyelination	Shaking pups in Springer Spaniels

lesion patterns either in the gray or in the white matter. However, be aware that combinations of white and gray matter lesions may occur. Recognizing these patterns focuses the neuropathological examination on certain groups of diseases.

- If depletion of neurons in a certain area is suspected, it is often useful to compare with sections of normal animals.
- The pattern of "intracellular storage" is not difficult to recognize. Neurons appear swollen and the nucleus is displaced by a cytoplasmic accumulation of abnormal, granular material.
- White matter degeneration (axons, myelin or both) is usually associated with pale staining (on HE) and variable degrees of a spongy state (to be differentiated

from spongy degeneration). Special histo- or immunohistochemical stains are useful to evaluate whether axons or myelin or both are affected.

- Swollen axons are a common finding in all types of CNS diseases. When these spheroids are particularly large and occur in large numbers, they are indicative of a primary axonal pathology.
- For the differential diagnosis for a spongy state pattern consult Fig. 6.14. In the gray matter, the distinction between spongy degeneration and spongiform degeneration is important.
- For the differential diagnosis of the pattern of "malacia" consult Fig. 6.1.
- Grossly visible pallor and softness of the white matter is indicative of developmental myelin disorders.

8.1.3 Diagnosis

- The final step is to allocate the lesions to one of the major degenerative disease categories (neuronal, axonal or spongy degenerations, myelin disorders, storage diseases, spongiform encephalopathies, or selective symmetrical encephalomalacias) and then to one of the specific diseases listed in Tables 8.2–8.6. Based on the nature and distribution of the lesions, a morphological diagnosis can be made and, depending on the species/breed, the findings may fit one of the more common well known diseases. It is extremely helpful to consult published lists of inherited diseases for the respective species/breed, which are available in either neurology text books or on the internet (http://www.vet.cam.ac.uk/idid/http://sydney.edu.au/vetscience/lida/). The chances are good that the lesion has been described and previously characterized.

- When a degenerative condition is suspected at necropsy, it is important to correctly collect, freeze and store fresh tissues for later biochemical and genetic examination.

- As discussed in the chapter on toxic–metabolic diseases, it is not surprising that similar lesions can be caused by certain toxins or deficiencies targeting the same molecular mechanisms affected by genetic defects. Thus, it is important to keep in mind the possibility of a toxic–metabolic etiology (Chapter 6) when encountering one of the morphological patterns described in this chapter.

8.2 Degeneration of neurons

8.2.1 General aspects

In this section, we focus on degenerations of the neuronal cell body caused by an intrinsic inherited biochemical defect. Such a genetic defect can lead, for example, to deficient transcriptional regulation, aggregation and abnormal clearance of proteins, alterations of calcium homeostasis, activation of pro-apoptotic routes or an abnormal structure/function of a protein (such as an ion channel), all of which will eventually lead to death of the cell. The characteristic morphological hallmark of these diseases is degeneration and loss of neurons in specific anatomical structures. Consistent with the slowly progressive nature of these diseases, various stages of the process can be seen in the same section. It is usually the reactive changes consisting mostly of diffuse micro- and astrogliosis in the affected areas that indicate a lesion. Sometimes in advanced cases, there is macroscopically visible evidence of atrophy. Clinical signs reflect the affected neuronal populations. A traditional approach is

to classify neurodegenerative diseases according to neuroanatomical criteria thus to the specific cell population affected ("*system disorder*"), which also reflects the clinical presentation (Table 8.2). However, while many neurodegenerations appear to be restricted to a particular neuronal type, it is becoming more apparent that many affect several functionally different neuronal populations simultaneously and these are therefore classified as *multisystem neuronal degenerations*. Some disorders involve not only the CNS but also the peripheral and/or autonomic nervous systems. It must be stressed that combinations of primary axonal and neuronal lesions also occur. In addition, as explained in Chapter 1, we should remember that significant loss of neurons can lead to degeneration in the anterograde tracts emanating from these neurons or nuclei. In addition, primary axonal and neuronal lesions can also lead to retrograde neuronal changes. A list of well known hereditary (or probably hereditary) neuronal degenerations is presented in Table 8.2.

8.2.2 Motor neuron diseases

General features

Motor neuron diseases (MND) are degenerative disorders of the CNS affecting motor neurons of spinal cord, brainstem and motor cortex. Human MND subtypes are distinguished by their major anatomical site of degeneration. In **amyotrophic lateral sclerosis (ALS)**, the most common human motor neuron disease, there is involvement of upper and lower motor neurons, while in **progressive spinal muscular atrophy** and related syndromes the motor neurons in the spinal cord are primarily involved. The underlying molecular defect is known in some of these diseases. For instance mutations in the *superoxide dismutase (SOD 1) gene* in familial ALS suggest that neurons might die of oxidative stress. Transgenic mice expressing analogous SOD defects exhibit similar motor neuron lesions. In general all animals with MND show signs of weakness of the limbs, and muscles of the head with paresis and paralysis and progressive muscular atrophy. Because of severe neurogenic atrophy, these diseases are also named *spinal muscular atrophies* (SMA). Morphologically, all these conditions are similar. The motor neurons appear swollen, chromatolysis is a consistent finding starting focally and gradually involving all of the Nissl substance (Fig. 8.1). Affected neurons exhibit nuclear changes (Fig. 8.1) with peripheral eccentric displacement, flattening and pyknosis of the nucleus. Some neurons are eosinophilic, while others assume a glassy ghost-like appearance. Neuronophagia, neuronal depletion and marked gliosis are common features of advanced stages of MND

Table 8.2 Neuronal degenerations.

SUBTYPE	NAME OF DISEASE	SPECIES/BREED
Motor neuron disease (MND)	Hereditary canine spinal muscular atrophy	Brittany Spaniel
	Hereditary progressive neurogenic muscular atrophy	Pointer
	Familial motor neuron disease	Rottweiler dog
	Asymmetrical spinal muscular atrophy (SMA)	German Shepherd Dog
	Stockard's paralysis	Great Dane–Saint Bernard crossbreeds
	Hereditary progressive neurogenic muscular atrophy	English Pointer
	Hereditary neuronal abiotrophy	Swedish Lapland Dog
	Multisystem axonopathy and neuronopathy	Golden Retriever
	Multisystemic chromatolytic neuronal degeneration	Cairn Terrier
	Inherited motor neuron disease	Domestic cats
	Bovine SMA	Brown Swiss, Holstein, Friesian, Red Danish
	Hereditary porcine neuronal system degeneration	Pigs
	Lower motor neuron disease with neurofilamentous accumulation	Yorkshire pigs, Hampshire pigs
Cerebellar Purkinje cell degeneration	Cerebellar cortical abiotrophy (CCA) dogs	Scottish Terrier, Chow Chow, Airedale Terrier, Border Collie, Rough-Coated Collie, Lagotto Romagnolo, Beagle, Rhodesian Ridgeback, Australian Kelpie, Gordon Setter, Old English Sheepdog, Labrador Retriever, Finnish harrier
	CCA horses	Arabian horse, Gotland pony
	CCA bovines	Holstein, Shorthorn, Hereford, Angus
	CCA pigs	Yorkshire, Large White
	CCA sheep	Merino, Coriedale
	Hepatocerebellar degeneration,	Bernese Mountain Dog
	Olivopontocerebellar atrophy	Cats
	Striatonigral and cerebello-olivary degeneration,	Chinese Crested dog, Kerry Blue Terrier
	Late-onset progressive spinocerebellar degeneration	Brittany Spaniel
	Neonatal cerebellar ataxia (Banderas ataxia)	Coton de Tuléar
	Multisystem neuronal abiotrophy	Miniature Poodle
Cerebellar granule cell degeneration	Cerebellar granule cell degeneration	Border Collie, Coton de Tuléar, Bavarian Mountain Dog, Lagotto Romagnolo
Other neuronal degenerations	Multisystem neuronal degeneration	Cocker Spaniel
	Neuronal vacuolation and spinocerebellar degeneration	Rottweiler dog, Siberian Husky, Boxer dog
	Hypertonicity syndrome	Labrador Retriever

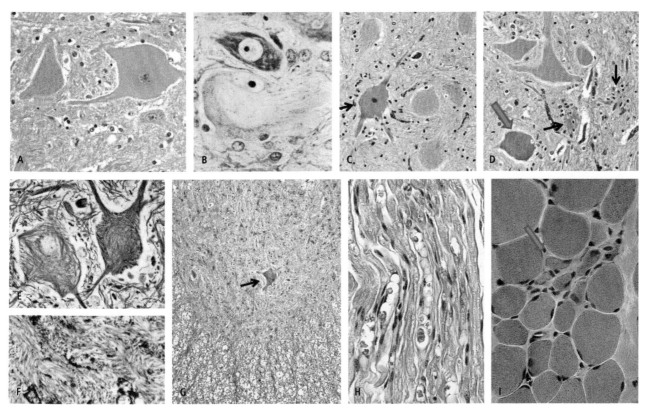

Fig. 8.1 Motor neuron disease (MND). A: Brown Swiss calf. Spinal cord. Spinal muscular atrophy (SMA). Ventral horn motor neuron with chromatolysis. HE. B: Cat. MND. Chromatolysis in motor neuron with eccentric nucleus and peripheral margination of Nissl substance compared with normal neuron. LFB-CEV. C: Calf. SMA. Spinal cord. Necrotic neuron attracting a microglial response. HE. D: Calf. SMA. One dark-staining acutely degenerating neuron (large arrow) and two glial nodules, one containing neuronal remnants (small arrows). HE. E: Cat. MND. Two motor neurons with abnormal accumulation of of agyrophilic fibrillary material (neurofibrillary accumulation) in cytoplasm, Holmes silver stain. F: Same cat as in E with cytoplasmic accumulation of neurofilaments. Electron micrograph. G: Dog. Chronic MND. Spinal cord. Massive loss of motor neurons and gliosis with only one surviving neuron. HE. H: Brown Swiss calf. SMA. Sciatic nerve. Acute Wallerian degeneration of some myelinated nerve fibers. HE. I: Brown Swiss calf. SMA. Skeletal muscle. Group fiber atrophy typical of neurogenic disease, HE.

(Fig. 8.1). Wallerian degeneration in the peripheral motor nerves and neurogenic atrophy of the muscles are also conspicuous features (Fig. 8.1). In several conditions, accumulation of abnormally phosphorylated neurofilaments in swollen degenerated motor neurons has been described (Fig. 8.1). This condition has been termed lower MND with *neurofibrillary accumulation* thought to be associated with abnormalities in the synthesis, catabolism or transport of the neurofilaments. However, it is also possible that this change is secondary to a primary axonal transport defect.

MND in small animals

Hereditary canine spinal muscular atrophy (HCSMA), a disease in Brittany Spaniels, is the best studied MND in domestic animals. HCSMA is an autosomal dominant inherited disorder, displaying varying degrees of severity ranging from mild exercise intolerance to tetraplegia. Atrophy of the tongue, masticatory and facial muscles

are also associated with the disease. In the accelerated form, which resembles **Werdnig–Hoffman disease** in children, abnormal axonal internodes are distended and a massive accumulation of neurofilaments is the most conspicuous lesion. The intermediate form, which shows nerve cell loss and smaller numbers of axonal swellings, resembles human juvenile MND forms. Both phenotypes exhibit growth arrest and axonal atrophy suggesting that motor axons failed to reach normal size as well an impairment of axonal transport resulting in an accumulation of neurofilaments. Other studies indicate a defect in neurofilament assembly. Recent studies suggest that the motor failure in HCSMA is due to a primary failure of neuromuscular synaptic transmission preceding nerve and muscle pathology.

Probably the longest known MND in veterinary medicine was **Stockard's paralysis** in Great Dane–Saint Bernard or Great Dane–Bloodhound crossbreeds with a complex mode of inheritance. A further example of MND is **familial motor neuron disease** in Rottweiler dogs, which resembles HCSMA in Brittany Spaniels and is associated with megaesophagus due to degenerating neurons in the nucleus ambiguus. **Hereditary progressive neurogenic muscular atrophy** in English Pointer pups is an autosomal recessive disease showing all the clinical hallmarks of motor neuron disease, but there is no actual loss of motor neurons but rather an accumulation of numerous membranous cytoplasmic bodies reminiscent of a storage disease. Other canine MNDs include a number of cases without genetic information including MND in the following breeds: Dobermann, Griffon Briquet Vendéen, Collie sheepdog, Pug, Dachshund, Fox Terrier and Saluki. A curiosity is an **asymmetric MND** with focal involvement of the cervical cord described in German Shepherd Dogs. MNDs have also been described in cats as sporadic cases sometimes with adult onset. The **inherited motor neuron disease** in domestic cats has an autosomal recessive mode of inheritance and is characterized by rapid early progression followed by stabilization of signs and prolonged survival times. The disease is associated with a deletion in the LIX1 gene, which is believed to be involved in RNA metabolism in motor neurons.

MND in large animals

Bovine spinal muscular atrophy (SMA) has been described in a variety of breeds. An autosomal recessive inherited bovine MND reminiscent of juvenile human MND was described in Brown Swiss cattle, while a phenotype resembling Werdnig–Hoffman disease in humans has been identified in Holstein–Friesian calves. Further affected breeds include Herefords and Red Danish cattle. A missense mutation in the 3-ketodihydrosphingosine reductase FVT1 has been proposed as a candidate mutation for bovine spinal muscular atrophy. A MND of suspected hereditary origin, **lower motor neuron disease with neurofilamentous accumulation,** has been described in Yorkshire and Hampshire breeds of pigs.

MND combined with degeneration of other systems

Multisystemic chromatolytic neuronal degeneration in Cairn Terriers is also termed **progressive neuronopathy.** The clinical signs suggest spinal muscular atrophy. Microscopically, chromatolytic changes are confined not only to motor neurons of the spinal cord and brainstem nuclei (including red nucleus), but involve also the thalamic and deep cerebellar nuclei. Ultrastructurally, chromatolytic neurons of the dorsal and ventral horns of the spinal cord show dispersion and loss of ribosomes accompanied by excessive numbers of mitochondria.

There is no evidence of actual neuronal loss. Interestingly, large numbers of chromatolytic neurons have also been found in spinal, autonomic and myenteric ganglia. In **hereditary neuronal abiotrophy** in Swedish Lapland dogs, an autosomal recessive disease, degenerative changes were not only found in motor neurons but also in spinal ganglia, Purkinje cells and deep cerebellar nuclei. Axonal damage was apparent in dorsal roots, dorsal funiculus of the spinal cord and spinocerebellar tracts, as well as in trigeminal, optic and vestibulocochlear nerves. A "dying back" phenomenon was suggested. This implies that the initial lesion occurs in the terminal portion of the axon and then proceeds retrogradely towards the neuronal cell body. In **multisystem axonopathy and neuronopathy** in Golden Retrievers, there is extensive motor neuron disease combined with a severe axonopathy in the spinal cord predominantly affecting the lateral and ventral columns. A similar distribution of degenerative lesions was found in pigs with **hereditary porcine neuronal system degeneration**.

8.2.3 Cerebellar degenerations

Purkinje cell degenerations

These diseases are also referred to as **cerebellar cortical abiotrophies (CCAs)**, and are probably the most common type of neurodegeneration in domestic animals, resulting from primary Purkinje cell loss. CCAs have been reported in many different dog breeds. The hereditary (mostly autosomal recessive) or at least familial nature of the disease has been shown in Scottish Terriers, Airedales, Border Collies, Rough-Coated Collies, Lagotto Romagnolos, Beagles, Rhodesian Ridgebacks, Australian Kelpies, Gordon Setters, Old English Sheepdogs, Labrador Retrievers, Chow Chows and Finnish Harriers. In addition, there are numerous case reports in other breeds. The disease is much rarer in cats, although hereditary feline CCAs have been recently reported. CCA is also well known in several cattle breeds (e.g. Holstein, Shorthorn, Hereford and Angus, in the latter associated with seizures) and sheep (Merino, Corriedale) breeds, Arabian horses, Gotland ponies and swine (Yorkshire, Large White). It is quite possible that there is considerable genetic overlap between the different CCAs described in various breeds and species, but there are certainly differences in onset, course and severity of the signs/lesions suggesting a spectrum of different disease mechanisms.

The clinical signs in cerebellar degeneration are usually quite dramatic and include cerebellar ataxia with head tremor, truncal ataxia, symmetrical hypermetria, spasticity and broad-based stance and gait. In general, cerebellar cortical degenerations have an early onset of clinical signs between weeks and months after birth, tending to progress, slowly or rapidly. Very early onset (**neonatal cerebellar cortical atrophy**) has been seen in Beagles, Samoyeds, Rhodesian Ridgebacks and Irish Setters (**hereditary quadriplegia and amblyopia**). Later clinical onset is not uncommon in dogs, for example in adult Gordon Setters and Old English Sheepdogs.

Neuropathological changes are similar in all CCAs. Purkinje cells are primarily affected with a progressive reduction in their population. There are variations in lesion distribution pattern within the cerebellum among the different CCAs, but the lesions generally occur earlier and/or are usually more severe in the vermis and paramedian lobes than in the lateral hemispheres. Purkinje cells show various stages of degeneration (e.g. chromatolysis, necrosis). In advanced cases, nearly all Purkinje cells may be lost and the cerebellum is grossly reduced in size (Fig. 8.2). See MRI Atlas. Secondary transneuronal retrograde degeneration and

loss of granule cells (which project on the Purkinje cells) is usually associated with Purkinje cell degeneration (Fig. 8.2). Other common changes secondary to Purkinje cell loss include shrinkage of the molecular layer in severely affected cerebellar areas, proliferation of so-called *Bergmann astrocytes* in folia where significant Purkinje cell loss has occurred (Fig. 8.2), empty basket cells and spheroids or "*torpedo*" formation (swollen Purkinje cell axons) in the granule cell layer and/or cerebellar white matter. Cerebellar nuclei are often gliotic, but obvious loss of neurons in these nuclei due to transynaptic neuronal degeneration is rare. In CCA in Scottish Terriers, there are also numerous polyglucosan bodies in the molecular layer. Putative retrograde neuronal degeneration in olivary nuclei from primary Purkinje cell loss has been described in Labrador Retrievers and in cats.

Breeding studies, pedigree analysis or segregation analysis in the majority of the reports describing multiple cases of cerebellar cortical abiotrophies have either suggested or established an autosomal recessive mode of

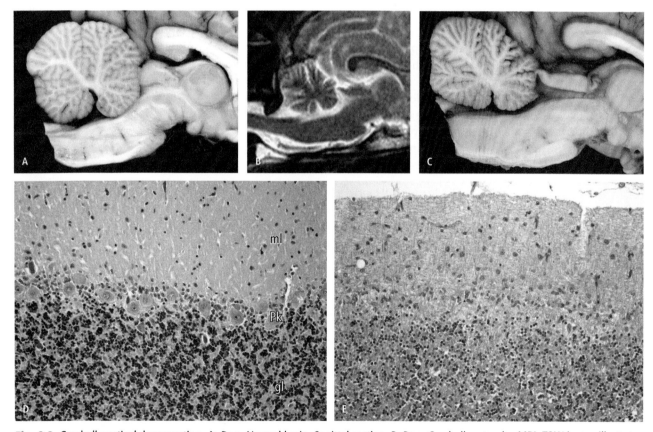

Fig. 8.2 Cerebellocortical degeneration. A: Dog. Normal brain. Sagittal section. B: Dog. Cerebellar atrophy. MRI. T2W image illustrates marked widening of CSF-filled sulci between atrophic cerebellar folia. C: Same dog as in B. Grossly, there is marked thinning of some cerebellar folia; compare to normal cerebellum in A. D: Dog. Histology of normal cerebellum. Cortex with intact Purkinje cells (ml, molecular layer; Pk, Purkinje cell layer; gl, granule cell layer). HE. E: Dog. Cerebellar atrophy. There is complete loss of Purkinje cells and gliosis in molecular layer, depletion of granule cells and atrophy of the molecular layer. HE.

inheritance. However, the underlying defect in most cerebellar cortical abiotrophies in domestic animals remains unknown. In CCA of Arabian horses, a mutation has been recently found affecting expression of MUTYH, a DNA-repairing enzyme, which has been implicated in human Parkinson's disease. It remains to be shown at the molecular level whether some of the animal cerebellar cortical degenerations are comparable in molecular terms to the group of human spinocerebellar ataxias caused by triplet nucleotide repeats. The triplet (CAG) repeat disorders have inserts in certain CNS genes leading to altered function and neurotoxic effects of the corresponding proteins. In Finnish Harriers a mutation in the SEL1L gene has been discovered, which is thought to lead to endoplasmatic reticulum stress. In CCA in Staffordshire Terriers and Pit Bull Terriers, Purkinje cell degeneration is associated with **ceroid lipofuscinosis**, in which the neuronal storage process predominantly targets the Purkinje cells (see Section 8.5.2). A further variation is **hepatocerebellar degeneration** in Bernese Mountain Dogs, a phenotypic replica of the human disorder. In Rhodesian Ridgebacks, CCA has been associated with coat color dilution.

A special case is the **neonatal cerebellar ataxia (Banderas neonatal ataxia)**, an autosomal recessive hereditary disease caused by a mutation in the GRM1 gene (which codes for the metabotropic glutamate receptor 1) in Coton de Tuléar dogs, showing severe cerebellar signs soon after birth, which may stabilize without further deterioration. In these dogs, no histological changes were found despite severe clinical signs. Electron microscope studies in these puppies revealed loss of synaptic terminals, varicosities in the parallel fibers and lamellar bodies in Purkinje cells.

Combined degeneration of Purkinje cells and other systems

In **olivopontocerebellar atrophy (OPCA)** in cats with progressive cerebellar signs, loss of Purkinje cells, basket cells, Golgi cells, stellate cells and granule cells was observed. Pontine nuclei and the olivary complex were also severely depopulated. Dominantly inherited late-onset OPCAs observed in humans are caused by expanded triplet repeats in one of the *ataxin* genes. However, characteristic ubiquitinated nuclear inclusions as well as Purkinje cell axon torpedoes, as observed in human OPCA, were absent in cats. Whether the condition in cats is sporadic rather than genetic remains to be confirmed.

Striatonigral and cerebello-olivary degeneration is an autosomal recessive disease in Kerry Blue Terriers and Chinese Crested Dogs. In addition to degeneration of Purkinje cells, there is severe neuronal loss with cavita-

tion of the olivary nuclei, neuronal loss and gliosis in the substantia nigra and acidophilic neuronal degeneration in the caudate nucleus. A suspicion of increased functional demand on caudate neurons and Purkinje cells was suggested by mitochondrial enlargement in their dendrites. The disease is related to a defect in the canine gene, which is homologous to the *Park2 gene*, a defect associated with an hereditary form of Parkinson's disease in people.

Late-onset progressive spinocerebellar degeneration in Brittany Spaniels is clinically characterized by excessive hypermetria in the front limbs (*saluting disease*). Dogs between 8 and 11 years of age are affected. There is a major loss of Purkinje cells, associated with bilateral and symmetrical neuronal degeneration in sensory neuronal systems of the medulla oblongata and spinal cord, together with secondary axonal degeneration. Accumulation of phosphorylated neurofilaments appears to precede Purkinje cell degeneration.

In **multisystem neuronal abiotrophy** in Miniature Poodles, CCA is combined with degenerative changes throughout the cerebral cortex.

Cerebellar granule cell degeneration

A few familial/hereditary conditions have been described in a small number of canine breeds, in which there is primary **cerebellar granule cell degeneration**.

Neuropathologically, this degeneration is characterized by progressive loss of granule cells, thinning of the granule cell layer and astrogliosis (Fig. 8.3). In Collies, the condition was suspected to be associated with a

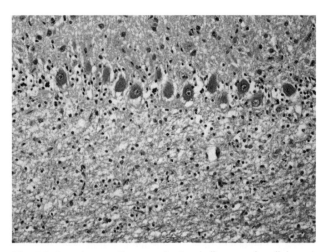

Fig. 8.3 Dog. Lagotto Romagnolo. Cerebellar granule cell degeneration. The Purkinje cell layer is intact, but there is massive depletion of granule cells (compare to Fig. 8.2D). HE.

defect in potassium ion channels, and recent descriptions in a family of Border Collie dogs suggested similarities with the homozygous weaver mouse. An inbred metabolic error in granule cells was suspected in a Brittany Spaniel and in Bavarian Mountain Dogs. A congenital immune-mediated response against granule cells was proposed in Coton de Tuléars and Lagotto Romagnolos affected by granule cell atrophy, because of diffuse invasion by T cells in the lesions.

Acquired cerebellar degeneration

As discussed in Chapter 6, certain plant poisons can cause Purkinje cell degeneration in herbivores.

8.2.4 Other neuronal degenerations

Multisystem neuronal degeneration in Cocker Spaniels

An inherited **multisystem neuronal degeneration** was found in young Cocker Spaniels that showed slowly progressive neurological signs with ataxia and mental deterioration. Pathologically, the lesions consisted of diffuse neuronal loss and gliosis in the septal nuclei, globus pallidus, subthalamic nuclei, substantia nigra, mesencephalic tectum, medial geniculate bodies and the cerebellar and vestibular nuclei. Axonal degeneration and demyelination were also found. Pedigree analysis strongly suggests a hereditary cause for this disease.

Neuronal vacuolation and spinocerebellar degeneration in dogs

Neuronal vacuolation and spinocerebellar degeneration was originally described in Rottweiler dogs from 3–8 months of age. A similar condition has been seen in Boxers, Siberian Huskies and mixed breed dogs. Clinically, there is weakness and ataxia in the pelvic limbs progressing within weeks to severe generalized ataxia, tetraparesis and laryngeal paralysis. Intracytoplasmic neuronal vacuolation and mild spongiform change have been found in the cerebellar nuclei and in nuclei of the extrapyramidal system, thalamus, ventral and dorsal horns of the spinal cord as well as in spinal ganglia and ganglia of the autonomic nervous system (Fig. 8.4). In some areas there is also both neuronal chromatolysis and degeneration (Fig. 8.4). Vacuolation, neuronal degeneration and axonal torpedoes can be seen in Purkinje cells in advanced cases. The gray matter changes are accompanied by Wallerian-like degeneration in the ventromedial and dorsolateral white matter tracts of the spinal cord. There are also changes in the PNS with Wallerian-like degeneration. Neuronal vacuolation and spinocerebellar degeneration is inherited but the mode of transmission remains to be determined. There is no accumulation of prion protein as in transmissible spongiform encephalopathies (see Section 8.6), no abnormalities have been found at the

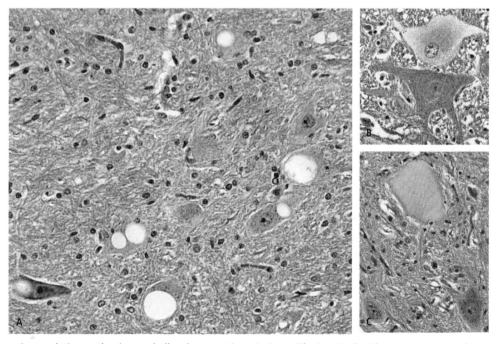

Fig. 8.4 Neuronal vacuolation and spinocerebellar degeneration. A: Dog. Siberian Husky. There are intracytoplasmic neuronal and parenchymal vacuoles in brainstem neurons. HE. B: Dog. Rottweiler. Peripheral chromatolysis in a brainstem neuron. HE. C: Same dog as in B. A necrotic neuron. HE.

level of presynaptic membranes, and ubiquitin inclusions or markers for apoptotic neurons are absent.

Hypertonicity syndrome in Labrador Retriever dogs

Male Labrador Retrievers between 2 and 16 months of age showed extreme generalized muscle stiffness associated with continuous motor unit activity in the electromylogram (EMG), which ceased under anesthesia. Histologically, diffuse gliosis was found in the spinal cord gray matter, reticular formation and basal nuclei. Neuronal numbers were decreased in specific Rex lamina of the cord. The **hypertonicity syndrome** in Labrador Retrievers is thought to be an X-linked hereditary condition.

Alzheimer's disease (AD)-like lesions.

Probably the most important group of neurodegenerations in people comprises **Alzheimer's disease** (AD) and other forms of presenile dementia. In AD, there is an accumulation of *β-amyloid protein*, which is derived from a normal neuronal precursor protein, and becomes transformed into an insoluble conformation consisting of amyloid fibrils. β-Amyloid is concentrated in *senile plaques* (focal accumulations) and around blood vessels (*congophilic angiopathy*) and appears to be toxic for neurons particularly in the cerebral cortex. An additional finding are the so-called *neurofibrillary tangles* (NFT) in neurons, which are derived from the τ (tau) protein, a microtubule-associated molecule. Such changes are also found in the brains of mentally normal elderly people but in AD the lesions are far more widespread and start at an earlier age. Familial predisposition for AD has been linked to defects in certain genes coding for proteins called *presenilins*.

Age-associated "dementia" has also been recognized in dogs, although the cognitive decline is clinically less well defined in this species. A true clinical and pathological correlate to AD has not been found in dogs or in other domestic animals. Nevertheless, while NFT are very rare in dogs, congophilic angiopathy and diffuse but not neuritic amyloid plaques occur in elderly dogs (see Chapter 1), and according to some studies their extent may correlate with declining cognitive functions. Such a correlation has also been reported with decreasing neuronal numbers in certain nuclei. These lesions in dogs are considered to be an important model for AD and have been used in experimental treatment and prevention studies.

8.3 Axonal degenerations

Neurons are the largest cells in the body some with their axons extending over enormous distances. Since all metabolites are produced in the cell soma, elaborate mechanisms evolved to transport materials away from (*anterograde*) or towards (*retrograde*) the cell body. Such mechanisms include molecular motors (e.g. *dynein*, *kinesin*) transporting a variety of metabolites along tracks provided by the cytoskeleton. In view of the high complexity of this system it is not surprising that a multitude of defects occur. In this group of diseases, the axon is primarily involved with either sparing or retrograde degeneration of its soma. They are generally multisystem disorders because axons from widely diverging neuronal populations are usually simultaneously affected. Typically, young animals are affected. The signs have an insidious onset and usually start in the hind limbs and progress relentlessly until animals become severely incapacitated. Proprioceptive deficits with preservation of nociception are frequent findings. Depending on the affected systems, a marked cerebellar clinical component may be apparent.

Morphologically, we distinguish two major groups: 1) axonopathies which look like Wallerian degeneration and therefore manifest themselves primarily in the white matter and 2) axonal diseases with conspicuous focal swellings of the axon (axonal spheroids). This change can be found in the white matter but when such swelling begins at the distal end of the axon (where they synapse with their target neurons) the lesions are most obvious in the gray matter.

The distinction between these groups is not always clear since, in several conditions, features of more than one subgroup may be present and in some conditions also neuronal cell bodies are affected. A list of well known axonal diseases in presented in Table 8.3.

8.3.1 Wallerian-like degenerative axonopathies

In the CNS, axonal necrosis, segmentation of myelin with removal of myelin and axonal debris by hematogenous macrophages over the whole length of an axon distal to a site of injury is called *Wallerian-like degeneration* (see Chapter 1). Many degenerative axonopathies exhibit the typical morphological features of Wallerian-like degeneration. Microscopic lesions consist of diffuse axonal and secondary myelin degeneration in ascending or/and descending fibers, thus usually involving multiple anatomical systems (*multisystem axonal degeneration or MAD*). Astrogliosis, axonal swelling and status spongiosus with macrophage invasion are common. The primary insult is not known in most of these diseases in animals. The initial lesion may be either in the proximal or distal parts of the axon, or in different sites simultaneously. In some of these conditions it appears that the

Table 8.3 Axonal diseases.

SUBTYPE	NAME OF DISEASE	SPECIES/BREED
Wallerian-like axonal degeneration	Hereditary ataxia	Smooth-haired Fox Terrier, Jack Russell Terrier, Ibizan Hound
	Sensory ataxic neuropathy	Golden Retriever
	Labrador Retriever axonopathy	Labrador Retriever
	Peripheral and central axonopathy	Birman cat
	Degenerative myelopathy of large breed-dogs	German shepherd, Boxer, Rhodesian Ridgeback, Chesapeake bay retriever, Hovawart, Siberian Husky, Bernese mountain dog
	Degenerative myelopathy	Pembroke Welsh Corgi
	Bovine progressive degenerative myeloencephalopathy	Brown Swiss cattle
	Degenerative axonopathy in neonatal calves	Friesian Holstein cattle
	Inherited progressive spinal myelinopathy	Murray Grey cattle
	Degenerative axonopathy	Tyrolean Grey cattle
	Familial degenerative neuromuscular disease	Gelbvieh cattle
	Central peripheral axonopathy	Rouges des Prés cattle
	Myelopathy	Holstein X Gir cattle, Merino sheep
Axonopathy with axonal swelling	Neuroaxonal dystrophy	Rottweiler dog, Papillon, Chihuahua, Collie sheepdogs, Jack Russell Terrier; tricolored Domestic Shorthair cat, Domestic Shorthair cat, Siamese cat; Suffolk, Merino sheep
	Equine degenerative myeloencephalopathy (EDME)	Morgan, Mongolian, other breeds
	Giant axonal neuropathy	German Shepherd Dog
	Central axonopathy	Scottish Terrier
	Progressive axonopathy	Boxer dog
	Segmental axonopathy	Merino sheep

most distal parts of the axon are the first to degenerate, possibly as a result of a metabolic defect in the neuronal cell body. This defect presumably makes it difficult for the cell to support its most distal parts, neurons being exceptionally large cells with processes extending over many centimeters or even meters in large animals. Thus, in ascending tracts (e.g. spinocerebellar tracts) the lesions are more severe in the cervical spinal cord and in descending tracts (e.g. rubrospinal tracts) in the lumbar cord. This concept of *dying back axonopathy* has been studied in toxic models such as organophosphate intoxication. The lesions become particularly conspicuous where affected axons are in functional bundles or tracts and therefore many of these diseases are classified as myelopathies (spinal cord degenerations), or myeloencephalopathies when involvement of the brain also is found. Both motor and sensory systems can be involved. This is reflected in the clinical presentation in which abnormalities of gait with weakness and incoordination prevail.

A prototype of MAD is illustrated in Fig. 8.5. There is bilaterally symmetrical loss of axons and myelin with reactive gliosis in selected areas of the white matter of the spinal cord. The lesions are usually visible on HE sections as pale staining and hypercellularity and become much more obvious with myelin- and/or axon-specific stains (Fig. 8.5). All these different diseases differ from each other mainly with respect to their clinical course,

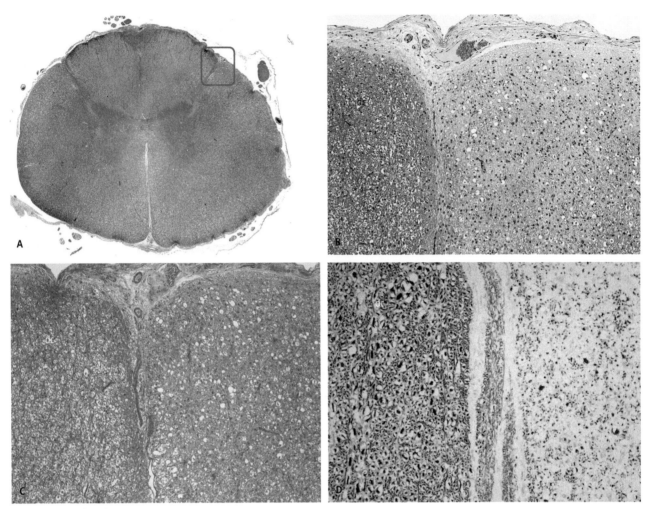

Fig. 8.5 Wallerian-like degeneration. Tyrolean grey cow. Degenerative axonopathy. A: Transverse section of spinal cord. There is a bilaterally symmetrical loss of white matter in lateral and ventral columns with replacement by astrogliosis in most severely affected areas. Box indicates area shown in subsequent images. LFB-HE. B: Loss of myelin and marked gliosis in affected area, sharply demarcated from adjacent normal dorsal column. HE. C: Same site as in B. There is a diffuse loss of myelin staining. LFB-HE. D: Same site. There is marked axonal loss as compared to adjacent dorsal column white matter. Bielschowsky silver stain.

the distribution of the lesions in the spinal cord and whether there is additional neuropathology in other structures of the CNS or PNS. Examples of such diseases are presented below.

Hereditary multisystem axonal degenerations (MAD) in small animals

In **hereditary ataxia** in Smooth-Haired Fox Terriers and Jack Russell Terriers there is involvement of ventral and lateral columns especially in the cervical cord (spinocerebellar tracts) and central auditory pathways with numerous axonal spheroids in the dorsal nuclei of the trapezoid body, cochlear nuclei and their connecting

tracts (Fig. 8.6). Thus there are some features of neuroaxonal dystrophy as described in Section 8.3.2. Degeneration of spinal nerve root and nerves can also be present. Pedigree studies in Jack Russell Terriers suggested that more than one gene defect may be involved. A very similar lesion distribution pattern has been found in families of Ibizan Hounds, in which the mode of inheritance appears to be autosomal recessive.

In **sensory ataxic neuropathy** in Golden Retrievers there is degeneration of central and peripheral axons. Proprioceptive fibers are most severely affected. Affected dogs show decreases in mitochondrial ATP production rates and respiratory chain enzyme activities and muscle changes typical of mitochondrial pathology. A deletion

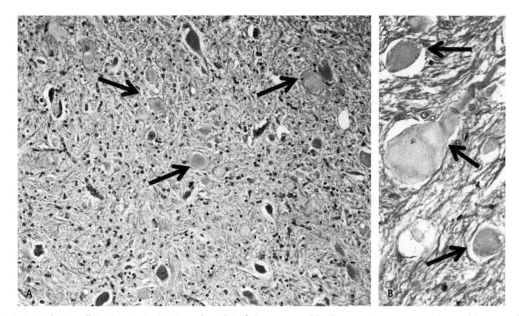

Fig. 8.6 Ataxia in Jack Russell Terrier. A: Brain. Dorsal nuclei of the trapezoid body contains numerous dystrophic axons (arrows) and there is prominent gliosis. HE. B: Multiple axonal spheroids (arrows) in auditory tract. HE.

in the mitochondrial tRNA (Tyr) gene is the causative mutation.

Labrador Retriever axonopathy is thought to be a recessively inherited condition with clinical signs of spasticity and progressive gait problems starting soon after birth. In addition to extensive myelopathy, all animals show aplasia or hypoplasia of the corpus callosum, cerebellar involvement and olivary neuronopathy.

Late-onset spinal cord degeneration has also been described in small-breed dogs. A late-onset hereditary condition in Pembroke Welsh Corgies (PWC) called **degenerative myelopathy of PWC dogs** is an autosomal recessive condition of late onset with progressive ataxia and weakness in elderly dogs. There is symmetrical systemic degeneration of ascending as well as descending long tracts in the spinal cord. A mutation in the superoxide dismutase (SOD) 1 gene has been found. Since SOD1 mutations are present in about 2% of all human ALS cases (see Section 8.2.2 on motor neuron diseases) degenerative myelopathy of PWC dogs was considered to be similar to ALS in humans. However, there is no loss of motor neurons in degenerative myelopathy, although there appears to be aggregation of SOD1 protein in neurons as in certain forms of human ALS and murine experimental models.

Peripheral and central axonopathy in Birman kittens is a suspected hereditary multisystem degeneration with a distribution pattern of the lesions suggestive of a distal axonopathy. Both the central nervous system and peripheral nerves are involved.

Degenerative myelopathy (DM) of old dogs

Degenerative myelopathy is a rather common condition that affects predominantly large breeds, in particular German Shepherd Dogs. Other affected breeds are Boxers, Rhodesian Ridgebacks, Chesapeake Bay Retrievers, Hovawarts, Siberian Huskies and Bernese Mountain Dogs. At this stage it is not clear whether all the reported cases called DM represent one and the same disease. Common to all is the late onset, slow progression of spinal signs and Wallerian-like degenerative lesions in the spinal cord.

Typically, signs consistent with weakness and ataxia of the hind limbs begin at the age of 7 years or older with an insidious onset and progressive deterioration over several months to years. DM in large dogs is also known as **chronic degenerative radiculomyelopathy** because nerve roots may also be involved, which may explain the clinical hyporeflexia sometimes recorded. It may be difficult to distinguish such PNS lesions from age-related changes (see Section 1.3.8). Different from the hereditary conditions described above, lesions in the spinal cord of large dogs with DM are more diffuse, not as sharply defined and often not symmetrical. In longitudinal sections, the lesions do not always seem to be continuous. Mild numbers of axonal swellings and demyelination are found in all funiculi of the spinal cord, being most prominent in the mid and caudal thoracic segments. In advanced cases, lesions become also visible in the lumbar and cervical areas. The dorsolateral and ventromedial columns appear to be the

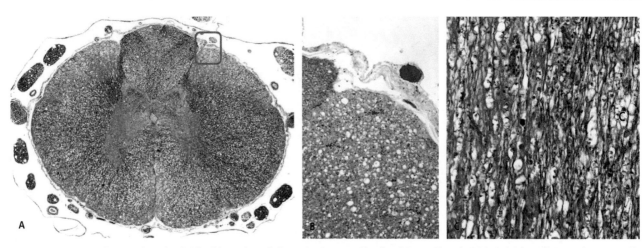

Fig. 8.7 Degenerative myelopathy (DM) of large-breed dogs. A: German Shepherd Dog. Chronic DM. Spinal cord. Note the generally bilateral but not totally symmetrical loss of myelin staining most severe in the dorsolateral and ventromedial columns. There is also myelin loss and vacuolation in both ventral and dorsal nerve roots. LFB-HE. Box indicates area described in B. B: Marked vacuolation and gliosis of white matter. HE. C: Longitudinal section of dorsolateral column with severe patchy loss of myelinated fibers (areas of axonal loss and demyelination are stained pink). HE-LFB.

most consistently affected area (spinocerebellar, corticospinal, rubrospinal and reticulospinal tracts). In advanced cases bilateral, more or less symmetrical focal areas of intense degeneration and gliosis are found in these areas (Fig. 8.7). The lesions can be particularly well seen in longitudinal sections of the cord. Neuronal degeneration and loss may occur in the vestibular and red nuclei.

In most cases of DM in large dogs, the disease appears to be sporadic and may be acquired. Because of immunohistochemical evidence for immunoglobulin and complement deposition in spinal cord lesions, and detection of oligoclonal bands in the CSF, some authors suggested that this condition is associated with a disturbed immune response. While some studies indicated that vitamin E deficiency may be involved, others showed that the gene of the canine α-tocopherol transfer protein is normal. Genetic factors could play a role in view of the higher incidence of DM in specific breeds. One study in a family of Siberian Huskies suggested hereditary transmission. The same mutation as in DM in PWC dogs described above was found in a population of large dogs with DM, but the association between the SOD1 mutation and the phenotype of DM was weak. This was thought to be due to age-related incomplete penetrance, but could also indicate that DM in PWC and DM in large dogs are unrelated conditions. Recently, another SOD1 mutation was found in Bernese Mountain Dogs with DM. It remains to be seen whether all the conditions collectively called DM in various breeds are pathogenetically related.

MAD in large animals

Bovine progressive degenerative myeloencephalopathy or **bovine weaver syndrome** is an autosomal recessive hereditary condition in Brown Swiss cattle known in many parts of the world. All spinal cord funiculi and many tracts in the brainstem are severely affected. Lesions have also been found in sensory nerves and myoneural junctions. Dystrophic axons are present in the cerebellar granule cell layer and there is patchy loss of Purkinje cells. The number of synapses in the cerebral cortex appears to be decreased. Ultrastructural changes may suggest a disturbance of axoplasmic transport and subsequent axonal degeneration.

Spinal cord degeneration has been reported in Friesian–Holstein cattle (**degenerative axonopathy of neonatal Friesian–Holstein calves**) with clinical onset soon after birth. In so called **inherited progressive spinal myelinopathy** in Murray Grey cattle, axonal lesions are also associated with chromatolyis in the red nucleus, various brainstem nuclei and spinal cord gray matter. In **central peripheral axonopathy** in Rouges des Prés cattle, peripheral nerves are clearly involved and the lesions are more severe in the distal than in the proximal parts of the axons. In addition, there are also prominent dystrophic axons in certain brainstem nuclei, which is a feature of neuroaxonal dystrophy (see Section 8.3.2).

Axonal degenerations occur in Holstein–Gir and Gelbvieh cattle. The latter is associated with myopathy, nephropathy and PNS lesions and thought to be caused by hereditary hypovitaminosis E. A **degenerative axonopathy** in Tyrolean Grey cattle (Fig. 8.5) is associated with a translationally silent variant in the mitofusin 2 gene (*MFN2*). A spinal cord degeneration of unknown origin with onset of signs between 5 months and 2 years of age has been described in Merino sheep.

Acquired long tract degenerations

As mentioned in Chapter 6, axonal degeneration of long tracts may also result from intoxications and deficiencies.

8.3.2 Axonopathies with prominent axonal swelling

Neuroaxonal dystrophy (NAD) in small animals

The term neuroaxonal dystrophy is used for the morphological alterations of axons leading to swelling, atrophy and/or degeneration. A prototypic change is the *axonal spheroid*, a localized swelling of the axon with distal atrophy and secondary myelin degradation. NADs in humans make up a group of inherited or acquired neurodegenerative diseases with infantile and juvenile forms. The axonal changes start at the preterminal portions of the axon and in the synaptic terminals resulting in axonal transport impairment. Therefore, dystrophic axons in NAD are mostly found in the nuclei of the gray matter in the brain and spinal cord (**Fig. 8.8**). Degeneration of the axon progresses proximally, eventually resulting in death of the neuronal cell body. In addition to the gray matter changes there is often also degeneration of white matter tracts. Electron microscopy studies have shown that dystrophic axons contain tubulovesicular structures as well as accumulations of smooth membranes, membranous aggregates reminiscent of myelinic and residual bodies, and a few neurofilaments.

NAD is best known in young Rottweilers, although it has also been described in Chihuahuas, Collie sheepdogs, Papillons and Jack Russell Terriers. Typically, in **Rottweiler NAD** signs start at the age of 1 year with hypermetria of the front limbs, and progress to a full cerebellar syndrome over 1–2 years. Sensory systems are predominantly affected with dystrophic axons in areas such as the nucleus thoracicus, dorsal horns of the spinal cord, dorsal column nuclei, sensory trigeminal nucleus, cerebellar granular layer, vestibular nuclei and geniculate bodies. Sometimes there is loss of Purkinje cells in the vermis and flocculus. Dystrophic axons appear swollen, eosinophilic, homogeneous or granular, and contain variable amounts of ubiquitin–immunoreactive deposits as well as numerous synaptic proteins. Ubiquitination indicates involvement of the intracellular protease degradation system. In Chihuahuas and Papillons with NAD, dystrophic axons are also widespread in the white matter of the brain. NAD in the sensory relay nuclei of the brainstem has been found in English Cocker Spaniels with primary metabolic vitamin E deficiency and retinal pigment epithelium dystrophy. An autosomal recessive infantile form of NAD with severe neurological dysfunction already present at birth occurs in Beagles and is similar to human infantile NAD.

NAD in tricolored Domestic Shorthair cats, an autosomal recessive disease, is associated with inner ear abnormalities. Mild cerebellar atrophy with Purkinje cell and granule cell loss can be present. Multiple spheroids are found in the olivary, cerebellar and lateral cuneate nuclei, brainstem tegmentum and the spinal cord. They are also seen in some white matter tracts, dorsal roots and spiral ganglion and can contain a PAS-positive core. Ultrastructurally, the swollen axons are covered by a thin myelin sheet. Feline NAD of unknown genetic background has been described in Domestic Shorthair and Siamese cats (Fig. 8.8).

NAD in horses

Equine degenerative myeloencephalopathy (EDME) was originally reported in North America but has been since recognized in several European countries. The disease occurs sporadically in many breeds but clusters have been described. The underlying cause is currently thought to be an hereditary defect (a familial predisposition was noticed earlier in some breeds such as Morgan and Mongolian horses), which predisposes to pathology related to an environmental or nutritional factor. In this respect an association between EDME and vitamin E deficiency has been demonstrated in several studies. Low vitamin E serum concentrations appear to be critical in the first months of life. Clinical signs usually start at the age of 6 months but later onset has also been observed. There is ataxia and tetraparesis. Dystrophic axons with neuronal degeneration are encountered in the thoracic nucleus of the spinal cord, the medial and lateral (accessory) cuneate and gracilis nuclei (Fig. 8.8D). Large spheroids and neurons may undergo vacuolar degeneration. In addition, there is extensive Wallerian-like degeneration in the spinal cord white matter, particularly in the dorsal spinocerebellar and in the ventromedial tracts (Fig. 8.8C). Excessive lipofuscin pigment accumulation is prominent in endothelial cells, neurons and

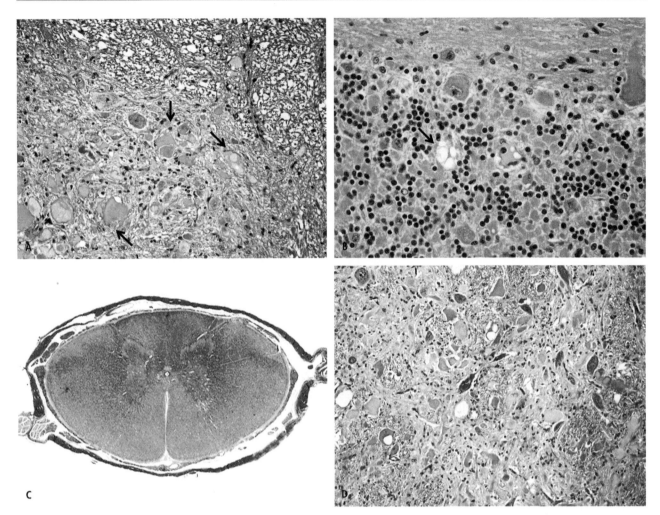

Fig. 8.8 A: Cat. Neuroaxonal dystrophy. Large numbers of eosinophilic swollen dystrophic axons (arrows) in the accessory cuneate nucleus. HE. B: Same cat as A, cerebellar cortex. There are numerous dystrophic axons throughout the granule cell layer and one has also vacuolar degeneration (arrow). HE. C: Quarter Horse. EDME. Thoracic cord segment T8. Bilateral and symmetrical axonal loss and paler myelin staining in dorsal spinocerebellar and ventromedial tracts. LFB-HE. D: Lusitano horse. EDME. Accessory cuneate nucleus. Large numbers of swollen and vacuolated axons and necrotic neurons and mild astrogliosis and microgliosis. HE.

macrophages in affected nuclei. Remember that in all domestic animal species relatively large numbers of spheroids and degenerating neurons can be found in increasing concentrations with age in the lateral cuneate nucleus without causing clinical symptoms.

NAD in sheep

Typical NAD has been described in 4–7-month-old Merino lambs and in Suffolk sheep of 1.5 and 5 months of age that developed a progressive ataxia finally becoming recumbent. It is considered to be hereditary. Lesions are similar to those observed in Rottweilers and primarily involve afferent systems involved in proprioception.

Acquired NAD

(NAD)-like lesions with numerous swollen axons throughout the neuraxis occur in various intoxications as discussed in Chapter 6.

Giant axonal neuropathy in German Shepherd Dogs

First reported in humans, **giant axonal neuropathy (GAN)** is a generalized disorder of cytoplasmic intermediate filaments affecting the peripheral nervous system particularly, but also the brain and spinal cord in advanced cases. Giant axons accumulate neurofilaments.

This is similar to neuroaxonal dystrophy, in which mitochondria and organelles also accumulate.

GAN has been described in young adult German Shepherd Dogs showing hind limb weakness and ataxia with progressive loss of patellar reflexes and placing reactions. GAN in German Shepherd Dogs is characterized by swollen axons containing excessive and disorganized neurofilaments in the spinal cord, mainly at the distal portions of long neuronal fiber tracts but also in the PNS. The fasciculus gracilis and dorsal spinocerebellar tracts are affected only in the cranial cervical spinal cord while the lateral corticospinal tract is principally involved in the lower thoracic and lumbar spinal cord. Myenteric and sympathetic axons are also affected.

Central axonopathy in Scottish Terriers

A **central axonopathy**, which differs from previously reported NAD in dogs, has been described in Scottish Terrier puppies from three different but related litters. Clinical signs consisted of severe whole body tremor and ataxia first detected at the age of 10–12 weeks. Signs worsened with activity and excitement and diminished during rest or sleep. Neuropathological examination revealed primary axonal damage and secondary vacuolation and gliosis in the white matter of the spinal cord, brain stem, cerebellum and cerebrum. Many axons in the lateral and ventral columns had an enlarged diameter without signs of fragmentation. Dystrophic axons were prominent in the brainstem nuclei, thalamus, cerebellum and cerebral white matter. Their myelin sheaths appeared thin. The condition is probably hereditary but the mode of transmission is not known.

Progressive axonopathy in Boxer dogs

Progressive axonopathy in Boxer dogs is clinically characterized by hind limb ataxia starting around 3 months of age as well as signs of skeletal muscle denervation. CNS and PNS are both affected. Spheroids and axonal degeneration are prominent in the lateral and ventral funiculi of the spinal cord, in several brainstem nuclei, cerebellar white matter and optic pathways. The autonomic nervous system is also affected and distal limb muscles show varying degrees of neurogenic atrophy. In the PNS, paranodal axonal swellings occur in the extradural spinal nerve roots, most consistently in the lumbar region. The occurrence of proximal axonal swelling of nerve roots, together with distal hypoplasia suggests impaired transport of neurofilaments that are major determinants of axon growth. Further immunochemical studies that focused on cytoskeletal proteins such as tubulin, neurofilaments, actin and fodrin, confirmed that defects in slow axonal transport are involved

in the pathogenesis of this disease. An axonopathy sharing more similarities to the progressive axonopathy of Boxers than to the polyneuropathy of Rottweilers has been described in a Rottweiler pup.

Segmental axonopathy in Merino sheep

Segmental axonopathy in Merino sheep becomes clinically manifest with progressive ataxia at 3.5–6 years of age. Microscopically, cerebellar abiotrophy is accompanied by widespread segmental axonal ballooning, or spheroid formation, in the white matter of the brain and spinal cord as well as in the PNS. This condition, which is inherited and thought to be due to a cytoskeletal defect, is distinct from other neuroaxonal dystrophies observed in sheep.

8.4 Myelin disorders

In this group we distinguish between disorders with severe destruction of the myelin sheaths, often also leading to loss of axons, and diseases with insufficient or retarded production of myelin. These diseases are listed in Table 8.4.

8.4.1 Leukodystrophies

Definition

Leukodystrophies are disorders of myelin synthesis and maintenance affecting bilaterally symmetrical selective areas of the white matter, with destruction of myelin and eventually axons. In most human leukodystrophies myelin, is initially formed to a variable extent but subsequently degenerates soon after birth. Microscopically, axons lacking sheets are admixed with numerous macrophages, containing myelin debris, and reactive astrocytes. In animals, similar lesions occur, which are mostly ill characterized in molecular terms. The diseases listed here below include a very heterogeneous collection of lesions, which can be broadly classified under the heading "leukodystrophy" or "*myelinolytic diseases*". Common to all are bilaterally symmetrical areas of massive degeneration of the white matter, which is often macroscopically visible. The distribution pattern of the lesions is often selective or even bizarre and therefore difficult to explain by a general defect at the level of myelin metabolism.

Necrotizing myelopathy

Necrotizing myelopathy is an autosomal recessive disease, which has been described in young Afghan Hounds, Kooikers and sporadically in Miniature Poodles with rapidly progressing spinal signs. Lesion distribution is bizarre: there is bilaterally symmetrical lysis

Table 8.4 Myelin disorders.

SUBTYPE	NAME OF DISEASE	SPECIES/BREED
Leukodystrophy	Cavitating leukodystrophy	Dalmatian dog, Labrador Retriever
	Necrotizing myelopathy	Afghan dog, Kooiker dog, Miniature Poodle
	Leukomyeloencephalopathy	Rottweiler dog, Leonberger dog
	Globoid cell leukodystrophy	West Highland White & Cairn Terrier, Australian Kelpie, Irish Setter
	Leukodystrophy	Crossbred Maltese dog
	Fibrinoid leukodystrophy	Labrador Retriever, Merino sheep
	Progressive ataxia	Charolais cattle
	Oligodendroglial dysplasia	Bull Mastiff
Myelin dysgenesis	Dysmyelination	Chow Chow, Weimaraner dog, Lurcher dog, Samoyed dog, Bernese cattle dog, Siamese cats
	Shaking pups	Springer Spaniel
	CNS hypomyelination	Rat Terrier
	Congenital tremor	Jersey, Holstein–Friesian, Angus, Shorthorn, Hereford cattle
	Congenital tremor type AIII	Landrace pig
	Congenital tremor type AIV	Saddleback pig
	Congenital bovine spinal dysmyelination	Brown Swiss cattle

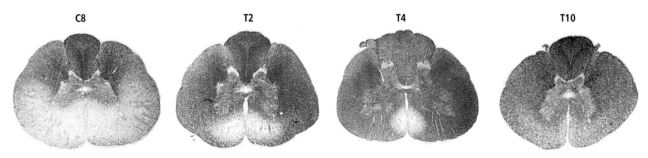

Fig. 8.9 Afghan dog myelopathy. Spinal cord. Bilaterally symmetrical leucomyelomalacia with a unique and distinctive distribution pattern (cord segments C8, T2, T4, T10). LFB. (Reproduced with permission from Dr. Alexander de Lahunta.)

of white matter in the whole circumference of the mid-thoracic cord with tapering of the lesions cranially and caudally involving only ventral or dorsal funiculi in cervical and lumbar segments (Fig. 8.9). Rarely, there is some focal involvement of the brainstem. The fasciculus proprius is relatively spared. Destruction of white matter is associated with invasion of macrophages and vascular proliferation. The initial lesion appears to be splitting of the myelin sheath along the intraperiod line. Gray matter involvement is uncommon involving the dorsal nuclei of the trapezoid body and periphery of the ventral horns.

Leukoencephalomyelopathy

Rottweiler and Leonberger dogs with **leukoencephalomyelopathy** show slowly progressive ataxia between 1.5 and 4 years of age. There are destructive lesions of the white matter in the spinal cord and brainstem (Fig. 8.10), generally in a bilaterally symmetrical pattern, but at some levels of the cord lesions are clearly asymmetrical. See MRI Atlas. The myelin is primarily affected with initial preservation of axons (Fig. 8.10). There is demyelination and remyelination, ultrastructurally confirmed because many axons are covered by very thin myelin sheaths. Although this is clearly a myelin lesion, in the spinal cord only certain areas of the lateral columns are affected, suggesting that the primary defect may be located in neurons, leading to defects in axonal signals required for normal myelination.

Globoid cell leukodystrophy

Globoid cell leukodystrophy or **Krabbe's disease** occurs as an autosomal recessive disorder in people, dogs (West Highland White Terrier puppies and some other breeds such as Beagle, Australian Kelpie, Bluetick and Irish Setters) and sporadically in cats. It is a lysosomal storage disease resulting from *galactocerebroside beta-galactosidase* deficiency (see Section 8.5). There is marked degeneration and loss of white matter in the cord and brain (Fig. 8.11). Perivascular accumulation of "globoid cells", large macrophages filled with PAS-positive storage material, is characteristic of globoid cell leukodystrophy (Fig. 8.11).

Hereditary "cavitating" leukodystrophy

Hereditary cavitating leukodystrophy, transmitted by autosomal recessive inheritance has been described in Dalmatian dogs between 3 and 5 months of age. A similar disease has been seen in Labrador Retrievers.

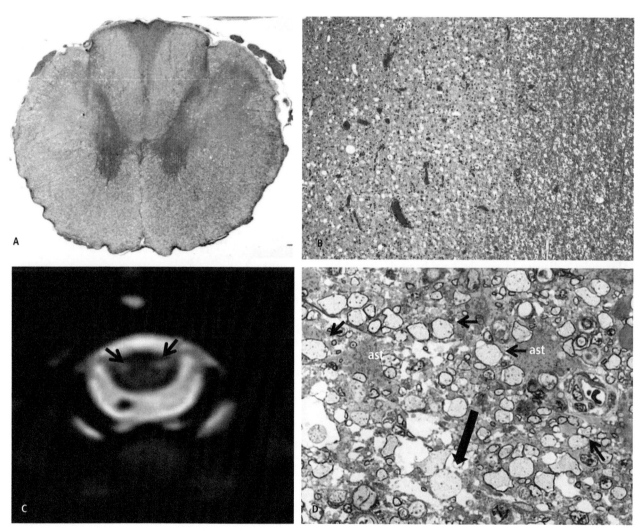

Fig. 8.10 Dog. Leonberger. Leukoencephalomyelopathy. Spinal cord. A: Bilaterally symmetrical areas of myelin degeneration in the lateral columns. HE-LFB. B: Spinal cord. Sharply delineated area of pale staining and hypercellularity in the spinal cord white matter. HE. C: Spinal cord. MRI. T2W transverse slice revealing bilateral areas of hyperintensity corresponding to the areas of myelin degeneration in A. D: White matter spinal cord. Transverse section. There are intact axons in various stages of demyelination (large arrow) and axons with a very thin myelin sheet (small arrows) indicating remyelination. There are several reactive astrocytes (ast). Semithin section. TB stain.

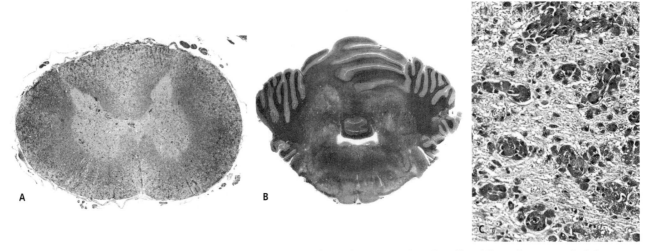

Fig. 8.11 Dog. West Highland White Terrier. Globoid cell leukodystrophy. A: Spinal cord. Diffuse bilaterally symmetrical degeneration with demyelination of the peripheral areas of the spinal cord white matter. HE. B: Cerebellum. Marked symmetrical loss of white matter in brainstem and cerebellum. LFB-HE. C: Perivascular accumulation of large macrophages containing myelin debris ("globoid cells"). PAS.

Particularly the white matter of the cerebrum (centrum ovale), most prominently in the occipital lobes, is affected with malacia progressing to cavitation of the affected areas. The subcortical fibers are spared. Microscopic lesions are found in the white matter of the basal nuclei and ventral horns of the cord. Initially, there is degeneration of myelin with sparing of the axons.

Fibrinoid leukodystrophy

Very rare cases of **fibrinoid leukodystrophy**, also named **Alexander's disease** in people, have been described in male, black Labrador Retriever littermates, a Scottish Terrier, a Miniature Poodle, a Bernese Mountain Dog and Merino sheep. There is involvement of the cerebral white matter but also of other areas. In fibrinoid leukodystrophy, the myelin lesions are associated with *Rosenthal fiber* formation. These are string-like depositions of brightly eosinophilic amorphous ovoid bodies especially perivascularly and below the pia and ependyma (Fig. 8.12A). They contain alpha beta crystalline, GFAP and ubiquitin. A mutation of the GFAP gene as in people was not found in Merino sheep with Alexander's disease.

Leukodystrophy in crossbred Maltese dogs

In **leukodystrophy** of crossbred Maltese dogs changes are mainly found in cerebellum and spinal cord. In addition to myelinolytic lesions there are areas of intense astrogliosis in the white matter, which appear to precede myelin breakdown.

Progressive ataxia in Charolais cattle

Progressive ataxia in Charolais cattle starts with ataxia at the age of about 8 months. Signs are progressive and,

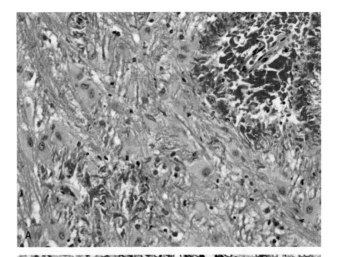
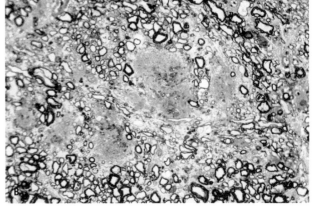

Fig. 8.12 Dog. Alexander's like disease (fibrinoid leukodystrophy). A. Distinctive eosinophilic staining of Rosenthal-like fibres in astrocytic foot processes lining blood vessels and in the neuropil, which contains many abnormally large hypertrophied astrocytes. HE. B: Cow. Charolais ataxia. Brain. Semithin section illustrating focal areas in the white matter devoid of myelinated fibers surrounded by normally myelinated axons. TB.

if the animal is supported, end with paralysis after 1–2 years. The lesions are very characteristic. The white matter of spinal cord and brainstem is interspersed with round or oval areas, which remain pale following staining for myelin or axons (Fig. 8.12B). At higher magnification, a finely granular or fibrillar structure can be demonstrated. Ultrastructurally the areas are composed of disorganized myelin sheaths and hypertrophied oligodendrocytic processes. It is suspected that initially normal myelin becomes unstable and degenerates due to an as yet unknown genetic defect. A similar lesion has been seen in **oligodendroglial dysplasia** in Bull Mastiff dogs.

8.4.2 Myelin dysgenesis

This is also called hypomyelinogenesis or retarded myelinogenesis. Histologically, the two forms are very similar, but in the course of time the symptoms of hypomyelinogenesis remain unchanged whereas in retarded myelinogenesis they resolve and eventually disappear. Dysmelinogenesis is well known in a variety of species and breeds. The symptoms are severe tremors of the whole body (e.g. trembling lambs and piglets, "congenital tremor"), which increase with excitement and disappear at rest.

Dysmyelination in small animals

In Chow Chows, Springer Spaniels, Weimaraners, Lurchers, Samoyeds, Bernese Cattle Dogs, Siamese cats and some other dog breeds hereditary (or suspected hereditary) forms of dysmyelination have been reported. The cause is a congenital defect at the level of structural myelin proteins and/or metabolic defects of the oligodendrocyte. **Shaking pups** (Springer Spaniels) have an X-linked recessive defect with mutations in the proteolipid protein and DM-20 protein resulting in abnormal oligodendrocyte differentiation and formation of immature myelin. Inadequate myelination/dysmyelination is visible macroscopically, the white matter assuming a grayish translucent appearance (Fig. 8.13B). On HE sections there is pallor of the white matter. Depending on the particular disease some areas may be more affected than others. Special myelin stains and especially semi-thin sections and electron microscopy help to define the defect (Fig. 8.13C,D,E,F). As a rule, the PNS is normally myelinated. In some conditions

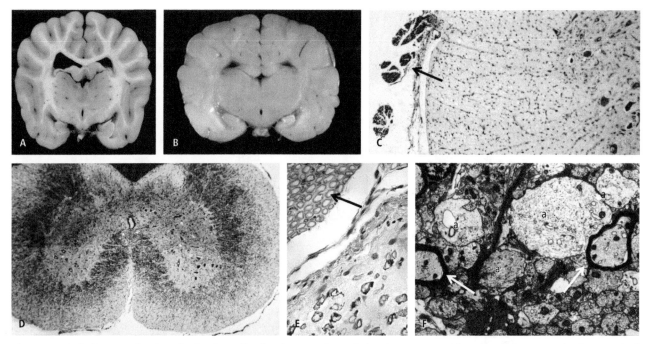

Fig. 8.13 A-C: Hypomyelination. Lack of myelin development in a Dalmatian puppy with congenital tremor. A: Age-matched normal brain at same level showing distinct contrast between grey and normal white matter. B: Bilaterally symmetrical lack of white matter development. C: Complete lack of myelin staining in the spinal cord in contrast to normally myelinated spinal nerve roots. LFB. D-F: Dysmyelination. Dog. Chow Chow. Spinal cord. D: Defective myelin formation in peripheral layers of spinal cord. LFB. E: Semithin section of same dog as in D. There are few myelinated fibers in contrast to adjacent spinal nerve fibers (arrow), all of which are normally myelinated. Toluidin blue stain. E: Electron micrograph of the lesion in D reveals that most axons (a) are naked or have only very thin myelin sheaths compared with other normally myelinated axons (arrows).

such as in the male shaker pups of Springer Spaniels, animals exhibit severe neurological signs for their (short) life, in others such as in Chow Chows, animals gradually myelinate normally ("retarded myelination") and become clinically normal. **CNS hypomyelination** in Rat Terriers is associated with a *congenital goiter* and a mutation in the *thyroid peroxidase gene*.

Dysmyelination in large animals

This condition, commonly referred to as **congenital tremor**, has been described in calves from a number of bovine breeds (e.g. Jersey, Angus, Shorthorn, Hereford). **Congenital bovine spinal dysmyelination** in American Brown Swiss cattle and crossbreeds is characterized by congenital recumbency with spasticity and opisthotonus. The myelin lesions affect the dorsomedial, dorsolatereral and ventromedial columns in the cord and are also associated with axonal degeneration. The disease is caused by a missense mutation in the SPAST gene, whose human ortholog is associated with **hereditary spastic paraplegia**.

In swine, a sex-linked condition has been described in Landrace and Landrace crosses (**congenital tremor type AIII**) and an autosomal recessive disease in Saddleback pigs (**congenital tremor type AIV**), in which myelin is thought to be unstable and is therefore prone to degeneration soon after synthesis.

Viral-induced dysmyelination

Abnormal myelination similar to the hereditary conditions discussed here above can be induced by intrauter-ine transplacental viral infections. These diseases are covered in Chapter 3 on inflammatory diseases.

Astrocytic hypertrophy of the white matter

An autosomal recessive disease occurs in Gordon Setter puppies starting with weakness and continuous vocalizing at a few weeks of age, which progresses rapidly to recumbency. The only change found is a diffuse morphometrically confirmed hypertrophy of the astrocytes predominantly in the white matter of the CNS.

8.5 Storage diseases

8.5.1 Lysosomal storage diseases

Mechanism

Due to a congenital defect at the level of the lysosomal hydrolase enzyme system, certain cellular molecules cannot be degraded and recycled and thus accumulate in the lysosomes. Common to most storage diseases in man and animals is the early onset of progressive neurological symptoms.

The primary enzymatic defect can be localized at different levels, e.g. a mutation in the enzyme itself, a post-translational modification, a defective transporter protein or a defective activator protein. As a result, there is progressive accumulation, or "storage", of non-degradable material in lysosomes in the affected cells. Depending on the specific molecular defect, several specific cell and tissue types in the body can be involved. Skeletal/connective tissue abnormalities, for example, in

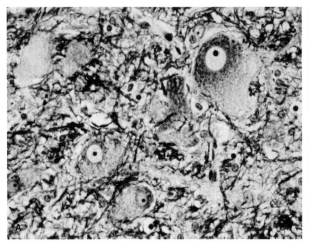
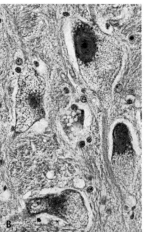
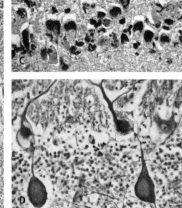

Fig. 8.14 Lysosomal storage diseases. A: Neurons in GM1 gangliosidosis with massive cytoplasmic accumulation of lysosomes containing storage material with displacement of Nissl substance and the nucleus. LFB-CEV. B: Alpha-mannosidosis. The storage material exhibits a distinct granular appearance within densely packed lysosomes. HE. C: A lipid stain confirms the neuronal accumulation of lipid storage material. Sudan black. D: Axonal "torpedos" of affected cerebellar Purkinje cells in a storage disease. Bielschowsky silver stain.

Table 8.5 Lysosomal storage diseases.

DISEASE TYPE	NAME	ENZYME DEFECT	SPECIES/BREED
Glycoproteinoses	Fucosidosis	α-L-fucosidase	English Springer spaniel
	Mannosidosis	α-mannosidase	Domestic short hair cat (DSH), Domestic long hair cat Persian cat, Aberdeen-Angus cattle, Murray grey cattle, Galloway cattle
		ß-mannosidase	Nubian goat, Salers calves
	Galactosialidosis	neuraminidase-β-galactosidase	Schipperke dog
Sphingolipidoses	GM1 gangliosidosis	ß-galactosidase	Siamese cat, DSH, Korat cat, English Springer spaniel, Beagle, Portuguese water dog, Friesian cattle, Suffolk cross sheep
	GM2 gangliosidosis	ß-hexosaminidase	DSH, Korat cat, Pointer dog, Yorkshire pigs
		activator protein	Japanese spaniel
	Globoidcell-leukodystrophy	ß-galactocerebrosidase	West Highland white terrier (WHWT), Cairn terrier, Beagle, Poodle, DSH, Dorset sheep
	Gauchers disease	glucocerebrosidase	Sydney silky terrier
	Niemann-Pick disease	sphingomyelinase cholesterol-esterification	Balinese cat, Siamese cat, Boxer dog, DSH
Mucopolysaccharidoses	MPSI (Hurler)	α-L-iduronidase	DSH, Plott hound
	MPSII (Hunter)	iduronate-2-sulfatase	Labrador retriever
	MPS III (San Filippo)	sulfamidase	Wire-haired-dachshund, Nubian goat
	MPS VI (Maroteaux-Lamy)	arylsulfatase B	Siamese cat
	MPS VII (Sly)	ß-glucuronidase	Mixed breed dog

(*Continued*)

Table 8.5 (*Continued*)

DISEASE TYPE	NAME	ENZYME DEFECT	SPECIES/BREED
Glycogenoses (Oligosaccharidoses)	type Ia (von Gierke)	glucose-6-phosphatase	Canine toy breeds
	type II (Pompe)	α-1.4-glucosidase	Lapland dog, DSH, Shorthorn beef cattle, Braham cattle, Corriedale-sheep
	type III (Cori)	amylo-1.6-glucosidase	German shepherd dog, Akita dog
	type IIIa	glycogen-debranching-enzyme	Curly coated retriever
	type IV (Anderson)	glycogen branching enzyme	Norwegian forest cat
	type VII	phosphofructokinase	English Springer spaniel, American Cocker spaniel
Proteinoses	Ceroid-lipofuscinosis	range of defects	Pit bull terrier, Staffordshire terrier, American Bulldog, Irish setter, English setter, Tibetan terrier, miniature dachshund and other dog breeds, Siamese cats, Devon cattle, South Hampshire, Borderdale and Ramboulliet sheep, Nubian goat

mucopolysaccharidosis may also indirectly cause neurological signs by compressing nervous tissues.

When neurons, which cannot regenerate, are affected by a lysosomal storage disease, severe progressive neurological deficits are eventually fatal.

Classification and morphology

Depending on the specific enzyme defect, the accumulated material can consist of glycolipids, carbohydrates, proteins etc. Accordingly, storage diseases are classified as **glycoproteinoses**, **sphingolipidoses**, **mucopolysaccharidoses**, **glycogenoses** and **proteinoses**. Within these major groups, the storage diseases are then named according to either the storage product, the name of the discoverer or just a number. Table 8.5 lists some examples of storage diseases.

Neuropathological features are easy to recognize. Storage in neurons is characterized by massive cytoplasmic accumulation of granular or vacuolar-like inclusions with dislocation of other cell organelles (Fig. 8.14). The neurons appear swollen. Lesions are usually widespread but some areas can be more severely involved

than others. Other cell types such as glial, endothelial and choroid plexus epithelial cells can be affected depending on the type of storage defect. Secondary changes are axonal swellings (Fig. 8.14D) *meganeurites*, which are fusiform enlargements of the initial axon segment and loss of synapses and dendritic spines. Loss of neurons and atrophy of certain populations also occurs in some storage diseases. In mannosidosis, there is also deficient myelination and axonal degeneration in the white matter. A special case is globoid cell leukodystrophy (galactosylceramidase 1 deficiency), in which the storage disease leads to severe degeneration of the white matter with the perivascular accumulation of large distended macrophages ("globoid cells") (Fig. 8.11C).

Many different storage diseases have been identified in animals; in several types their biochemical and genetic defects have been elucidated (Table 8.5). In routine examination from biopsy tissue, the biochemical identification of the storage product can be partially identified by special stains and lectin binding patterns. Electron microscopy can also help to identify the specific defect, but specific characterization requires biochemical and molecular biological examination. For an increasing number of conditions DNA tests are available for animals.

8.5.2 Neuronal ceroid lipofucsinoses (NCL)

Definition and mechanism

Neuronal ceroid lipofucsinoses are a special group of storage diseases characterized by accumulation of autofluorescent lipofuscin pigment-like material, with characteristic ultrastructural lamellar profiles, in neurons and other cells of the body, followed by cell degeneration. In people, NCL were classified into infantile, late infantile, juvenile (**Batten disease**) and adult (**Kuff's disease**) types, according to the age of onset and the ultrastructural morphologic features of the storage material. Current classification of human NCL is based on eight main genetic forms (CLN1–8). In contrast to most other storage diseases, the underlying pathogenesis of NCL has not been entirely clarified. Some studies suggested that the primary defect in NCL may involve mitochondria rather than lysosomal catabolism.

NCL in domestic animals

NCL occurs in domestic animal species including several dog breeds (such as Pit Bull Terriers, Staffordshire Terriers and Irish Setters), Siamese cats, Devon cattle, South Hampshire, Borderdale and Ramboulliet sheep. The molecular genetics are being characterized in a rapidly increasing number of these diseases. For example, a frame shift in the TPP1 gene (the ortholog of human

CLN2) has been found in Miniature Dachshunds with NCL, a mutation in the CLN8 gene in English Setters and in the cathepsin D gene in American Bulldogs. Tibetan Terriers with late-onset NCL have a truncating mutation in ATP13A2. NCL in American Staffordshire Terriers has been linked to sulfatase deficiency (a lysosomal enzyme) resulting from an arylsulfatase G mutation. However, as in people, it is not always clear whether lysosomal catabolism is involved in NCL. In sheep, a large portion of the storage material consists of subunit c of mitochondrial ATP synthase.

Animals affected by NCL are usually young adults (about 1–2 years of age) at the start of clinical signs, although some dogs may be much older at onset. As in other storage diseases, accumulation of abnormal material in neurons is easily detected (Fig. 8.15B,C). A special feature is the autofluorescence of this material under UV light (Fig. 8.15C). NCL is usually associated with severe progressive atrophy of involved areas which can be seen on MRI or macroscopically (Fig. 8.15A). See MRI Atlas. In the American Staffordshire Terriers and American Staffordshire Terrier–Pit Bull Terrier crosses, storage primarily affects Purkinje cells and certain thalamic nuclei leading to thalamic and cerebellar atrophy.

8.5.3 Lafora's disease

People

Lafora's disease is another special type of storage disease with accumulation of polyglucosan as small and large inclusions in neuronal cell bodies and dendrites. In

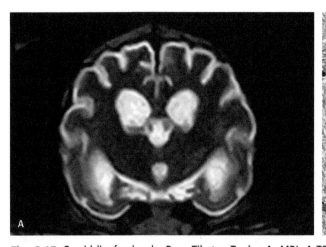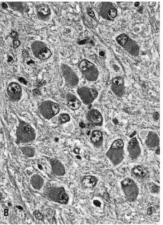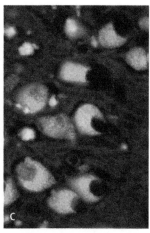

Fig. 8.15 Ceroid lipofuscinosis. Dog. Tibetan Terrier. A: MRI. A T2W transverse image of cerebral atrophy associated with neuronal ceroid lipofuscinosis with marked distension of sulci filled with CSF and dilated ventricles from the brain atrophy. B: Dog. Dachshund. Swollen neurons in hippocampus. HE. C: Autofluorescence of ceroid lipofuscin storage material in hippocampal neurons. UV emission.

people, the disease depends on defects in the genes coding for *laforin* (a phosphatase) and *malin* (ubiquitin ligase), which control proteins that affect glycogen metabolism.

Canine Lafora's disease

In dogs, the disease has been described as an inherited problem in Beagles, Basset Hounds and Miniature Rough-Coated Dachshunds. In the latter, the genetic defect has been identified as the first *triplet repeat disorder* to be discovered in domestic animals. In contrast to humans, in dogs the clinical signs start late in life with (as in children) myoclonus epilepsy. The neuronal inclusions have a characteristic morphology allowing diagnosis from HE sections and electron microscopy (Fig. 8.16). Polyglucosan bodies are sometimes found in the brain of aging dogs and cats not associated with Lafora's disease.

8.5.4 Acquired lysosomal storage diseases

These have been reported to result from ingestion of plant toxins. These toxins affect lysosomal enzymes by various herbivorous species as discussed in Chapter 6.

8.6 Spongiform encephalopathies

8.6.1 Transmissible degenerative diseases

From a pathological view, spongiform encephalopathies (SE) are clearly degenerative diseases with sym-metrical, slowly evolving non-inflammatory lesions in the gray matter. Some human SE are hereditary diseases, and SE in small ruminants are under tight genetic control. However, SE of domestic animals as well as of humans can be transmitted to other animals at least under experimental conditions and are therefore called: **transmissible spongiform encephalopathies (TSE)** (Table 8.6).

TSE are progressive lethal diseases with very long incubation periods (years) with a spongy state of the CNS in the absence of inflammation. The development of the disease is associated with a conformational change of a normal GPI-anchored cellular protein called *prion protein*, abbreviated PrP^c (c stands for cell), which undergoes a conformational change resulting in the accumulation of a protease-resistant isoform called PrP^d (d stands for disease). This accumulation is visible as amyloid fibrils in histological plaques, which occur in certain human and experimental TSE diseases. These *scrapie-associated fibrils* (SAFs) can also be seen by electron microscopy following density gradient centrifugation of homogenized brain. Thus the pathogenesis is similar to other so-called *protein conformation disorders* such as Alzheimer's disease (see Section 8.2.4). Unique to TSE is that the accumulated amyloid can transmit the disease to other animals. The prion theory postulates that PrP^d, also called *prion*, is capable of initiating its own replication by acting as a template for further PrP^c molecules to become abnormally folded. Thus, according to the prion theory the infectious agent of TSE

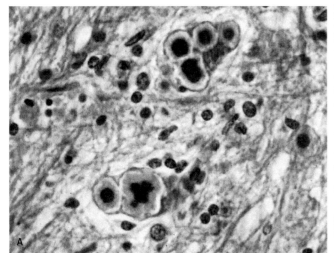
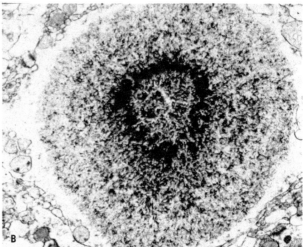

Fig. 8.16 Lafora's disease. Dog. Basset Hound. Thalamus. A: Typical Lafora body intraneuronal inclusions with a solid dark centre and outer light halo. HE. B: Ultrastructurally, the inclusions consist of an electron-dense core surrounded by a fibrillar matrix. Electron micrograph. (Reproduced with permission from Dr Schwarz-Porsche.)

Table 8.6 Tansmissible spongiform encephalopathies.

SPECIES	DISEASE; TRANSMISSION
Human	Creutzfeldt-Jakob disease (CJD), sporadic, familial Kuru, food borne (cannibalism) Variant CJD, food borne infection (BSE) Gerstmann-Stäussler-Scheinker (GSS), hereditary Familial fatal insomnia (FFI), hereditary
Small ruminants	Classical scrapie, natural infection Atypical scrapie, transmission mode unknown
Cattle	Classical bovine spongiform encephalopathy (BSE), food borne infection Atypical BSE, transmission mode unknown
Mink	Transmissible mink encephalopathy, food borne infection (scrapie?)
Zoo ungulates	BSE, food borne infection
Domestic cats, zoo felids	Feline spongiform encephalopathy, food borne infection (BSE)
American mule deer/elk	Chronic wasting disease (CWD), natural infection

consists solely of protein. Genetics of the PrP gene and experiments with transgenic mice lend support to the prion theory. The major argument against it is the existence of strain-dependent variation. How exactly the PrP^d accumulation leads to vacuolation of neurons is not clear.

As a result of the bovine spongiform encephalopathy (BSE) outbreak in the late twentieth century, these TSEs received enormous attention of the media, politics and consequently research funding organizations, fostering an immense flood of scientific information. As a result of eradication measures, the incidence of TSEs declined rapidly back to pre-BSE levels, again being very rare diseases of limited economic importance but remaining a public health issue.

8.6.2 Neuropathology of TSE

The basic neuropathology of TSE is very similar in all these conditions both in humans and animals. The major differences between species and between TSE strains within a species, apart from the length of incubation time, only relate to the distribution of the lesions in the CNS and to the morphology and biochemical profiles of the PrP^d accumulations. The morphological hallmark of TSE is *spongiform change* of specific areas of the gray matter, which is always bilaterally symmetrical. This lesion consists of vacuolation of the neuropil, which can readily be detected at low power magnification (Fig. 8.17A,B). These vacuoles are rather uniform in size, well delineated and they appear empty. Ultrastruc-

turally, the vacuoles are located in neuronal cell processes. The neuroanatomical localization of spongiform change depends on the species and TSE strain. In BSE, this change is predominant in the brainstem with the nucleus of the solitary tract and the spinal trigeminal nuclei as the first consistently affected areas.

In scrapie, lesion distribution depends on the strain. In feline spongiform encephalopathy (FSE), spongiform changes are invariably found in the caudate nucleus, but they are widespread and also often encountered in the thalamus, cortex and brainstem. Spongiform change may sometimes be confused with spongy degeneration, brain edema and postmortem degeneration (see Fig. 6.14 for differential diagnosis of spongy state in the CNS).

The second hallmark of TSE is *vacuolation of neuronal cytoplasm*. This change is exceedingly rare in conditions other than TSE and rarely occurs in postmortem degeneration. However, few intracytoplasmic neuronal vacuoles are a frequent finding in the brainstem and midbrain of normal ruminants. Neuronal vacuoles can vary in size, they can be single or multiple and are frequently not associated with neuronal degeneration (Fig. 8.17C). Neuronal vacuoles are mostly empty; occasionally granular or amorphous inclusions may be found within them. Neuronal vacuolation occurs in areas of predilection. In BSE, the most important locations are the vestibular nuclei, followed by the reticular formation, parasympathetic nuclei of the vagus and nuclei of the hypoglossus nerve. In scrapie, the TSE of small ruminants, brainstem nuclei are also frequently affected. In

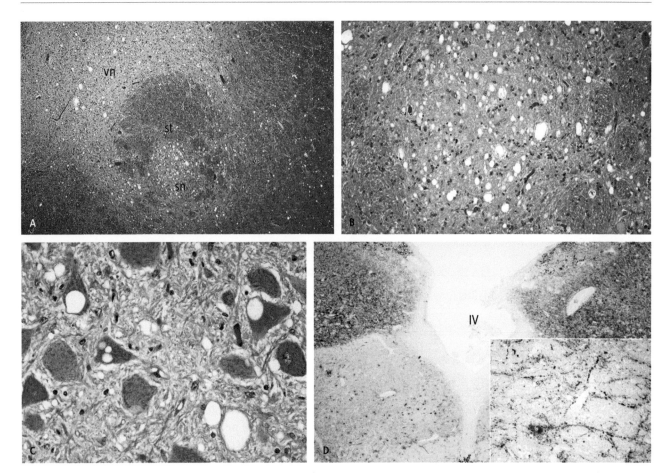

Fig. 8.17 Spongiform encephalopathy. Cow. BSE. A: There is a characteristic gray matter localization of a spongy state (sn, solitary tract nucleus; vn, nucleus vagus; st, solitary tract). HE. B: A higher magnification of the spongiform change with associated astrogliosis. HE. C: Intracytoplasmic neuronal vacuolation in a brainstem nucleus. HE. D: Immunohistochemical visualization of PrP^d accumulation with a bilaterally symmetrical pattern of distribution (IV, fourth ventricle). IHC Inset: typical linear PrP^d pattern of localization. IHC.

feline spongiform encephalopathy, neuronal vacuoles are mostly found in the nuclei of the caudal brainstem, red and vestibular nuclei.

In bovine spongiform encephalopathy (BSE), neuronal loss may occur in the lateral vestibular nucleus. Astrocytic proliferation is typically found in areas undergoing spongy degeneration (Fig. 8.17B). Gliosis is not restricted to the areas of spongiform degeneration or neuronal vacuolation, however, but frequently also involves other areas in a widespread fashion. In fact, in some scrapie forms, astrogliosis is much more prominent and precedes the vacuolar changes. Some investigators believe that astrocytosis in TSE may be a primary change and not merely a reaction to neuronal damage.

Bilaterally symmetrical PrP^d accumulation is generally found in areas where spongiform changes occur. Using immunohistochemistry for PrP^d most immunoreactive material is found in the neuropil between neurons (Fig. 8.17D). The material appears to be associated with cell processes, assuming a fibrillar and linear pattern (Fig. 8.17D, inset). Some material is amorphous and aggregates in plaques. Plaques are frequently seen in the cerebellum of sheep with scrapie. The amount of material varies between cases and does not necessarily correlate with the extent of the lesions.

8.6.3 TSEs in domestic animals

Scrapie

The oldest known TSE is **scrapie** in sheep and goats. More than 20 different scrapie strains are known, which differ from each other only in respect to the length of the incubation time and the distribution pattern (lesion profile) of the spongiform lesions. Scrapie in small ruminants is a naturally occurring disease usually with a low incidence within a herd. There is a clear genetic predisposition in sheep associated with polymorphisms at the level of at least three codons in the prion protein gene. In scrapie, there is replication of the infectious agent in the lymphatic tissues prior to invasion of the CNS. There is also considerable replication of the agent in the placenta, which accounts for vertical transmission, probably during the perinatal period, as well as horizontal transmission through contaminated pastures. Clinically, animals show ataxia with hypermetria, tremor and pruritis.

Atypical scrapie

In the frame of vast surveillance schemes for TSE in Europe, in the wake of the BSE epidemic, **"atypical" scrapie** was first identified in 1998 in Norwegian sheep and, therefore, this condition is also called Nor98. By active surveillance, similar cases have been detected in Europe since 2002 and, in some European countries, the numbers of atypical cases even exceed those of classical scrapie cases. There are several differences from classical scrapie. Atypical scrapie animals are generally older and the salient clinical sign, whenever reported, is ataxia whereas pruritus and wool loss are not observed. As a rule, single animals within a herd are affected and, at present, although atypical scrapie can be experimentally transmitted, natural transmission between animals has not been shown. From the neuropathological point of view, in contrast to classical scrapie, lesions and PrP^d deposits are mostly very mild in the brainstem, but most pronounced in the cerebellum.

BSE

More than 200 000 cases of **bovine spongiform encephalopathy (BSE)** have been diagnosed since 1985. BSE was transmitted by animal protein supplements in the form of meat and bone meal (MBM). Interruption of the chain of infection by prohibiting feeding of animal proteins to ruminants and later to all farm animals lead to a remarkable decrease of BSE incidence. The disease is now nearly eradicated. BSE had also spread to about 10 other animal species, mostly sporadic cases in antelopes in zoological gardens, but also to domestic cats and captive felides causing **feline spongiform encephalopathy (FSE)**, and to humans (**variant CJD**) mostly in the UK.

Atypical BSE

By means of active surveillance for BSE, at least two **atypical forms of BSE** have been detected in cattle: the L-type (BASE) and the H-type, where L and H refer to the lower and higher molecular mass of PrP^d, respectively, in the Western blot. Affected cattle are generally

older than in classical BSE. Reliable information on neuropathology and PrP deposition patterns is very limited.

8.7 Spongy degenerations

8.7.1 Definition and general morphological features

The morphological hallmark of these diseases is spongy state in the CNS. This change may be more or less severe and affects either gray or white matter or both, as always in degenerative diseases, in a bilateral and symmetrical fashion (Fig. 8.18). Basically, the spongy state is due to cytotoxic edema. Fluid accumulates predominantly in astrocytes as a result of disruption of osmoregulation and also in the white matter between myelin lamellae with splitting and ballooning of the myelin sheets.

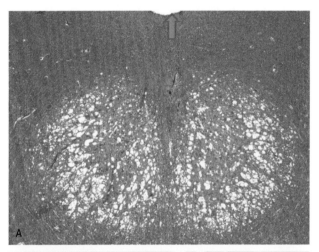

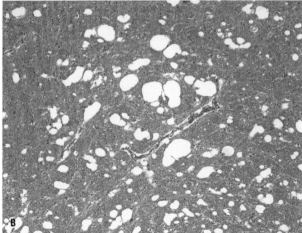

Fig. 8.18 Spongy degeneration. A: Norfolk Terrier pup with bilaterally symmetrical severe spongy state in the oculomotor nuclei (aqueduct depicted by arrow). HE. B. Dog. Spongy degeneration of gray matter with sharply defined empty vacuoles and no reactive changes. HE.

The vacuoles in the tissue are sharply delineated and empty (Fig. 8.18). Often there is neither degeneration of neurons/axons nor of the white matter; apart from astrocytic hypertrophy described in some conditions, reactive changes are usually lacking, at least in the early stages of the disease. In severe cases with a long clinical history, destructive lesions, presumably resulting from compression or poor perfusion, may occur, with degeneration of neurons, axons and myelin and even frank malacia. Reactive changes in this case consist of invasion of macrophages, vascular proliferation and gliosis. Thus, morphologically there may be some overlap between this group of diseases and the selective symmetrical encephalomalacias (SSEs) (Section 8.8) depending on the severity and stage of the disease. In the case of white matter involvement there may some resemblance to leukodystrophies (Section 8.4.1). In several reports, the term *spongiform* degeneration has been used to denote the lesions. The term: "spongiform" should really be reserved for the TSEs discussed in Section 8.6.

It is important to differentiate spongy degeneration from spongiform encephalopathy and various lesions of the white matter associated with status spongiosus (see Fig. 6.14).

Spongy degenerations are listed in Table 8.7.

8.7.2 Spongy degeneration in branched-chain organic acidurias
Organic acidurias in people

In people, these diseases have been known for a long time as **spongy degeneration of van Bogaert-Bertrand type** or **Canavan's disease**. Later, such lesions were recognized to be associated with a group of metabolic diseases, the so-called *branched-chain organic acidurias*. The latter result from an abnormality of specific enzymes involving the catabolism of branched-chain amino acids (leucine, isoleucine, valine). Maple syrup urine disease (MSUD), isovaleric acidemia (IVA), propionic aciduria (PA) and methylmalonic aciduria (MMA) represent the most common human organic acidurias.

Congenital neuraxial edema/spongy degeneration in cattle

Spongy degeneration of the CNS has been recognized as an autosomal recessive hereditary disease in Hereford cattle since the 1960s and was originally named **congenital cerebral edema** or **hereditary neuraxial edema**. The lesions affect the gray and white matter and are severe. Later it was shown that this lesion in Hereford and red poll cattle was caused by a *branched-chain keto acid decarboxylase* deficiency, also named **maple syrup urine disease**. In addition **citrullinemia**, an inherited aminoacidopathy, has been recognized in Friesian calves with *argininosuccinatesynthetase* deficiency. The latter induces accumulation of citrulline and subsequent spongy degeneration.

Organic acidurias in dogs

As in cattle, *organic acidurias* have also been discovered in small animals. **L-2-hydroxyglutaric aciduria (L-2-HGA)**, a hereditary neurometabolic disorder, has been described in Staffordshire Bull Terriers and West Highland White Terriers; it also occurs in people. In dogs, an analogous mutation has been found in *the L-2-hydroxyglutaric acid dehydrogenase* gene. Marked spongy

Table 8.7 Spongy degenerations.

SUBTYPE	DISEASE	SPECIES/BREED
Organic acidurias	L-2-Hydroxyglutaric aciduria	West Highland White Terrier, Staffordshire Bull Terrier
	Methylmalonic/malonic aciduria	Labrador Retriever
	Maple syrup urine disease	Hereford, Red Poll cattle
	Citrullinemia	Holstein-Friesian cattle
Mitochondrial encephalopathy	Canine spongiform leukoencephalomyelopathy	Shetland Sheepdog, Australian cattle dog
Unknown cause	Familial cerebellar ataxia with hydrocephalus	Bull Mastiff
	Spongy degeneration with cerebellar ataxia	Malinois dog
	Congenital status spongiosus	Gelbvieh cattle

changes predominantly affect the gray matter of the cerebral cortex, thalamus, cerebellum and brainstem. **Methylmalonic and malonic aciduria** has been observed in Labrador Retrievers with spongy degeneration.

8.7.3 Spongy degenerations of other causes

Dogs and cats

In **canine spongiform leukoencephalomyelopathy** in Shetland Sheepdogs and Australian Cattle Dogs, spongy degeneration of the white matter has been linked to a missense mitochondrial DNA mutation in cytochrome b. In humans, there are also certain mitochondrial encephalopathies (see Section 8.8.2) targeting the white matter with spongy degeneration (e.g. **Kearns-Sayre syndrome**).

Spongy degeneration of unknown cause has been described in sporadic cases or small, perhaps familial, clusters in several dog breeds and cats. Predominantly gray matter involvement has been reported in Malinois, Saluki and Bull Mastiff puppies and in Birman, Persian and Shorthair kittens. Spongy degeneration of the white matter has been seen in Silky terriers, Samoyed puppies, Labrador Retrievers , Border terriers and Egyptian Mau kittens and adult Ragdoll cats. In Bull Mastiffs (**familial cerebellar ataxia with hydrocephalus**), Malinois (**spongy degeneration with cerebellar ataxia**) and Border terriers (spongiform leukoencephalomyelopathy) the disease is hereditary. We have seen sporadic cases in other dog breeds, Domestic Shorthair cats and rabbits. A common clinical manifestation is congenital tremor: animals show a generalized body tremor which increases with excitement and disappears at rest. The spongy changes in all these conditions varies in severity and distribution pattern.

Cattle

Congenital status spongiosus of Gelbvieh-cross cattle is probably a genetically transmitted disease, which is not associated with organic aciduria.

Toxic–metabolic causes of spongy degeneration

In view of the fact that many different insults may compromise the function of astrocytes to support water homeostasis in the brain, it is not surprising that a number of toxic–metabolic conditions can induce very similar lesions; these are discussed in Chapter 6.

8.8 Selective symmetrical encephalomalacias (SSE)

8.8.1 General morphological features

Neurological syndromes characterized by sharply defined areas of encephalomalacia in a bilaterally symmetrical fashion in selective anatomical areas of the brain and spinal cord have been described in several animal species (Table 8.8) and humans, mostly in juvenile individuals. We prefer the term SSE to distinguish these diseases from enterotoxemias and other acquired forms, called focal symmetrical encephalomalacia (FSE). The pathology of these diseases is quite characteristic, consisting of focal symmetrical areas of malacia in specific gray matter areas of the CNS (Fig. 8.19). The lesions vary in intensity from spongiosis to cavitation of the tissue. Interestingly, in areas of malacia, neurons are frequently spared. Reactive changes include vascular proliferation, astrogliosis, and sometimes perivascular mononuclear cuffing. Astrocytes can be vacuolated. Consult Fig. 6.1 for the differential diagnosis of malacia in the CNS.

8.8.2 Mitochondrial encephalopathies in people and similar lesions in animals

Leigh syndrome

Mitochondrial protein defects have been frequently associated with muscle diseases in people and animals (mitochondrial myopathies). Such defects are also the

Table 8.8 Selective symmetrical encephalomalacias (SSE).

SUBTYPE	DISEASE	SPECIES/BREED
Mitochondrial (possibly)	Hereditary polioencephalomyelopathy	Australian Cattle Dog
	Alaskan Husky encephalopathy	Alaskan Husky
	Subacute necrotizing encephalopathy	Yorkshire Terrier
	Multifocal symmetrical necrotizing encephalomyelopathy	Angus cattle
	Multifocal subacute necrotizing encephalomyelopathy	Simmental cattle
	Encephalomyelopathy	Simmental/crosses

cause of a variety of brain or PNS lesions in people and in domestic animals, as shown in Sections 8.3.1 (sensory ataxic neuropathy in Golden Retriever dogs) and 8.7.3 (canine spongiform leukoencephalomyelopathy). In **Leigh syndrome** in children, focal symmetrical encephalomalacia is associated with molecular defects in respiratory enzymes of mitochondria. Other confirmed human mitochondrial encephalopathies with gray matter disease are MELAS (Mitochondrial encephalomyopathy, lactic acidosis, and stroke-like episodes), MERRF (myoclonic epilepsy with red ragged fibers) and Alper's syndromes.

SSE in small animals

Sporadic cases of selective symmetrical encephalomalacia have been reported in several dog breeds and in cats. In **hereditary polioencephalomyelopathy** of Australian Cattle Dogs, lesions occur in the brainstem and cerebellar nuclei, and gray matter of the spinal cord (most severely in segments C7–T1) (Fig. 8.19C). Electron microscopy reveals abnormally high numbers of swollen mitochondria in astrocytes.

In **Alaskan Husky encephalopathy**, macroscopic cavitating, bilaterally symmetrical, malacic lesions are consistently found in the thalamus (Fig. 8.19A,B). Other affected areas include the caudate nucleus, putamen, midbrain, pons, medulla, base of the cerebral sulci and midline cerebellar gray matter as well as sometimes the cervical spinal cord white matter. In the lesions, there is spongiosis, vascular proliferation, astrogliosis and in some lesions perivascular invasion with inflammatory cells (Fig. 8.19D). Neurons may be remarkably preserved within severely affected areas. Reactive astrocytes are occasionally vacuolated. Very similar lesions occur in **subacute necrotizing encephalopathy** in Yorkshire Terriers. In the latter, evidence was claimed for mito-

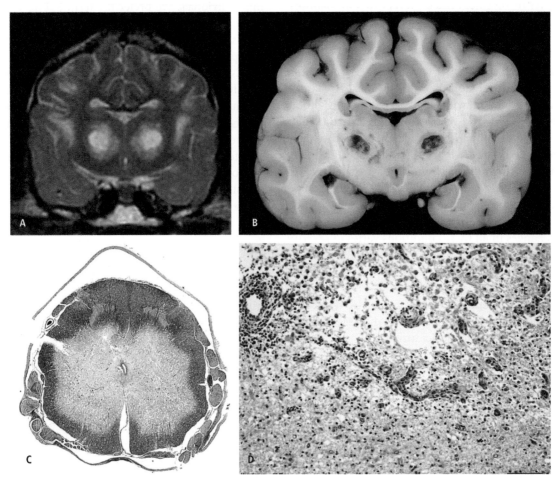

Fig. 8.19 Selective symmetrical encephalomalacia. A. Dog. Alaskan Husky encephalopathy (AHE). Brain: MRI. T2W image with distinctive characteristic bilaterally symmetrical areas of malacia in thalamus. B: Dog. AHE. Corresponding transverse slice through the thalamus with bilateral cystic encephalomalacia. C: Australian Cattle Dog. Spinal cord. Hereditary polioencephalomyelopathy. There are bilaterally symmetrical areas of myelomalacia. LFB-HE. D: AHE. Histology of the thalamus with malacia, infiltration of gitter cells, neovascular proliferation, mild perivascular mononuclear cell cuffing and marked reactive gemistocytic and fibrillary astrocytosis. Morphologically intact neurons can be found in these lesions. HE.

chondrial abnormalities, namely reduced activity of respiratory chain complexes I and IV. However, while morphological changes have been seen in mitochondria in several of these conditions, all efforts to identify unequivocal biochemical and/or molecular biological mitochondrial defects, similar to those in Leigh syndrome have been unsuccessful.

SSE in large animals

Angus calves which developed ataxia, nystagmus, tetanic spasms and episodic convulsions at 2–6 weeks of age died within 1 week after the onset of clinical signs. The **multifocal symmetrical necrotizing encephalomyelopathy** in Angus calves affected the parasympathetic vagal nucleus, lateral cuneate and olivary nuclei in the medulla oblongata and sometimes the spinal cord, substantia nigra and cerebellar peduncles.

In **multifocal subacute necrotizing encephalomyelopathy** in Simmental calves and Simmental-crosses, such lesions were most consistently located in the olivary nuclei but also in other brain regions and in the thoracic spinal cord.

A similar condition, **encephalomyelopathy** of Simmental and Simmental-cross calves, a more protracted disease, occurs in 5–12-month-old animals in New Zealand, Australia and the US, with ataxia, dullness and emaciation developing over up to 6 months. The encephalomalacic lesions are found in the basal nuclei, brainstem and spinal cord gray matter. Abnormal mitochondria are found in muscle tissue but not in the CNS. A similar syndrome has been seen in Limousin cattle in Great Britain, but in these animals there is more involvement of the white matter.

Acquired FSE

As discussed in Chapter 6, bilaterally symmetrical areas of encephalomalacia occur in a number of conditions caused by intoxications and deficiencies, notably in small ruminants. Consult Fig. 6.1 for the differential diagnosis of malacia.

8.9 Degenerative diseases of the peripheral nervous system and muscle

In recent years, enormous progress has been made in the recognition, description and molecular genetics of diseases of the peripheral nervous system and muscle in domestic, mostly small animals. The diagnosis of these diseases requires in-depth neurological assessment, including electrodiagnostic testing and specialized histological, histochemical, immunohistochemical and ultrastructural techniques. Below, we very briefly review a few aspects of classification and nature of these dis-

eases. The reader is referred to the specialized literature for further information. Whenever a suspicion of a neuromuscular disease exists, appropriately sampled material should be retained and stored for subsequent evaluation by specialized laboratories. Routinely FF-PE tissue can reveal some changes but is replete with artifacts and mostly inadequate for a specific diagnosis.

8.9.1 Degenerative polyneuropathies

The classification and diagnosis of degenerative diseases of the PNS is based on several criteria: histopathological changes, distribution pattern of the lesions (either proximal or distal parts of the nerves are primarily involved), whether sensory or motor nerves are involved and whether there are additional lesions in the spinal cord and brain. Several degenerative polyneuropathies in dogs appear to be distal axonopathies, with degeneration beginning at the distal end of the nerve fibers. An important clinical presentation in this respect is laryngeal paralysis. Animals with motor and mixed polyneuropathies present with progressive weakness and neurogenic atrophy of the muscles. Sensory nerve involvement is characterized by ataxia and abnormal sensation, sometimes leading to automutilation. Another distinguishing feature is whether axons or myelin sheaths are primarily involved. In routine diagnostic work on HE sections from FF-PE tissue, axonal degeneration, demyelination, fiber loss and Schwann cell proliferation can be detected in all these conditions. A precise diagnosis, however, requires both specialized expertise and correct tissue sampling, storage and processing.

8.9.2 Degenerative myopathies

An impressive spectrum of hereditary muscle diseases occurs in domestic animals; these are clinically characterized by exercise-induced weakness, muscle atrophy or sometimes hypertrophy and muscle pain. All these diseases have been described in specific breeds, mostly in dogs and cats. Many of these are functional disorders, but several are associated with degenerative changes in the muscle tissue, which can be seen in muscle biopsies. Among these, **muscular dystrophies** are an important group, particularly in dogs but also in cats associated with hereditary *dystrophin deficiency*, dystrophin being a major muscle protein. In addition, mutations of other muscle proteins (e.g. alpha 2 laminin, sarcoglycan complex) have been identified. Histologically, there is degeneration and regeneration of muscle fibers with reactive changes, and atrophy and sclerosis in advanced stages. These dystrophin deficiencies in dogs and cats are very similar to their human counterparts and have been developed as important animal models for pathogenesis and therapy.

Metabolic myopathies result from inborn metabolic defects. In **mitochondrial myopathies**, there is massive proliferation and enlargement of mitochondria in tissue sections leading to a typical pattern called *red ragged fibers* (RRFs). **Lipid storage myopathies** are characterized by accumulation of lipid droplets. **Muscular glycogen storage diseases** occur in small animals and are quite common in horses resulting from mutations in the glycogen synthase I gene. The disease can be diagnosed by finding amylase-resistant PAS-positive inclusions in type II fibers; it does not necessarily cause clinical signs but appears to predispose the animal to other muscular problems such as **exercise-induced rhabdomyolysis** (leading to *myoglobinuria*). The latter is characterized by acute muscle fiber necrosis, the pathogenesis of which is complex. A particularly severe form of rhabdomyolysis is **equine atypical myopathy**. Exertional rhabdomyolysis also occurs in racing Greyhounds and sled dogs. Further examples of rare myodegenerative diseases in small animals, which can be diagnosed on biopsies, are **nemalin myopathy** (nemalin rods in muscle fibers), **myofibrillar myopathy** with desmin storage in muscle fibers and **centronuclear-like myopathy**.

Further reading

Motor neuron diseases

Da Costa RC, Parent JM, Poma R, de Lahunta A. Multisystem axonopathy and neuronopathy in Golden Retriever dogs. J Vet Intern Med 2009;23:935–939.

Fyfe JC, Menotti-Raymond M, David VA, Brichta L, Schäffer AA, Agarwala R, Murphy WJ, Wedemeyer WJ, Gregory BL, Buzzell BG, Drummond MC, Wirth B, O'Brien SJ. An approximately 140-kb deletion associated with feline spinal muscular atrophy implies an essential LIX1 function for motor neuron survival. Genome Res 2006;16:1084–1090.

Green SL, Westendorf JM, Jaffe H, Pant HC, Cork LC, Ostrander EA, Vignaux F, Ferrell JE Jr. Allelic variants of the canine heavy neurofilament (NFH) subunit and extensive phosphorylation in dogs with motor neuron disease. J Comp Pathol 2005;132:33–50.

He Q, Lowrie C, Shelton GD, Castellani RJ, Menotti-Raymond M, Murphy W, O'Brien SJ, Swanson WF, Fyfe JC. Inherited motor neuron disease in domestic cats: a model of spinal muscular atrophy. Pediatr Res 2005;57:324–330.

Krebs S, Medugorac I, Röther S, Strässer K, Förster M. A missense mutation in the 3-ketodihydrosphingosine reductase FVT1 as candidate causal mutation for bovine spinal muscular atrophy. Proc Natl Acad Sci U S A 2007;104:6746–6751.

Cerebellar degenerations

Brault LS, Cooper CA, Famula TR, Murray JD, Penedo MC. Mapping of equine cerebellar abiotrophy to ECA2 and identification of a potential causative mutation affecting expression of MUTYH. Genomics 2011;97:121–129.

Flegel T, Matiasek K, Henke D, Grevel V. Cerebellar cortical degeneration with selective granule cell loss in Bavarian mountain dogs. J Small Anim Pract 2007;48:462–465.

O'Brien DP, Johnson GS, Schnabel RD, Khan S, Coates JR, Johnson GC, Taylor JF. Genetic mapping of canine multiple system degeneration and ectodermal dysplasia loci. J Hered 2005;96:727–734.

Urkasemsin G, Linder KE, Bell JS, de Lahunta A, Olby NJ. Hereditary cerebellar degeneration in Scottish terriers. J Vet Intern Med 2010;24:565–570.

Other neuronal degenerations

Geiger DA, Miller AD, Cutter-Schatzberg K, Shelton GD, de Lahunta A, Schatzberg SJ. Encephalomyelopathy and polyneuropathy associated with neuronal vacuolation in two Boxer littermates. Vet Pathol 2009;46:1160–1165.

Vanhaesebrouck AE, Shelton GD, Garosi L, Harcourt-Brown TR, Couturier J, Behr S, Harvey RJ, Jeffery ND, Matiasek K, Blakemore WF, Granger N. A novel movement disorder in related male Labrador Retrievers characterized by extreme generalized muscular stiffness. J Vet Intern Med 2011;25:1089–1096.

Alzheimer disease

Cotman CW, Head E. The canine (dog) model of human aging and disease: dietary, environmental and immunotherapy approaches. J Alzheimers Dis 2008;15:685–707.

Insua D, Suárez ML, Santamarina G, Sarasa M, Pesini P. Dogs with canine counterpart of Alzheimer's disease lose noradrenergic neurons. Neurobiol Aging 2010;31:625–635.

Wallerian-like axonal degenerations

Awano T, Johnson GS, Wade CM, Katz ML, Johnson GC, Taylor JF, Perloski M, Biagi T, Baranowska I, Long S, March PA, Olby NJ, Shelton GD, Khan S, O'Brien DP, Lindblad-Toh K, Coates JR. Genome-wide association analysis reveals a SOD1 mutation in canine degenerative myelopathy that resembles amyotrophic lateral sclerosis. Proc Natl Acad Sci U S A 2009;106:2794–2799.

Baranowska I, Jäderlund KH, Nennesmo I, Holmqvist E, Heidrich N, Larsson NG, Andersson G, Wagner EG, Hedhammar A, Wibom R, Andersson L. Sensory ataxic neuropathy in golden retriever dogs is caused by a deletion in the mitochondrial tRNATyr gene. PLoS Genet 2009;5(5):e1000499. Epub 2009 May 29.

Jäderlund KH, Orvind E, Johnsson E, Matiasek K, Hahn CN, Malm S, Hedhammar A. A neurologic syndrome in Golden Retrievers presenting as a sensory ataxic neuropathy. J Vet Intern Med 2007;21:1307–1315.

March PA, Coates JR, Abyad RJ, Williams DA, O'Brien DP, Olby NJ, Keating JH, Oglesbee M. Degenerative myelopathy in 18 Pembroke Welsh Corgi dogs. Vet Pathol 2009;46:241–250.

Rohdin C, Lüdtke L, Wohlsein P, Jäderlund KH. New aspects of hereditary ataxia in smooth-haired fox terriers. Vet Rec 2010;166:557–560.

Degenerative myelopathy in old dogs

Coates JR, Wininger FA. Canine degenerative myelopathy. Vet Clin North Am Small Anim Pract 2010;40:929–950.

Johnston PE, Barrie JA, McCulloch MC, Anderson TJ, Griffiths IR. Central nervous system pathology in 25 dogs with chronic degenerative radiculomyelopathy. Vet Rec 2000;146:629–633.

Kamishina H, Oji T, Cheeseman JA, Clemmons RM. Detection of oligoclonal bands in cerebrospinal fluid from German Shepherd dogs with degenerative myelopathy by isoelectric focusing and immunofixation. Vet Clin Pathol 2008;37:217–220.

Wallerian-like degeneration in large animals

Drögemüller C, Reichart U, Seuberlich T, Oevermann A, Baumgartner M, Kühni Boghenbor K, Stoffel MH, Syring C, Meylan M, Müller S, Müller M, Gredler B, Sölkner J, Leeb T. An unusual splice defect in the mitofusin 2 gene (MFN2) is associated with degenerative axonopathy in Tyrolean Grey cattle. PLoS One 2011;6(4): e18931.

Moisan PG, Steffen DJ, Sanderson MW, Nietfeld JC, Finley MR, Grotelueschen DM, Andrews GA, Johnson G, Williamson L, Rushton SD, Hall DG, Harmon BG. A familial degenerative neuromuscular disease of Gelbvieh cattle. J Vet Diagn Invest 2002;14: 140–149.

Timsit E, Albaric O, Colle MA, Costiou P, Cesbron N, Bareille N, Assié S. Clinical and histopathologic characterization of a central and peripheral axonopathy in Rouge-des-prés (Maine Anjou) calves. J Vet Intern Med 2011;386–392.

Neuroaxonal dystrophy

Aleman M, Finno CJ, Higgins RJ, Puschner B, Gerocota B, Ghohil K, LeCouteur RA, Madigan JE Neuroaxonal dystrophy in Quarter horses JAVMA 2011;239:823–833.

Fyfe JC, Al-Tamimi RA, Castellani RJ, Rosenstein D, Goldowitz D, Henthorn PS. Inherited neuroaxonal dystrophy in dogs causing lethal, fetal-onset motor system dysfunction and cerebellar hypoplasia. J Comp Neurol 2010;518:3771–3784.

Jolly RD, Johnstone AC, Williams SD, Zhang K, Jordan TW.Segmental axonopathy of Merino sheep in New Zealand. N Z Vet J 2006;54: 210–217.

McLellan GJ, Cappello R, Mayhew IG, Elks R, Lybaert P, Watté C, Bedford PG. Clinical and pathological observations in English cocker spaniels with primary metabolic vitamin E deficiency and retinal pigment epithelial dystrophy. Vet Rec 2003;153:287–392.

Nibe K, Kita C, Morozumi M, Awamura Y, Tamura S, Okuno S, Kobayashi T, Uchida K. Clinicopathological features of canine neuroaxonal dystrophy and cerebellar cortical abiotrophy in Papillon and Papillon-related dogs. J Vet Med Sci 2007;69:1047–1052.

Leukodystrophies

Fletcher JL, Williamson P, Horan D, Taylor RM. Clinical signs and neuropathologic abnormalities in working Australian Kelpies with globoid cell leukodystrophy (Krabbe disease). J Am Vet Med Assoc 2010;237:682–688.

Kessell AE, Finnie JW, Manavis J, Cheetham GD, Blumbergs PC. A Rosenthal fiber encephalomyelopathy resembling Alexander's disease in 3 sheep. Vet Pathol 2012;49:248–254.

Morrison JP, Schatzberg SJ, De Lahunta A, Ross JT, Bookbinder P, Summers BA. Oligodendroglial dysplasia in two bullmastiff dogs. Vet Pathol 2006;43:29–35.

Oevermann A, Bley T, Konar M, Lang J, Vandevelde M.A novel leukoencephalomyelopathy of Leonberger dogs. J Vet Intern Med 2008;22:467–471.

Sisó S, Botteron C, Muhle A, Vandevelde M. A novel leukodystrophy in a dog. J Comp Pathol 2005;132:232–236.

Dysmyelination

Millán Y, Mascort J, Blanco A, Costa C, Masian D, Guil-Luna S, Pumarola M, Martin de Las Mulas J. Hypomyelination in three Weimaraner dogs. J Small Anim Pract 2010;51:594–598.

Pettigrew R, Fyfe JC, Gregory BL, Lipsitz D, Delahunta A, Summers BA, Shelton GD. CNS hypomyelination in Rat Terrier dogs with

congenital goiter and a mutation in the thyroid peroxidase gene. Vet Pathol 2007;44:50–56.

Thomsen B, Nissen PH, Agerholm JS, Bendixen C. Congenital bovine spinal dysmyelination is caused by a missense mutation in the SPAST gene. Neurogenetics 2010;11:175–183.

Yaeger MJ, Majercik K, Carter M, Rothschild M. An autosomal recessive, lethal, neurologic disease of Gordon Setter puppies. J Vet Diagn Invest 2000;12:570–573.

Lysosomal storage diseases

Abitbol M, Thibaud JL, Olby NJ, Hitte C, Puech JP, Maurer M, Pilot-Storck F, Hédan B, Dréano S, Brahimi S, Delattre D, André C, Gray F, Delisle F, Caillaud C, Bernex F, Panthier JJ, Aubin-Houzelstein G, Blot S, Tiret L. A canine arylsulfatase G (ARSG) mutation leading to a sulfatase deficiency is associated with neuronal ceroid lipofuscinosis. Proc Natl Acad Sci U S A 2010;107: 14775–14778.

Haskins M. Gene therapy for lysosomal storage diseases (LSDs) in large animal models. ILAR J 2009;50:112–121.

Lohi H, Young EJ, Fitzmaurice SN, Rusbridge C, Chan EM, Vervoort M, Turnbull J, Zhao XC, Ianzano L, Paterson AD, Sutter NB, Ostrander EA, André C, Shelton GD, Ackerley CA, Scherer SW, Minassian BA. Expanded repeat in canine epilepsy. Science 2005; 307:81.

Sisó S, Navarro C, Hanzlícek D, Vandevelde M. Adult onset thalamocerebellar degeneration in dogs associated to neuronal storage of ceroid lipopigment. Acta Neuropathol 2004;108:386–392.

Warren CD, Alroy J. Morphological, biochemical and molecular biology approaches for the diagnosis of lysosomal storage diseases. J Vet Diagn Invest 2000;12:483–496.

Spongiform encephalopathies

Aguzzi A, Calella AM.Prions: protein aggregation and infectious diseases. Physiol Rev 2009;89:1105–1152.

Jeffrey M, González L. Classical sheep transmissible spongiform encephalopathies: pathogenesis, pathological phenotypes and clinical disease. Neuropathol Appl Neurobiol 2007;33:373–394.

Jeffrey M, McGovern G, Sisó S, González L. Cellular and sub-cellular pathology of animal prion diseases: relationship between morphological changes, accumulation of abnormal prion protein and clinical disease. Acta Neuropathol 2011;121:113–134.

Seuberlich T, Heim D, Zurbriggen A. Atypical transmissible spongiform encephalopathies in ruminants: a challenge for disease surveillance and control. J Vet Diagn Invest. 2010;22:823–842.

Surguchev A, Surguchov A. Conformational diseases: looking into the eyes. Brain Res Bull 2010;81:12–24.

Vidal E, Acín C, Foradada L, Monzón M, Márquez M, Monleón E, Pumarola M, Badiola JJ, Bolea R. Immunohistochemical characterisation of classical scrapie neuropathology in sheep. J Comp Pathol 2009;141:135–146.

Wemheuer WM, Benestad SL, Wrede A, Wemheuer WE, Brenig B, Bratberg B, Schulz-Schaeffer WJ. Detection of classical and atypical/Nor98 scrapie by the paraffin-embedded tissue blot method. Vet Rec 2009;164:677–681.

Spongy degenerations

Li FY, Cuddon PA, Song J, Wood SL, Patterson JS, Shelton GD, Duncan ID. Canine spongiform leukoencephalomyelopathy is associated with a missense mutation in cytochrome b. Neurobiol Dis 2006; 21:35–42.

Penderis J, Calvin J, Abramson C, Jakobs C, Pettitt L, Binns MM, Verhoeven NM, O'Driscoll E, Platt SR, Mellersh CS. L-2-hydroxyglutaric aciduria: characterisation of the molecular defect in a spontaneous canine model. J Med Genet 2007;44: 334–340.

Scurrell E, Davies E, Baines E, Cherubini GB, Platt S, Blakemore W, Williams A, Schöniger S. Neuropathological findings in a Staffordshire bull terrier with l-2-hydroxyglutaric aciduria. J Comp Pathol 2008;138:160–164.

Skvorak KJ. Animal models of maple syrup urine disease. J Inherit Metab Dis 2009;32:229–246.

Windsor P, Agerholm J. Inherited diseases of Australian Holstein-Friesian cattle. Aust Vet J 2009;87:193–199.

Selective symmetrical encephalomalacias

Baiker K, Hofmann S, Fischer A, Gödde T, Medl S, Schmahl W, Bauer MF, Matiasek K. Leigh-like subacute necrotising encephalopathy in Yorkshire Terriers: neuropathological characterisation, respiratory chain activities and mitochondrial DNA. Acta Neuropathol 2009; 118:697–709.

Brenner O, Wakshlag JJ, Summers BA, de Lahunta A. Alaskan Husky encephalopathy – a canine neurodegenerative disorder resembling subacute necrotizing encephalomyelopathy (Leigh syndrome). Acta Neuropathol 2000;100:50–62.

Filosto M, Tomelleri G, Tonin P, Scarpelli M, Vattemi G, Rizzuto N, Padovani A, Simonati A. Neuropathology of mitochondrial diseases. Biosci Rep 2007;27:23–30.

Philbey AW, Martel KS. A multifocal symmetrical necrotizing encephalomyelopathy in Angus calves. Aust Vet J 2003;81:226–229.

Degenerative diseases of the PNS and muscles

Coates JR, O'Brien DP. Inherited peripheral neuropathies in dogs and cats. Vet Clin Small Anim 2004;34:1361–1401.

Dixon PM, Hahn CN, Barakzai SZ. Recurrent laryngeal neuropathy (RLN) research: where are we and to where are we heading? Equine Vet J 2009;41:324–327.

Shelton GD. Routine and specialized laboratory testing for the diagnosis of neuromuscular diseases in dogs and cats. Vet Clin Pathol 2010;39:278–295.

Shelton GD. What's new in muscle and peripheral nerve diseases? Vet Comp Orthop Traumatol 2007;20:249–255.

Shelton GD, Engvall E. Canine and feline models of human inherited muscle diseases. Neuromuscul Disord 2005;15:127–138.

Index

Page numbers in *italics* refer to figures and those in **bold** to tables, but note that figures and tables are only indicated when they are separated from their text references.

Veterinary Neuropathology: Essentials of Theory and Practice, First Edition. Marc Vandevelde, Robert J. Higgins, and Anna Oevermann.
© 2012 John Wiley & Sons, Ltd. Published 2012 by John Wiley & Sons, Ltd.